Nurses of a Different Stripe

Nurses of a Different Stripe

*A History of
the Columbia University School of Nursing
1892–1992*

GARY GOLDENBERG

*Columbia University School of Nursing
New York*

Columbia University School of Nursing
630 West 168th Street, New York, NY 10032

© 1992 by Gary Goldenberg
and the Columbia University School of Nursing
All rights reserved

Library of Congress Catalog Card Number: 91-77490
ISBN 0-9631670-0-6
Printed in the United States of America
99 98 97 96 95 94 93 92   5 4 3 2 1

Designed by Tanya Krawciw

To Brenda Wineapple

The field is wide;
you must set no limits to your usefulness.

Anna C. Maxwell
Founder, School of Nursing

Contents

Foreword

by Mary O. Mundinger, Dr.P.H.
Dean, Columbia University School of Nursing

When Anna Maxwell set her firm mind on the establishment of the School of Nursing in the cold, clear winter and spring of 1892, she was one in a long line of creative, indomitable spirits who brought their dreams to fruition in the last years of a century. With the centennial of this venerable School, we also celebrate 500 years of American progress, professional achievements, and womenfolk on the move.

In 1492 Columbus sailed to North American shores, sent and funded by a woman, Queen Isabella of Spain. The same year Leonardo da Vinci drew a flying machine, surely a flight of fancy well before its time.

One hundred years later, in 1592, Shakespeare produced three timeless dramas — *Two Gentlemen of Verona*, *King Richard III*, and *Titus Andronicus*. In Holland, windmills were used for the first time to drive mechanical saws. In Pisa, Galileo was forced to leave his university position after disproving the accepted belief that objects fall to the ground at speeds proportionate to their body weights.

In 1692 the first calculating machine that could multiply and divide was invented in Germany, and in America the first witch trials began. This clear scientific dissonance on opposite sides of the ocean reflects how isolated from each other the world's peoples still were.

In 1792 our fledgling nation began the construction of the White House and the U.S. Capitol, the New York Stock Exchange was founded, and Eli Whitney invented the cotton gin, inadvertently reinforcing the institution of slavery by creating a demand for more bodies to plant cotton. In the same year Denmark became the first nation to ban slavery.

In 1892, just a generation after slavery was abolished in America and the year that the Russian, Dmitri Ivanovski, pioneered the science of virology, American industry grew exponentially; Union Carbide, Shell Oil, General Electric, Maxwell House, Spalding, Wrigley Gum, Coca-

Cola and Hormel Food were established. The same year the University of Chicago, the University of Rhode Island, and Ithaca College were founded. Adirondack State Park, still the nation's largest forest preserve, was created, the Sierra Club was established, and the first gasoline tractor was invented. Chicago's elevated train — the Loop — was opened, as was Ellis Island.

In New York City in the early days of that year, as Anna Maxwell sought to develop a curriculum, hire instructors, and select students for her new school, another major development was born a few blocks north: The cornerstone was laid for the Cathedral of St. John the Divine.

Although Anna Maxwell was a reasonably religious woman, the real connection between the Columbia School of Nursing and the Cathedral occurs on another level. When construction of the Cathedral was begun, our nation was the lucky beneficiary of the artistry of Italian stonemasons. From generation to generation these skilled men passed on their art, one that was unchanging and highly valued, but inadequately recognized or recompensed. Today, a century later, the Cathedral is still under construction. It is rich and beautiful in tradition, dynamic and responsive in its service to people, and at risk of losing the talents of the stonemason artisans who have all but disappeared. The Columbia School of Nursing is in a period of similar growth, celebration, pride, and concern for the disparity between availability of and need for our artisans — the valued but still inadequately recognized professional nurses.

As we move into our second century, we enter a time of breathtaking opportunities for nursing in general and for our school in particular. We continue to lead the profession in practice excellence, and collaboration with our physician colleagues has never before been so promising and so necessary. The students we are privileged to teach are among the nation's most promising citizens. They will make a difference in health care well into the next millennium.

Eighteen-ninety-two was a rich beginning. It has taken a century for the School to flourish in research as well as in practice and teaching, but we are on our way. We welcome change and the dynamism of the profession, and we owe a great debt to the good and true and feisty women who laid our groundwork for us.

Gary Goldenberg has performed a magnificent service for our more than 8,000 alumni in writing this perceptive and riveting book. He has made the historical connections in tracing the School's progress (or lack of it), understood the professional issues, unearthed the perfect quotes to paint a colorful picture, and been exhaustive and careful in his research. We thank him for this wonderful centennial gift.

Acknowledgments

During my college years, medicine was my main passion. (Nursing never crossed my mind — it was a "soft" science, something that women did.) I eventually discovered that I would rather write about medicine than practice it. Which led me to a graduate program in journalism and then, in 1981, to Mae Rudolph's staff in the Office of Public Information at the Columbia University College of Physicians & Surgeons. One of my first tasks at P&S was to take over the fledgling journal, *SNC* (an acronym for the School of Nursing at Columbia). Slowly, I learned the fine art of journalism. I also learned, working with then-Dean of Nursing JoAnn Jamann and her faculty, that nursing was refreshingly humanistic, holistic, and patient-centered (qualities I had found lacking in medicine), and that it had unlimited scholarly potential. The experience was priceless.

After a few years at P&S, I decided to try my hand as a freelancer, largely because Mae and JoAnn agreed to be my first clients, letting me continue as *SNC* editor. JoAnn's successor, Mary Mundinger, upped the ante, granting me the resources to expand and redesign the journal, which we renamed *The Academic Nurse* to reflect the School's new professional emphasis. One of our first projects was a series of articles tracing the history of the School, culminating with the 1992 centennial.

Pleased with the response to the series, Mary asked me to write this book. No problem, I thought. I would revise Eleanor Lee's two histories of the School, conduct a few interviews and, one-two-three, it would be done. However, the more I delved into the subject, into the various archives, into the lives of the students and faculty and alumni, the more I realized that this story was endlessly rich and complex, that it could not be told without addressing so many topics tangential to nursing education, from the rise of hospitals to the rise of urban America, from the Victorians to the Progressives, from wars to epidemics, from the civil rights to the students' to the women's movements.

xiv *Acknowledgments*

Above all, this is a story of resilience and perseverance. In America, a relatively young nation, it is exceptional when any institution celebrates a centennial. In nursing — a "female" profession in a male-dominated industry and society — it is all the more remarkable. From year one to year one hundred, the School of Nursing has had to struggle for recognition and respect, for curricular and financial independence, and at times for its very existence. Rarely has it had the opportunity to focus exclusively on the education of nurses and the development of nursing science. (Early on, I jokingly named this project, *One Hundred Years of Servitude,* a title that in many ways turned out to be quite appropriate.) The School's foes have been many: self-protective physicians, conservative hospital administrators, reactionary politicians, myopic military officials — and nurses and women themselves, caught up in the orthodoxy of professional and social roles. Its friends have been many, too, from all walks of life, which is why the School is around to celebrate its one-hundredth anniversary.

I have been fortunate to witness ten of those years through my own eyes and the rest through the writings and reminiscences of generations of students and faculty. It has been a most illuminating journey.

I have many people to thank for making *Nurses of a Different Stripe* possible:

First of all, Mary Mundinger, who asked me to write this history, and then let me be. What more could a writer ask?

The individuals who reviewed — and immeasurably improved — my manuscript: Mae Rudolph; Sarah Cook, associate dean for academic and clinical affairs at the School of Nursing; Lucie Kelly, former professor of nursing and public health at Columbia; Robin Roy, director of development and alumni affairs at the School of Nursing; and Keville Frederickson, president of the Columbia University–Presbyterian Hospital School of Nursing Alumni Association (Chapters 19 and 21).

Those involved in the book's production: Tanya Krawciw, designer; Kristin Warbasse (administrative assistant to the dean of nursing), proofreader; WLCR New York, typesetters; and Maple-Vail Book Manufacturing Group, printers.

Phyllis Di Filippo, administrator of the Alumni Association, and Martin Collins, administrative aide in P&S Central Records, who were especially helpful by giving me free access to their files.

Current and former Columbia-Presbyterian staff members (who suffered my endless requests for this and that over the years): Bea Bennis,

Cheryl Francis, Elisabeth Gay, Earl Lewis, Isis Primus, Helen Rodrigues, and Kathy Thompson.

Elizabeth Wilcox, longtime Columbia-Presbyterian Medical Center photographer.

Richard Zucker and Susan Parker, former directors of Public Interest at Presbyterian Hospital, who were instrumental in my freelance career.

The students, faculty, and alumni of the School of Nursing.

Mom and Dad, whose love and support has been constant and generous.

Lastly, Brenda Wineapple, professor of English at my undergraduate alma mater, Union College, Schenectady, N.Y. Graham Greene once wrote that in every childhood there's a moment when a door opens and lets the future in. Fifteen years ago, as a confused biology major, I happened upon her course in major American authors, in which she spoke of "original versions of reality." From her teachings and our conversations, I discovered original versions of my own reality, that I had other options, other talents, that I *could* combine my seemingly incompatible interests in science and literature. Thank you, for letting the future in.

Nurses of a Different Stripe

1

Without Regard to Race, Creed, or Color

> In...the pre-Maxwellian era, the male wards were in
> the exclusize charge of casual convalescent patients,
> plumbers or brass-fitters perhaps, who by the grace of
> custom were somewhat ironically known as "orderlies."
> Their bedside notes...were extremely brief and served
> better as examples of phonetic spelling than as scientific
> observations of value.
>
> W. Gilman Thompson, M.D.
> (Commencement exercises, 1911)

A CENTURY AFTER AMERICA won freedom from British tyranny, it remained enslaved to illness and injury. Like a runaway locomotive, the Industrial Revolution roared through the eighteenth century, reshaping the social and economic landscape. Migrants and immigrants crowded into urban centers in search of an ideal, transforming quiet cities into dangerous, unsanitary megalopolises — perfect incubators of cholera, typhoid, influenza, tuberculosis, pneumonia, and diphtheria. Farms gave way to toxic and mechanized factories, which routinely crippled and killed. And farmhouses gave way to crowded tenements, where malnutrition and diarrhea devastated the young. Up to one-half of all infants did not survive their first year. Adults generally did not live to celebrate their forty-first birthday.

The well-to-do fared relatively well, of course. Not only were they isolated from the rigors of everyday life, they were able to afford the luxuries of a lengthy recovery and the ministrations of a private doctor or nurse. Although health care providers of the day had few truly beneficial weapons in their therapeutic armamentarium, they could at least offer patients rest and quiet, nourishment, cleanliness, and tender care — enough in many cases to give the body's natural defenses a fighting chance. Patients were lucky if that was all their caregivers offered. Doctors relied heavily on emetics, cathartics, and bleeding to adjust the body's equilibrium—the idea was to provoke, not alter, the fundamental systems of recovery. People with febrile illnesses, such as typhus and puerperal fever, were given liberal doses of brandy and whiskey or, later, perilous coal-tar derivatives. No one was safe from these "cures," not even a president of the United States. In 1850 Zachary Taylor was slowly drugged, bled, and blistered to death after developing a case of gastroenteritis from a Fourth of July meal of iced milk and chilled cucumbers. Women suffered terribly at the hands of so-called healers. A difficult delivery was a virtual death sentence, particularly if the physician resorted to cesarian section, the most dangerous surgical procedure of the day. Because of the certainty of doctor-to-patient infection, women had a better chance of survival if they performed the operation *themselves,* according to an 1887 study in the *American Journal of Medical Science.* The primitiveness of medicine in the mid-1800s led Oliver Wendell Holmes, the prominent Harvard physician, to declare that "if the whole materia medica, as now used, could be sunk to the bottom of the sea, it would be all the better for mankind—and all the worse for the fishes."

Average city dwellers, with no money to lavish on physicians, were saved the added insult of iatrogenic illness when they took sick. But they suffered all the same. Far from the tighter-knit communities of rural America or their foreign homelands, they could no longer rely on the support and care of family and friends, nor could they afford a lengthy recovery. Someone had to earn the rent or mind the children and keep the house.

The growing legions of single men suffered even more. They could turn only to the almshouse, the last resort of the rootless and the penniless, where the care was limited to ineffective medicines (usually alcohol products) and the ministrations of untrained and meagerly paid "nurses"—casual criminals and vagrants who had climbed a rickety "clinical ladder" from patient to keeper to caregiver. At the very least, the almshouse was a place where one could find a meal and a bed, yet often at the cost of an infection or two.

Hospitals that offered any semblance of organized medical and nursing care were rare in mid-century, and few people entrusted their lives to these institutions. "No self-respecting woman ever thought of having her baby in a public hospital," Charles Rosenberg writes in *The Care of Strangers: The Rise of America's Hospital System.* "A mid-nineteenth century student might think his teacher to be excessively fussy if he prohibited spitting in the wards. Infection and cross-infection were frequent. Several diseases became so common in hospitals that they were known as 'hospital diseases': erysipelas, pyemia, septicemia, and gangrene." Hospital nurses (except in some religious orders) were little better than their almshouse counterparts. Mostly from the tough charwoman class, they rightly regarded their chores as distasteful drudgery, and many numbed themselves with drink. They occupied the lowest rung in a lowly institution.

Slowly, a rational system of health care evolved. On the distant shores of wartorn Crimea, a young Englishwoman named Florence Nightingale shamed her nation, the world's richest and strongest, into providing the barest minimum of care for its fighting men. With a staff of only thirty-eight nurses, Nightingale transformed a 3,000-bed, vermin-infested, excrement-coated death house into a respectable hospital by introducing the most basic sanitary and nursing measures. The death rate plummeted from 60 percent to just over 1 percent. Thousands of lives were saved. And the modern English hospital system was born.

The lesson of the Crimea was not lost on the Confederate and Union armies, which established formidable hospital systems of their own during the Civil War. The North alone created more than 200 hospitals with 137,000 beds, treating one million men with a death rate below 10 percent. Again, the hospitals could tie their success not to any advance in medical therapeutics but to cleanliness, nutrition, warmth, and ventilation.

As in the Crimea, women also participated in this great health care experiment, though usually in menial roles. A few were commissioned nurses with modest training; most, however, were wives and sisters of the soldiers—untrained and unreliable, oblivious to the military mindset of rules and regulations. Military physicians, unwilling to distinguish between the trained and untrained, largely ignored and scorned the whole lot. The women had committed the sin of invading man's domain.

The stage was now set for the rise of America's hospital system. Heretofore, most Americans had gone from cradle to grave without seeing the inside of a hospital—only 120 existed at the time of the first national survey in 1873. But the Civil war, through the first-person accounts of returning warriors and the popular writings of Walt Whitman and Louisa May Alcott (both of whom served as nurses for the North), exposed the citizenry to the possibilities of institutional care. Equally important, the shared experience of the war united a diverse group of social activists—physicians, philanthropists, clergymen, teachers, and lawyers—in a crusade for hospital reform, led by upperclass women. All were convinced that the military hospital experiment, with some modifications, could be duplicated in peacetime. Physicians, too, eagerly joined the movement, recognizing in hospitals a place where they could gain prestige and power and money (from referrals and student fees). Finally, clergymen fell in line, seeing organized

4 Nurses of a Different Stripe

health care as a fitting extension of their traditional role as helper of the poor.

Curiously, one major player was missing from the reform movement, the federal government, which limited its post-war health care obligations to freedmen, merchant sailors, and a small class of professional soldiers. The enormous administrative and logistical framework of the military hospitals vanished soon after the last shots were fired, passing the burden of establishing a civilian health care system to state and private hands.

Among those hands was James Lenox, a wealthy New York philanthropist. Discerning that the city's six existing general hospitals were inadequate for the burgeoning population, now one million, Lenox persuaded a number of prominent citizens to erect another institution, which would become The Presbyterian Hospital in the City of New York. He originally intended it to be run by Presbyterians for Presbyterians, keeping it within the faith, which was not at all uncommon among religious orders of the time. Lenox, however, was impelled by one of the Hospital's founding physicians, Oliver White, to broaden its mission. According to Presbyterian physician and historian, Albert Lamb, White "was once called to care for an old, respected colored servant of a prominent family in his neighborhood. He found her in urgent need of hospital care, but because of her race he could not secure a bed for her in any hospital of his choice. Hotly indignant, he told Mr. Lenox that he hoped someday that there would be a hospital 'broad enough to admit patients without any regard to color or creed.' Mr. Lenox immediately accepted the idea as a fundamental principle for the Presbyterian Hospital."

Presbyterian's motto, which was engraved on a tablet placed conspicuously near the front entrance, thus became: "For the Poor of New York Without Regard to Race, Creed or Color."

Sparing no expense, Lenox commissioned Richard Hunt, New York's most renowned architect, to transform the block bounded by Fourth (Park) and Madison Avenues and 70th and 71st Streets, site of the former Five Mile Post Farm, into the showcase of hospital architecture. Hunt's design was dominated by two four-story buildings, one with wards and private rooms for one hundred patients and another for offices, living quarters, and a chapel. The buildings were connected by covered corridors, topped with roof gardens, which soon became the rage in hospital design. Several smaller structures dotted the property, housing a mortuary, kitchen, laundry, heating plant, and horse-drawn ambulance. A few years later, the "Cottage"—or "Hut," as the nurses called it—was built to isolate patients with infectious disease, mostly erysipelas, a contagious disease of the skin and underlying tissues.

Although the masses were welcomed into the Hospital, they were segregated on the three upper floors, each of which contained two twelve-bed
wards. Most of the first floor was devoted to "comfortably furnished"
rooms for private patients, costing thirty to fifty dollars a week—a fortune to the average citizen. The rare ward patient with any savings was
charged five to seven dollars a week; all others stayed for free. The upper
floors also contained the operating rooms, whose washable hardwood
floors, high ceilings, and large windows (for good light and ventilation) were
the envy of all other hospitals. Pitch pine was used to line the stairways as
well as the dumbwaiter, laundry, and refuse shafts—an attractive but ill-
considered design, posing a constant fire hazard. One house officer was
known to sleep with his clothes on a nearby chair, like a fireman, ready to
escape the flames—a habit that proved most useful in 1889, when a cat-
astrophic fire destroyed most of the ward building.

As soon as the Hospital opened in October 1872, critics complained that
it was too isolated. Indeed, Presbyterian was located way uptown, on the
upper, unpaved reaches of Madison Avenue, an hour away from midtown
by horse-car. Public transportation to the site was limited. According to Seth
Milken, a Presbyterian physician whose parents built a house nearby, "Goats
roamed the streets in herds... In rainy weather, Father walked the wooden
planks to avoid the mud... Mother's friends said, 'You're going to the country.
We'll never see you anymore.'" Nearby, one could discern the beginnings
of Frederick Law Olmstead's Central Park, but it was still littered with
ramshackle squatter's huts, inhabited by hucksters and thieves and junk-
men. When the wind was right, patients would awaken to the roar of sea
lions housed in the park's new menagerie, six blocks to the south, which only
added to the remote feel of the neighborhood.

Indeed, the new institution was isolated—but for good reason. As nursing
historian Susan Reverby points out in *Ordered to Care,* "The siting of hospitals could be a political minefield, unless they were built in remote and
unpopulated areas or placed among the poor who had far less capacity to
make their objections felt. Quarantine hospitals were particularly unpopular—and on occasion destroyed by irate neighbors—but lay fears of
contagion shaped attitudes toward all hospitals." Furthermore, the Hospital's planners knew that the fast-sprawling city would eventually come
to them. Real estate prices would rise, forcing the removal of the area's
unsavory elements. And the park, once a threatening, lawless frontier, would
become a great public amenity, a place where convalescent patients could
take carriage rides to escape the tedium of a lengthy hospital stay.

Organizing a hospital from scratch, particularly the nation's showcase hospital, was an enormous task. The challenge of hiring and training personnel for housekeeping and maintenance, the pharmacy, the kitchen, and, above all, the nursing staff fell to Jane Stuart Woolsey. Well-educated and well-to-do, Woolsey and her three sisters—Abby, Georgianna, and Eliza—rose to prominence during the Civil War, devoting themselves wholeheartedly to the Union cause. In 1861, they joined the Woman's Central Association for Relief (precursor to the United States Sanitary Commission and, in turn, the American Red Cross), which was formed to furnish supplies, nurses, and other services not provided by the federal government. Later, they were among one hundred women sent by Elizabeth Blackwell, the foremost woman physician of her time, to hospitals in New York City for one month of nursing training.

During the war, Jane Woolsey served briefly in hospitals in New York, Rhode Island, and Washington, then assumed clinical and administrative duties at the large Barrack Hospital in Fairfax, Virginia. A tireless worker, she also supported a number of institutions dedicated to newly freed slaves, including the privately organized Freedman's Institute and the government's Freedman's Bureau. In Richmond, she opened the Lincoln Industrial School for Colored Women, which manufactured inexpensive clothing for sale to the poor. She also directed the Industrial Department of the Hampton Normal and Agricultural Institute for Negro Women.

As Presbyterian Hospital's Resident Directress, Woolsey wielded unusual administrative power for a woman of her time. "There was also to be a Superintendent whose duties were concurrent," wrote Albert Lamb, "but it is clear that Miss Woolsey was [the Superintendent's] superior and acted in the same capacity as the Executive Vice President does today. It also seems likely that the Managers created the position of Directress in order to secure her services...Miss Woolsey served without pay."

She was ably assisted by her sister Abby, officially the acting clerk, but in reality Jane's alter ego. Whenever business or illness took Jane away from her post, Abby took over. That included a long stretch in 1873 when Jane was hospitalized for rheumatic fever. Abby was instrumental in forming Bellevue's pioneering nursing school in 1873 and wrote several important books, including *A Century of Nursing, with Hints Toward the Organization of a Training School* (1876).

In a matter of months, the Hospital was running smoothly under Jane Woolsey's masterful command. She assembled a fairly efficient nursing corps, consisting of women of "a plainer type" with little formal training. Woolsey, like her peers, revered the "womanly" aspects of nursing. However, while she prized nurses who were disciplined and orderly, she also wanted practitioners with initiative, who were willing to ignore established rules and methods that hindered effectiveness and efficiency. It was an attitude destined to arouse controversy, no matter how splendid her record. From the very beginning, she earned the wrath of some of the younger doctors, who resented the power of this aristocrat and "lady superintendent." The older medical men begrudged her, too. Not only did they have to bend to the will of the lay Board of Managers, but also to a woman that the board had put in power. Later, when the managers and the physicians came into conflict, she was the obvious scapegoat. As Lamb recounted, "The matter came to a head when one of the doctors insisted on breaking a stringent rule by sending infectious cases to the wards. Miss Woolsey objected. The doctor and some of his colleagues then so openly opposed her that they were dropped by the Managers from the Medical Board. In turn, some of the other members resigned, and so did some of the Managers. Miss Woolsey presented her resignation, but at the insistence of the Board of Managers withdrew it for the time being."

The directress won, but not without paying a price. Woolsey, accustomed to deference and respect, was disquieted by the hostility of the medical staff and exhausted by the upheaval (as well as a recent bout of rheumatic fever and the lingering effects of her service in the Civil War). She resigned after one more year, in March of 1876, outwardly content that her task had been completed. But deep down Woolsey worried that her accomplishments were only temporal. In a heartfelt farewell letter, she counseled her staff:

> Do not count any service in His household as "menial service," if it is only the sweeping of a room, or the cooking of a mess of broth, or the emptying of a refuse bucket...
>
> Keep the standard of your work high. Despise a poor and cheap quality of work, mere eye-service and man-pleasing. Never give yourself to bad or deceitful conduct or the evasion of rules or of rightful authority... Try to make no mistakes, but if honest mistakes happen, as they sometimes will, bear the blame cheerfully ... rather then shifting the blame to someone else's shoulders. Despise and discountenance gossip and tattle. Never allow yourselves to tattle about your patients or listen to those who do. The involuntary confidence of the sick as to their diseases, their personal histories, their family life and troubles, are part of their misfortune...
>
> There is a large class of persons in the great public hospitals ... whose sickness is the direct result, not of misfortune, but of vice and shameful living. You have sometimes found it hard to work for such persons. This is natural...Be even more patient and gentle with this class... [Y]ou have nothing to do with their guiltiness, only their suffering—and the word or two that

you drop, or the mere sight of your good will and faithful care...may do them more good than you will ever know...

Avoid petty disputes and jealousies...Help each other...Bickerings and cross purposes in a household like this hinder business and work downward into discomfort and suffering for the sick...

Save your health. Your business is a very wearing and exhausting one. Economize labor by putting thought into it. Study over it and see how you can make it more systematic and thorough.

Woolsey left many legacies to Presbyterian, foremost among them high standards of nursing care and administration. Although the Board of Managers was slow to realize it, she demonstrated that good health care originated with a competent nursing staff, which in turn originated in a commitment to the *training* of nurses—a hospital could not expect to recruit a cadre of experienced nurses with only a handful of nursing schools in existence. Shortsightedly, the managers would wait another sixteen years before awakening to this truth. Records indicate that in 1880 the Medical Board and the managers' Committee on Nursing decided that the capacity of the Hospital did not warrant the initiation of a training school for nurses, despite the declining state of its nursing corps and the demonstrated success of organized training elsewhere. Sadly, Woolsey died in 1891, months before the creation of Presbyterian's own school for nurses.

Another of Woolsey's legacies was her successor, Hester Rafferty, head nurse and general guardian of the wards. Rafferty, trained entirely by Woolsey, "was highly intelligent in the performance of her duties, absolutely devoted to her work and most efficient and sympathetic in the execution of it," according to David Bryson Delavan, M.D., an early house officer. Reflecting a doctor's perspective of a good nurse, he added, "Best of all, she carried out the orders given to her with implicit fidelity."

Though the medical men won in the long run by pushing Woolsey into retirement, they—and their patients—suffered for their hubris. Delavan claimed that the young doctors, "blinded by their own self-importance, did not hesitate to oppose the Resident Directress, imperiled the very existence of the institution and actually set back its progress for many years." Whether the Hospital actually teetered at the edge of extinction is debatable, but conditions did deteriorate. Rafferty had neither Woolsey's leadership abilities nor mandate to lead. In the overcrowded, understaffed wards, the training of nurses virtually ceased. A new superintendent, Henry F. Carpenter, inherited Woolsey's administrative duties, though not her skills and sensibilities. For example, he foolishly restricted the staff's access to the pantry. "The actual success of the hospital work was interfered with by the fact that we were not in proper physical condition, so that our tempers as well as our digestions suffered," wrote Delavan.

Carpenter's arrival accelerated the deterioration of the nursing staff. Most of the nurses, Delavan complained, were inadequate and inexperienced, not up to the task of caring for the many severely ill patients. To his utter frustration, he was frequently awakened by night nurses to attend to the most trivial complaints. "During a particularly busy period," he recalled,

> I retired one night, greatly fatigued, having given strict orders not to be disturbed unless under urgent necessity. At 2:30 a.m. a female nurse aroused me, reporting that a private patient with "nerves" was "very bad" and needed me at once. Dressing with diligent haste, I repaired to the patient who greeted me with a radiant smile and said "Doctor, I waked up a little while ago and thought that if you would come down and sit by me and let me hold your hand, perhaps I could go to sleep again." Through the treachery of the nurse my appearance at the breakfast table that morning was greeted with the above quotation, shouted in gleeful chorus by the assembled internes.

By 1887 the nursing staff was in shambles, a shadow of the crew that Woolsey had assembled. "I was much perturbed by the poor character of the nursing and the impossibility of finding from the nurses' records what had been the real condition of the patients during the temporary absences of the Medical Staff," newly hired physician W. Gilman Thompson grumbled to the managers. The men's wards were especially pitiful, staffed as they were by untrained "orderlies" — none other than convalescent patients looking to make a few extra dollars. The orderlies' night reports are laughable. The entire entry for September 3, 1889, for a thirty-bed ward, read: "All patients slept good, most part of the night: nothing else to report." Other nighttime entries were: "Everything quiet" or "All patients slept well except Snyder, who coughed considerable." That the wards were full of acutely ill patients, stricken with such diseases as typhoid and pneumonia, led Thompson to suspect that the person who had slept most comfortably was the orderly. Thompson implored one orderly, an Irishman named McCarthy, to elaborate in subsequent reports. McCarthy obliged with such entries as: "C. had a splendid night's rest, in fact it was the best night he had experienced since he came here. All the other patients slept massive." Two nights later: "There is nothing special to report this morning as all the patients slept well and C. slept like a young goat." And then: "C. slept well, but he kept shouting and whistling in that state, otherwise he was very quiet... All the other patients slept well."

A frustrated Thompson told the managers, "I must decline to accept responsibility for what went on in my wards during my absence at night... I suggested that in several other hospitals so-called training schools for nurses had been established and were proving increasingly successful and valuable, and I thought the one thing to do was to establish such a school at the Presbyterian Hospital and replace the orderlies in the men's wards with trained nurses."

The proposal provoked considerable discussion among the managers. A year later, in October 1890, John S. Kennedy, Presbyterian's president, wrote to Thompson, "As soon as the new buildings [replacing ones destroyed by the fire of 1889] are completed, I hope we shall have a training school for nurses. I intend that the Presbyterian shall be the best hospital in every respect in this city and in this country, and I am sure that you and other members of the Medical Board will do everything in your power to make it so."

As Thompson later joked, the Training School's "real founder" was McCarthy, the ersatz orderly. "We simply could not stand him, or his kind, any longer."

The administration's decision to open a training school was also influenced by its successful encounters with pupils from the nursing schools at Bellevue, New York, and New York Post-Graduate hospitals, who had come to Presbyterian Hospital for clinical experience.

Lephe Callender, Post-Graduate Hospital class of 1889, recalled that she had "spent many months in the Presbyterian Hospital as head nurse in the medical ward. I also had a private patient there and did duty in the 'hut,' where erysipelas cases were isolated. We all dreaded duty in the hut... [We] often had very sick patients suffering with pneumonia which kept us busy with [flaxseed] poultices every two hours. The poultices had to be very light weight and hold together and be put on piping hot. While on duty... we were obliged to rise at 5 a.m. in order to make the 5:30 a.m. horse-car as we had to be on duty at 6:30 a.m."

Margaret Graham, Post-Graduate class of 1890, remembered that "our work included mopping and dusting the wards, and we had to have everything done, the patients bathed, beds made, and everything in readiness for inspection by 9:30 a.m. This did not leave much time for idling."

Graham's classmate, Margaret Anderson, recollected, "My first patient was in a private room. I did not know the name of one instrument, but I watched Dr. Sharp do the dressing. The next day I had the instruments ready on a nice clean towel and he looked at me and said, 'You will do.'"

In 1891 Presbyterian requested another seventy pupils from the Post-Graduate Hospital (which understandably declined, for the arrangement would have deprived the hospital of its most vital resource: a continual and inexpensive supply of nurses-in-training to staff its own wards). Obviously, the Board of Managers was pleased with the pupils, but the magnitude of the request suggests a last-minute effort to avoid the trouble and expense of opening a training school.

Around that time, the managers learned of a woman at St. Luke's Hospital who had achieved great success in the fledgling art of nursing education. Finally, Presbyterian Hospital's experiment in the training of nurses would begin.

2

The Education of Anna C. Maxwell

I should like to be your biographer, I am sure I could
make three or four fat volumes and then not tell half.

Edith Ambrose '94*
(from a letter to Anna Maxwell, 1926)

AFTER THE CRIMEAN WAR, a debilitated Florence Nightingale retreated to her sickbed, where she remained for the rest of her considerable life. Nonetheless, through her prolific writings and extraordinary influence in high places, she profoundly affected, for better and for worse, the course of nursing in her native Britain and around the world.

Nightingale's experience taught her that death and disease stemmed primarily from dirt and disorder. The way to health, therefore, was through cleanliness, proper ventilation, nutritious food, skilled nursing, and administrative order, all of which fostered nature's healing powers. The nurse, as guarantor of this environment, was central to the patient's recovery. Given her remarkable success in the Crimea, she had every reason to cling to her ideals, to reject the dangerous notions of medical therapeutics. However, throughout her life she clung to them zealously, to the point of dismissing scientific rationalizations for the cause and spread of disease. Even though she had based her own theories on objective research and statistical analysis, she could not accept such newly emerging ideas as germ theory and specificity of disease, "heresies" that undermined the very foundation of her world. In Nightingale's view, illness was a consequence of one's environment as well as one's behavior. "If chance alone determined whether an individual should intersect with a disease-causing microscopic particle, then sickness was bereft of meaning; it could play no

---

*Denotes year in which she was graduated from the School of Nursing.

monitory role in a world of moral order," explains historian Charles Rosenberg.

As keeper of the moral flame, a Nightingale nurse played the maternal role in the patient's surrogate home, the hospital, ruled of course by the physician-father. One of Nightingale's widely copied innovations was to rearrange the ward so that the nurse could constantly mind her "children" from a single vantage point. Accordingly, Nightingale stressed the motherly aspects of nursing and felt that women were specially suited to be nurses. Womanhood alone wasn't enough, however. Training was necessary to nurture and mold sympathetic but controlled and nonsentimental women. Nursing, to Nightingale, was no ordinary line of work; it was a secularized calling, to which one was bound by duties and obligations.

So that women would retain control over their livelihood, Nightingale's ideal training school fell under the command of a female hierarchy, equal to but separate from the male hierarchy of the hospital. Nurses should be loyal to physicians, she believed, but not servile. Her ideals were realized in 1860 with the creation of the training program for nurses at St. Thomas' Hospital in London, a prototype for schools around the world.

In creating a new profession Nightingale seemingly empowered women, freeing them from the bonds of familial demands. Nursing was added to the small list of occupations considered proper for women to undertake, including teaching and handiwork. However, it could be argued that late-eighteenth century nurses merely exchanged the shackles of one master for the shackles of another. Because of Nightingale's philosophy of nursing practice, nurses became "professional" mothers and housekeepers. Because of her philosophy of education, nurse-trainees became hospital-based apprentices instead of true students. Because of her religious-military background, nursing schools became convent-like and authoritarian. Because of her antebellum views of disease, cleanliness and order took on an almost mystical importance, at the expense of the profession's scientific advancement. And because of her gender-limited conception of the good nurse, nursing became a woman's occupation, a severe handicap in a man's world.

This is a late-twentieth century perspective, of course. In her time Nightingale's accomplishments were remarkable, her motivations understandable. Her theories and practices gave nurses the prerequisites for building a profession and, in the larger scheme, they gave society the prerequisites for a creating a health care system. It was progress in nursing, not medicine, that stimulated the organization of hospitals. Medical science had begun to flower, yet not enough to change the practice of health care or to warrant physician dominance or the construction of special facilities (most care — even surgery — still could be performed in the home). Physicians held no monopoly on therapeutic wisdom. They were, however, the first to seize the potential of scientific rationalism, which they artfully manipulated in their favor, fueling their swift climb to social, economic, and political power.

The birth of organized nursing in America can be traced to 1872, when New England Hospital for Women and Children in Boston opened the first graded course in nursing patterned after the Nightingale model, followed soon after by Bellevue, New Haven, and Massachusetts General hospitals. The schools' apparent success in producing quality practitioners led to the exponential proliferation of training programs throughout the country.* In 1880 there were only sixteen schools with 323 students; by 1893 there were 432 schools with 11,164 students. The exact numbers are disputed, but the consequences of uncontrolled expansion are not. In a sense, the training school concept was too successful. The limited autonomy enjoyed by many early Nightingale schools evaporated as hospital administrators came to recognize the immense value of a system that could fill their wards with inexpensive nurses-in-training, supervised by a small cadre of paid graduate nurses. Such an enterprise simply could not be left in someone else's hands. This trend was particularly deleterious in schools affiliated with small, rural hospitals, where education suffered terribly at the expense of service. They were Nightingale schools in name only. Lacking a stable financial base, many programs had to "sell" student services to hospitals and individuals, further undermining the possibilities of nursing education.

It was a long time before the first nursing schools had a measurable impact on hospital care. Only a handful of graduate nurses were employed by institutions; most were hired for private duty nursing, which offered a meager and unpredictable wage.

Twenty years after New England Hospital's bold experiment, Presbyterian Hospital established its own training program for nurses. Presbyterian's leaders, like others of their time, were administrators first and educators second. They, too, looked to a school as a cost-effective means of staffing the wards. Nonetheless, the Hospital's top officers — John S. Kennedy,

*Sheila Rothman, in *Woman's Proper Place*, argues that conditions at the hospitals did not improve appreciably, largely because most of their graduates were not hired by the hospitals. However, the addition of fairly intelligent, obedient, and capable students must have been an improvement over untrained and undisciplined nurses.

president of the Board of Managers; Frederick Sturges, vice president and chairman of the Training School Committee; and C. Irving Fisher, M.D., superintendent—demonstrated a serious commitment to nursing education. Otherwise they would not have asked Anna Caroline Maxwell to become the School's first superintendent, at an annual salary of $1,500. By 1892 she was widely recognized as a consummate educator and a wily administrator, a women who feared no man, a nurse who feared no physician. Had Kennedy, Sturges, and Fisher wanted a puppet superintendent, they would have looked elsewhere.

Anna C. Maxwell was born on March 14, 1851, in Bristol, N.Y., a small town in the Catskill mountains. Though little is known about the childhood of this brown-eyed, brown-haired girl, it apparently was ideal for the incubation of a nurse. From her father, John Eglinton Maxwell, she inherited a strong measure of military and religious discipline, from her mother, Diantha Caroline Brown, a pioneering spirit. John Maxwell, a member of a distinguished Scottish military family that included a governor-general of Newfoundland, was educated at the University of Edinburgh and ordained a Baptist minister. Anna's mother was a descendant of English pioneer stock who settled in North America in 1634.

When Anna was a small child, the family moved to King, Ontario, Canada, where her two younger sisters were born. She was kept well-sheltered from the outside world, educated primarily at home under her father's guidance and at the Ripley boarding school in Middleport, N.Y. (she was sent home at age fifteen, having grown too fast and too thin.)

The Maxwell home was always open to the needy and unfortunate, instilling in young Anna the quality of selfless caring. As a youngster she probably had read of the heroic wartime exploits of Florence Nightingale and Clara Barton, but what likely piqued her interest in nursing were the two years she spent caring for her invalid mother. Anna displayed a natural talent for nursing, which was first recognized by the family physician, who recommended that she seek employment in a hospital, presumably to support the family after John Maxwell's death. Anna agreed—she was no stranger to work. In earlier days, she had labored in some capacity to help her father meet household expenses. He reportedly had a weakness for books, and sometimes diverted the family's scant resources to their purchase.

In 1874, at the age of twenty-three, Anna Maxwell became an assistant matron at New England Hospital. Curiously, Maxwell, who had no formal training, was not accepted as a student at the hospital, which had recently opened the first general training school for nurses. Administrators there apparently thought she had more to give than to receive.

To another family, one without a tradition of self-effacing service, Maxwell's appointment might have been a social embarrassment. Though a few nursing pioneers had distinguished themselves, formal nurse training was still in its infancy and not yet widely respected. Indeed, the conditions Maxwell encountered at New England Hospital were hardly suited to a refined young woman. They demanded every bit of the fortitude and discipline she had absorbed from her parents. The nurses worked twelve-hour days with one afternoon off each week. Patients had to be carried up and down the stairs. "Instead of a stretcher, as we know it, a six-foot wicker basket with three handles on each side was used, and we had to stiffen our spines in order to reach the third floor with one hundred and eighty pounds weight aboard," Maxwell recalled. She was eventually transferred to the maternity ward, where the patients were lighter but the hours longer. There she learned to bathe babies, make beds, wash diapers, and administer douches.

Although overwhelmed with tasks, Maxwell wanted more responsibility. She chafed at the restraints placed on the nurses, who, for example, were barred from examining patients directly. "We were to judge when to summon the doctors by the cries of the patients," she wrote.

Maxwell earned praise for her work. Her final record reads: "capability recognized on every hand." But the fledgling nurse was seeking more than commendations. The education she had hoped for was sporadic and informal. "The doctors," she recalled, "did not approve of our knowing the object of treatment or the contents of the medicine given. In explanation they said that nurses would imagine the results if they knew what was expected."

Dissatisfied, she left New England Hospital in 1876 in search of a better brand of nursing. Her quest led her to Europe, and she considered entering Nightingale's school in London. Instead, two years later (what transpired in this interval is not known), she enrolled at Boston City Hospital Training School for Nurses, lured by the opportunity to work under Linda Richards, generally regarded as America's first trained nurse. "Under the guidance of Linda Richards ... a woman of rare intelligence with a vision of the future always before her," Maxwell recollected, "I was to learn the elements of scientific training."

As an "experienced" nurse, Maxwell was given advanced standing at Boston City Hospital. Since graduate nurses were hard to come by, anyone with a modicum of training or ability was quickly pushed up the clinical ladder. A footnote on her application reads that she "is to enter training school, not as probationer [beginning student], but at $10 per month and with a view on our part of promoting her to take charge of a ward." With more realistic expectations than her employers, she assumed command of a thirty-two-bed men's surgical ward. "Many of them recovered, despite our ignorance and the crude attention our limited time made possible," she wrote.

Maxwell was not yet a skilled nurse, but she could recognize quality care and would not tolerate anything less. When she was transferred to a thirty-bed women's medical ward, she revolted at the incompetence and indifference of two nurses of the "old type." "These 'ladies' changed their dresses at the noon recess and attempted to occupy rocking chairs most of the afternoon," she wrote. "The condition of the patients was unspeakable; bed sores, tangled hair, unclean heads and bodies." At Maxwell's urging, the nurses were replaced by two pupils.

Maxwell's lessons at Boston City Hospital were invaluable. "There was an infinite variety to learn," she recalled. She came to nursing school with high expectations, which were pushed even higher. On one occasion she was reprimanded by an attending physician for her ignorance of a patient's condition. "Who should know if the head nurse doesn't?" he scolded. "I realized then," she said, "that the head nurse must have a marvelous memory, unlimited intuition, and that she must be vigilant and omnipresent!" Although temperature charts were in use, bedside notes were not. "We were expected to have the mental equipment to carry all details in our heads. My first head nurse impressed upon me that it was a sin ever to forget anything connected with the sick."

Maxwell learned her lessons well — perhaps too well, her superiors sometimes thought. Once, when her ward was overflowing with deathly ill typhoid patients, she protested to the school office, only to be told to make do with what she had. What she had was a staff exhausted from overwork, aching from administering sponge baths to patients on low-slung beds. "I burst out with the remark, 'You are killing one set of women to make well another.' I wasn't dismissed for my impertinence, although I expected to be ... The next day, another pupil was sent."

But logic did not always prevail within hospital walls, Maxwell learned. There was no explaining, for example, why at Boston City Hospital the administrators were slow to install window bars to keep delirious patients from jumping to their deaths. And there was no understanding the irrational behaviors of the hospital's many malingerers, who would do almost anything to earn another day in bed and another warm meal—even suck blood from their gums and regurgitate it to fool their keepers.

"Imagine the responsibility of the nurses," she later remarked. Others could imagine the responsibility, but not why a woman of proper breeding would want to assume it. "The house staff was quizzical," Maxwell wrote. "Why had we chosen such disagreeable work? Did we ever expect to be received by our social friends after taking such a radical step?" Accustomed to deferential and undemanding nurses, physicians felt threatened by this capable and unusual young woman and twitted her about practicing medicine without a license. Friends impatiently demanded to know when she would study medicine or give up nursing altogether. To both, she replied that she wanted to be a good nurse, not a poor doctor.

Not everybody sought to deflect Maxwell's ambitions. George H. M. Rowe, M.D., Boston City Hospital's superintendent, stated: "I esteem her admirably fitted for the position of Superintendent of a Training School."

Taking Rowe at his word, Montreal General Hospital hired Maxwell in October 1880 to establish a training school. It was in dire need of her expertise. Despite its fancy name, it was a glorified almshouse, a place where the floors were littered with the innards of straw-stuffed mattresses, where damp linen was hung to dry throughout the wards, where ventilation pipes were choked with dirt, where tubercular patients had to endure pipe-smoking neighbors, where urine samples were left on the wards for days at a time, and where nurses slept in drafty old wards.

Unfathomably, the managers and doctors fought Maxwell's every move. She managed to convince them of the need for nurses' notes and to count sponges during abdominal surgery. The latter innovation, initially criticized, was adopted only after errant sponges led to several deaths. She also persuaded the doctors to build a laboratory for the examination of urine samples, only to find the plan scuttled because it inconvenienced medical students. Provisions for educating nursing students never materialized. After a fruitless six months, Maxwell resigned. The plan for a training school was deferred for a decade.

"The Montreal physicians must have been singularly unimpressionable and pigheaded, and must have possessed uncommon backbone, to have withstood Miss Maxwell," recalled a friend, the Reverend Henry Sloane Coffin, president of the Union Theological Seminary in New York, decades later. "Tall, commanding, incisive, the very incarnation of the principles of nursing which she inculcated, Miss Maxwell was an impressive and forceful person ... That early experience explains ... in part the firmness and the zeal to which to the end Miss Maxwell insisted on and fought for the public acknowledgement of the nurse's professional standing."

Frustrated but not demoralized by the Montreal experience, Maxwell journeyed across the Atlantic for a three-month tour of British hospitals. She returned to Boston in November of 1881 to begin one of the briefest private duty nursing careers on record. While on her first case, she was offered the superintendency of the Training School for Nurses at Massachusetts General Hospital, one of the oldest, most conservative, and wealthiest hospitals in the nation. Obviously, her reputation had not been tarnished by the events in Montreal.

Fortunately, the trustees of Massachusetts General were open to innovation, for Maxwell aimed to transform their view of nursing. Despite her relative youth and inexperience, she won them over with her "enthusiastic devotion for the cause of nursing education, reinforced by unusual personal charm," according to Sarah Parson's history of the school.

When the new superintendent arrived, she observed that the "apprenticeship model was in full sway." That was soon changed. Under Maxwell, the nurses' quarters were improved and enlarged, a night superintendent was added to secure better care for the patients and to free the superintendent for educational activities, extra staff were hired to relieve the pupils of heavy domestic chores (which she felt were hurting the popularity of the field), a library was opened, textbooks and anatomical charts were secured, and three weeks of vacation were procured. She also arranged lectures and bedside demonstrations by the house and attending staffs and lessons in cooking and massage. To distinguish her pupils, Maxwell designed a uniform of gingham cotton with a pattern of white and turquoise-blue checks.

But Maxwell did not need a uniform to publicize her innovations, which compelled the hospital's staff to take a fresh look at the practice of health care. Her lessons in massage elicited wide interest, prompting head nurses to request a course at their own expense and doctors to prescribe massages. With the assistance of a staff physician, she persuaded the hospital to extend its reach into the community and institute a followup system for discharged patients, which later evolved into one of the first visiting nursing services. And Maxwell challenged the status quo in the operating room, a grisly place fit only for men (or so they said). "The operating room nurse was presided over by a male nurse who had served in the Civil War," Maxwell recalled. "When I suggested introducing pupil nurses into the operating room, he told surgeons it would be accomplished only over his dead body. Six years later this was done, and he survived!" Impressed with the students' capabilities, the surgeons asked that the nurses be taught to dress wounds, and physicians from other wards began to ask for nurse assistants.

During her years at Massachusetts General, Maxwell earned a reputation for both forcefulness and diplomacy in dealing with people of authority, traits partly traceable to the influence of Linda Richards. Richards, who was trained by a physician (Susan Dimock), did not share the view of many early hospital reformers, namely upperclass laywomen, that doctors were their chief antagonists. In establishing the influential Boston City Hospital Training School, Richards deviated from Nightingale's tenet of maintaining a school's autonomy. "She believed it was important for nursing to succeed through its own merits rather than through the influence of" the reformers, notes nursing historian Ellen Baer.

Once again, in the spring of 1889, Maxwell was asked to rescue a training school, this time at St. Luke's Hospital in Manhattan. (She had applied for the superintendency of nursing at the prestigious new Johns Hopkins Medical Center, but that position went to Isabel Hampton Robb.) The scene was all too familiar: overworked nurses, little ventilation, unsanitary conditions. "Small wonder that some [of the nurses] lost their health as well as their courage!" she wrote. "Many brave souls, however, withstood these vicissitudes and reaped a rich reward in seeing the eyes of the blind opened to the importance of a thorough nursing education and of every human being's right to health." One of her accomplishments was to abolish the practice of twenty-four duty, which required pupils to remain with their patients day and night, catching what sleep they could on cots at the bedside. She remained at St. Luke's until the autumn of 1891. While there is little record of her performance, the administration deeply regretted her resignation and praised her "intelligent and earnest work." And there is no indication that Maxwell was disenchanted with her employers. Rather, from another part of town came the opportunity of a lifetime: to establish a nursing school at one of the city's most prestigious and richest institutions, the Presbyterian Hospital. According to colleague Florence Horne, "To bring nursing to the level of a profession was Miss Maxwell's one ideal in life." At Presbyterian, she would devote the rest of her life to the realization of that lofty ideal.

3

Maxwell's Ideal

All things being equal, women of superior education
and culture will be preferred.

School circular (1892)

IN A WAY, the Presbyterian Hospital benefited from its tardiness in establishing a training school. By 1892 nurse educators had been refining and revising their methods and learning from their mistakes for almost two decades. Equally important, Anna Maxwell, now forty, had come of age. "She knew exactly what she wanted," said Rev. Henry Sloane Coffin. "Miss Maxwell had thought out her ideal, could set forth her views with convincing clarity, and the trustees of the hospital and the physicians listened to her and let her have what she wished." Her first wish was to recruit the preeminent nursing staff and faculty of the day. That they were one and the same made her task harder, not easier. Nurses who could run a large ward with an undertrained staff (i.e., unschooled nurses, student nurses, male orderlies), who could effectively and efficiently teach, who could manage an endless stream of equipment and supplies (housekeeping and medical), and who could oversee each patient's diet were scarce and already gainfully employed.

From St. Luke's came a former pupil, Florence A. Horne, a new graduate. "Come up and help," she said to Horne, "the pneumonia patients are dying from lack of proper nursing care." Horne took charge of the men's medical wards and often substituted for the superintendent. Horne's classmate, Jane A. Osborne, was appointed head nurse in the accident ward. Several recent graduates of the Boston City Hospital Training School were hired, including Annie K. MacFarlane, Susanna W. S. Lyman (who succumbed to pneumonia the next year), and M.A.G. Libby (who died of meningitis within months). Rounding out the staff were N. Stuart Bussell of Newton Cottage Hospital, Helen G. Hill of Cumberland Street Hospital in Brooklyn, a Miss Brown of Utica Memorial Hospital, Eleanor Campbell of Hartford Hospital, and Isobel K. Cooper of St. Thomas' Hospital in London. Nora Anthony, a young nurse at Johns Hopkins associated with the esteemed surgeon William Osler, came in August to take charge of the operating theater.

With these young women, Maxwell swiftly reorganized the nursing service. "It impresses me ... that such an efficient organization, as I found it in 1895, could have been in existence for only 3½ years," wrote T. Stuart Hart, M.D., an intern during Maxwell's inaugural period. "Not only was the nursing good and efficient, but the cooperative spirit which existed between the School of Nursing, the internes, the medical staff and the superintendent was very extraordinary."

Presbyterian Hospital's Training School Committee, under the guidance of Frederick Sturges, met for the first time in April 1892. One of its first tasks was to approve a publicity circular, announcing a two-year program for "women desirous of learning the art of nursing." Only women between the ages of twenty-three and thirty-five were invited to apply. It is remarkable that anyone bothered. Students were expected to work from seven in the morning until seven in the evening. "Reasonable time" — amounting to one afternoon and a part of Sunday each week, plus three weeks of vacation each year — was allowed for study, exercise, rest, and worship. Pupils were provided room and board plus a nine dollar monthly stipend the first year, eleven dollars the second, yet a large portion of that income went toward uniforms, text books, and miscellaneous expenses.

Each applicant was required to complete a questionnaire and submit two letters of recommendation, one from "a responsible person, testifying to her good moral character," another from a physician testifying to her sound health. Maxwell wanted to know if the candidate was connected with any church, single or widowed, free of responsibilities at home, and had ever been enrolled in a nursing school. The circular warned that one's ability to read aloud, write legibly and accurately, keep simple accounts, and take lecture notes — qualities deemed "indispensable" for a student at the School — were tested during a one-month probationary period.

The superintendent made no secret of her aristocratic preferences. According to an early head nurse, Maxwell leaned toward Canadian applicants, believing they were better "material" and more practically raised. "Women not naturally adapted for the work are almost sure to find it irksome, or, at best, to regard it simply as a means of earning a livelihood and thus miss its most inspirational features," Maxwell wrote in the first edition of *Practical Nursing: A Text-Book for Nurses and a Hand-Book for All Who Care for the Sick* (1907), co-authored by Amy Pope, a member of the first class.

From the first, the School earned a reputation for being an elite—some would say elitist—institution. Perhaps so. But Maxwell, having witnessed too much mediocre nursing, wanted only the very best. As she wrote in an early annual report, she was preparing nurses for their "life work," a formidable goal that only the brightest and best late-nineteenth century women were likely to meet.

Maxwell's ideal nurse met specific physical, mental, and moral criteria, detailed in her book. "Unless a woman be possessed of perfect health, a strong constitution, unlimited physical endurance, and freedom from an excessively high nervous organization, she cannot give her best to this work," she wrote. Given the long hours, intense physical work, and hazardous conditions, this was perfectly reasonable. In the School's early years, the class ranks were thinned by typhoid, diphtheria, pneumonia, influenza, and measles. Deaths were not uncommon.

To maintain one's health, she recommended "strict obedience to the laws of hygiene," which included personal cleanliness, suitable clothing, exposure to fresh air, "sufficient rest, the avoidance of all causes of indigestion, and early attention to all slight ailments." She encouraged nurses to maintain "a diversity of interests, in order to keep their minds alert and enable them to provide entertainment for their patients." To promote good digestion, Maxwell suggested that nurses avoid "ward talk" at meals, which would only cause them to eat too quickly in anticipation of work that yet to be done, and "to direct the conversation to interesting topics of the day and amusing incidents that will divert the mind into new channels of thought." Maxwell took her own advice, rarely discussing professional matters in the Hospital's dining hall, where the most promising young interns were invited to share her table. "Those of us who sat at the staff table with her in the old Presbyterian days will never forget the way in which she kept the ball of conversation rolling with keen and swift repartee," recalled James Miller Alexander, M.D.

Maxwell didn't specify that applicants possess any particular knowledge, rather "a high order of intelligence and a desire to learn ... Nurses will find that there is no knowledge, even of subjects far removed from nursing, which may not prove useful." At the very least, a widely read nurse made for a "resourceful companion" to patients. "She was delighted when young women with college degrees began to apply," said Rev. Coffin. "She knew that during their years in training, nurses had too little time for wide reading. Consequently, she looked for those who ... had already acquired well furnished minds." Otherwise, Maxwell prized an orderly mind, meticulous habits, promptness, a good memory (which required cultivation), and acute perception (even more cultivation). "Nurses must be quick to observe minute details and equally quick to act intelligently on their observations," she noted.

Maxwell valued the moral qualities of courtesy, dignity, economy (as opposed to "extravagance"), personal neatness, self-control, sympathy, tact, truthfulness, unselfishness, and obedience. While Maxwell knew that disobedience had its place in any bureaucracy, she also knew that without distinct lines of authority and respect for authority hospitals would be impossible to manage. "The etiquette of the army is, to a certain extent, repeated in the hospital," she wrote. "Nurses are required to stand when speaking to those in authority, and to give precedence at all times not only to their superiors, i.e., the superintendents, doctors, head nurses, but also to their seniors in school." (Such deferential behavior had amazing staying power. Catherine Weiser '20 was chided by an instructor "for talking to a head nurse with my hands *not* behind my back." And as late as the early 1960s, Presbyterian nurses were expected to leap to attention when a doctor entered the room.) Maxwell's rules were also intended to protect students from the folly of youth. "There is probably not a graduate nurse of any intelligence who, on looking back after experience has broadened her views, has not felt both mortified and amused at some of the egotistical judgments of her days in training," she contended.

One could apply to the School by letter, although a personal visit was preferred. From Carrollton, Ga., Conyers Prichett submitted a letter of application, dated December 1899, informing the superintendent of her age (twenty-three), height (five feet, four inches) and weight (130 pounds), education (college degree), experience (eighteen months of teaching), and health ("perfect"). Prichett related, "I have no family," explaining that her parents were deceased and her brothers and sisters away on business or married. "I am anxious to have a profession and I believe I can make a success of nursing." As required, Pritchett solicited two letters of recommendation, one from her pastor, the Reverend W. E. Dozier, and another from her physician, B.C. Powell, a prominent member of the Carrollton County Medical Society. "I can say that she has been a consistent, active, and interested member" of my church, wrote Dozier. "She is a young lady of good education and native ability, and of high Christian character. She belongs to a most excellent family and her home training has been of the best sort." Powell stated "that she is physically stout, strong, and healthy. Mentally, she is of quick perception and considerably above the average. In her disposition, she is amiable, kind, and gentle. She is unquestionably honest, reliable, and deserving of any aid she may ask or any position she might aspire to." Pritchett evidently met Maxwell's exacting standards and was accepted into the class of 1903.

"Few girls forgot their first interview with [Maxwell]," recalled Rev. Coffin.

> Her questions probed deep. She was not interested in the colorless, the insignificant, the emotional, the mediocre. It was the vital, the energetic, the staunch for whom she sought. If she were to discipline personalities, she wished young women with personalities worth disciplining. She was sometimes accused of laying stress upon external qualities as agreeable manners, pleasant looks, social grace; these she considered, for they had value, but her eye was fixed on underlying qualities which indicated strength of character. Her judgment was vindicated again and again in the nurse whom she helped to produce.

Maxwell's admissions standards were not inflexible. Promising if flawed young women could gain admittance. Upon meeting Anne Dravo Van Kirk, the superintendent feared that she was too small to handle the arduous tasks of nursing. But Kirk pleaded, "Let me try, I'll manage," and was allowed to enroll in the class of 1896. She went on to become the superintendent of Mt. Sinai Hospital Training School and helped raise the standards of nursing education and practice.

Once accepted, a student was beholden to the School, even before she arrived at the Hospital. An early acceptance letter reads: "You are expected to hold yourself in readiness to come at once when telegraphed for ... You should report to me any illness or any change in your address, for however short a time." Students weren't truly accepted, however, until they satisfactorily completed the one-month probationary period and committed to twenty-three months of training. And they could be dismissed at any time for "inefficiency, misconduct, neglect of duty, or failure to develop qualities fitting the profession," according to the School bulletin.

Maxwell's new venture evidently filled a cavernous void. In only eighteen months, it received 536 inquiries from prospective students. Interest surged after the 1893 World's Columbian Exposition in Chicago (a celebration of the 400th anniversary of the landing of Columbus), which included the medal-winning "Exhibit of the Training Schools for Nurses of New York and Brooklyn," a detailed miniature medical-surgical ward. The exhibit, which Maxwell helped organize, was a milestone in nursing, demonstrating to the country at large what rigorous training could do for hospitals and patients. (Thousands more viewed the exhibit at the Paris Exposition of 1900, the first world's fair.) By the end of the School's first decade, well over 9,000 women had inquired about nursing education at Presbyterian, only one percent of whom were awarded the honor of studying under Maxwell.

The Presbyterian Hospital Training School for Nurses officially opened on May 1, 1892, with an enrollment of ten probationers (called "probies") plus six nurses already employed at the Hospital, who were given advanced standing and slightly higher monthly stipends. Annie E. Leonard, one of the six, was allowed a full year's credit; five others—Sarah K. Davis, Julia Rose, Josephine C. Martin, Camilla Salling, and Nellie B. Hurlburt ("understanding that another attack of erysipelas would rule her out")— were allowed six months' credit. Sixteen additional probationers were accepted at intervals during the year.

Despite the rigor of Presbyterian's admissions standards and Maxwell's keen eye for nurses-to-be, several pupils didn't make the grade. According to her first annual report, "two [of the first students] were found incompetent, and two have fallen out from disability." The following year, two more were dropped for "inefficiency" and another for ill health.

All nursing staff and students were housed in an unused ward on the top floor of the medical building, lowering Presbyterian's potential bed count to 256. The converted ward included a dining room and kitchenette, several two-bed cubicles for the students, single rooms for graduate nurses (Maxwell included)—and plenty of mice. Jimmy, the resourceful elevator man, was offered a bounty of one cent per mouse tail, which he redeemed by the dozens from C. Irving Fisher, the Hospital's superintendent. (It was Jimmy who, in the absence of the superintendent and the directress, had guided the evacuation of the Hospital during the fire of 1889.)

New enrollees were instructed to bring the following items: three dresses of light-colored gingham or calico, "plainly made"; six large white aprons; a pin ball, needle case, and thimble; one pair of boots, "one inch longer than foot, with square heels"; and additional plain clothing. "If the teeth are out of order in any way, they must be attended to before coming for the probationary month." Full-fledged pupils were required to obtain their own forceps, scissors, soft night shoes, a watch with a second hand, and a School uniform. Only one trunk was allowed, as storage space was limited. However, opportunities for usefulness were not.

4

No Little Things in Nursing

Miss Maxwell was clear that she had to train a young woman from the inside out—to give her complete self-mastery from her inmost emotions out to deftness in every motion of her hands and control of every muscle in her face.

Rev. Henry Sloane Coffin (1942)

HEALTH CARE CHANGED DRAMATICALLY in the final quarter of the nineteenth century. Stethoscopes, hypodermics, thermometers, and aseptic techniques came into routine use. Every new year produced another major scientific, diagnostic, or therapeutic advance: the discovery of the organisms that cause gonorrhea (1879), typhoid (1880), tuberculosis (1882), and cholera (1883); surgery for ectopic pregnancy (1883); prophylactic treatment of rabies (1885); diphtheria antitoxin (1891); the use of rubber gloves in surgery (1891); light therapy for skin diseases (1893); x-rays (1895); serological tests for typhoid (1896); the discovery of the role of mosquitoes in malaria (1897); and the bronchoscope (1898).

In this scientifically charged atmosphere, nurses had to know more than how to mop a floor or wash a diaper or make a bed, a reasoning reflected in Maxwell's early curriculum, which mixed the old (discipline, order, devotion) with the new (scientific rationalism).* "The love of nursing seems born in some women," she wrote. "The instinct of the Mother, one of our

---

* Maxwell was not ashamed of menial labor, however. "There is no disgrace in doing any form of manual work and it has been our proud tradition that nurses have raised so much of what has been called 'menial' to the rank of a science and art," she once commented. And in 1923, at the fiftieth anniversary pageant of the Massachusetts General Hospital Training School for Nurses, she proudly demonstrated how she used to teach proper mopping techniques.

highest attributes, is seldom missing in the true woman. But these natural gifts must be supplemented by nursing education and practical experience. We must keep pace with the spirit of scientific advance in medical education and medical science of the present day, without losing the personal interest, the human touch that distinguishes the devoted nurse."

Accordingly, her first annual report reads: "It is the aim of this school to furnish a thorough medical, surgical, and obstetrical training for its pupils, to give them the advantage of lectures, demonstration and practical experience... [and] above all, to inspire them with a reverence for their work, and the desire to carry with them, into whatever branch of nursing they enter, that true love for humanity, which makes the helpful and successful nurse."

Early lectures at the Training School, mostly delivered by the medical staff, were rich and diverse. The 1893-94 academic year revolved around the following lectures, totaling about forty hours:

Junior Lectures
(Tuesdays at 4 p.m.)

Hygiene of the Sick Room (4 lectures)
   Air: Causes of pollution and methods of testing the quality
      Ventilation and heating
   Water: injurious constituents and purification
Outline of Bacteriology (3 lectures)
   Prevention and limitation of certain diseases
   Sterilization and disinfections of the apartments, clothing, excreta, and
      disposal of the latter
Topographical Anatomy (7 lectures)
   Demonstration of the circulation of the blood
   Alimentary apparatus and renal organs in health and disease
      Care of the dead
Medical Lectures (6 lectures)
   General care and observation of patients, medical appliances, emergencies, etc.
   Temperature, pulse, and respiration
   Secretions and excretions
   Food and diet
   Nursing in febrile diseases, cold water baths, etc.
   Nursing in contagious diseases; use of stomach and nasal tubes
Surgical Lectures (8 lectures)
   Administration of anesthetics; care of the patient before, during, and after
      operation; emergencies, stimulation, feeding, etc.
   Principles of aseptic and antiseptic surgery; sterilization of dressings,
      disinfectants and their preparation; healing of wounds and inflammation

Surgical diseases; suppuration and abscess; septicemia and pyemia; erysipelas, tetanus, etc.

Prompt aid to the injured; artificial respiration

Gynecology (3 lectures)

Anatomy of pelvis, diseases of women; gynecological positions and instruments

General gynecological operations, with preparation and after care

Abdominal surgery; preparation and after care; position of patients; vomiting; pain; tympanitis; dressing; catheterization; enemata; and hypodermic administrations

Senior Lectures
(Thursdays at 4 p.m.)

Obstetrics

Outline of anatomy and nursing in diseases of nose and throat

Outline of materia medica

Eye and ear: outline of anatomy, care in health and disease

Care of children (including infant feeding)

Care of nervous cases with rest cure

Care of the insane

Anatomy and care of the skin: nursing and diseases of the skin

Symptomatology: nervous system, heart, and respirative organs, abdominal organs

Instruction in practical bandaging and in urinalysis with demonstrations

The pupils were quite fortunate to learn—assuming that after a long day of ward duty they were still sentient—from some of the finest physicians in the city, including Andrew J. McCosh, Walter B. James, F. P. Kinnicutt, and W. Gilman Thompson. It is interesting to note that the hygiene lecture was delivered by a doctor of divinity, the Reverend Thomas Wall, the Hospital's former superintendent and current chaplain, reflecting the lingering moral-religious influence in health care.* (This was, after all, a *Presbyterian* hospital.) Another nonmedical man, Elias T. Green, lectured on materia medica. Maxwell gave additional talks and demonstrations. Lessons in Swedish massage and a course in cooking for invalids at the New York Cooking School on 23rd Street rounded out the curriculum. Students studied from Clara Weeks Shaw's *Textbook of Nursing for the Use of Training Schools, Families and Private Students* (1885) and had access to a variety of books and periodicals in the Training School library.

Over the next few years, clinical experiences were arranged at Sloane Maternity, the Foundling Asylum, Marion Street Maternity, the New York

---

* According to Rev. Coffin, Maxwell was "reticent when it came to her own most sacred beliefs and feelings. Nor was she conventionally devout, although she prized proper religious observances."

Asylum for Lying-in Women, and, later in the decade, Willard Parker Hospital for Contagion and the Scarlet Fever and Diphtheria Hospital. That so many affiliations were allowed speaks well of Presbyterian's managers. Most hospital administrators frowned upon outside experience for student nurses — unless it could generate income — fearing that it would breed institutional disloyalty or inflate operating expenses (from having to hire replacements). But added experience did produce a better nurse, a fact that more and more administrators were learning. "We hear constantly from Trustees and Managers of institutions, other than hospitals, the remark, 'Hereafter our Matron must be a Graduate Nurse,'" wrote Maxwell in her 1899 annual report.

Most of the pupils' time, it must be remembered, was consumed by ward duty, otherwise known as "practical work." They comprised the bulk of the nursing staff (forty-one of sixty-two nurses), which on an average day was charged with the care of 168 inpatients, 37 dispensary visitors, and 6 emergency cases, leaving little time for homework. It would have been more accurate — though less politic — to have called the pupils apprentices. After all, they paid no tuition and received a meager salary (termed a stipend) in exchange for working long hours at the feet of the master craftsmen, the graduate nurses. Caught in a netherworld, somewhere between academia and industry, student nurses seemed to have the worst of both. They were students, but their academic year was far longer than that of other professional schools, with no time off for major holidays and just three weeks of vacation. They studied, but they also toiled up to sixty hours a week, roughly 25 percent more than the average industrial laborer. They attended lectures, but what did they absorb after nine hours of ward duty? They took regular quizzes, but not when the wards were too hectic. They were assigned enormous responsibilities, involved in matters of life and death, yet they were also treated like children. They were required to live within the Hospital's walls, could not receive visitors, could not marry, and could not come and go freely (a multicolored pegboard, called the "peggy," was employed to keep track of the young women). "That immortal pedagogue, Wackford Squeers, Esq., of Dotheboys Hall [the ignorant and brutal character from Dickens' *Nicholas Nickleby*] could not have devised a set of rules better calculated to preserve decorum, elevate the spirit and make pleasant the lives of the pupils than those framed for the new Training School for Nurses of the Presbyterian Hospital," observed a bitingly sarcastic writer for the *New York Herald*. Students complained (anonymously) to the paper about a variety of regulations governing their living quarters, including ones prohibiting them from moving furniture or displaying any personal effects.

Remarkably, Presbyterian's pupils had it far better than most. Students in small rural hospitals, which far outnumbered their large urban counterparts, spent most of their time cleaning floors, windows, furniture, patient rooms, wards, tubs, and equipment, even after the probationary period ended. Little time was wasted teaching them abstract concepts they supposedly would never use. Such institutions had few, if any, full-time instructors or regular clinical rotations. As late as 1912 about half of all training programs still did not have a single paid instructor and half did not have a library.

Like all other nurses-in-preparation, Maxwell's pupils made beds and gave bed pans, and they scrubbed and they dusted. But the similarity with their rural counterparts ends there. Each took charge of six to ten patients as well as the medicine, linen, and supply closets. "Each pupil... cares for her own patients, remaining with them as a rule long enough to observe the cases fully," wrote Maxwell. "She has the care of the bed, the nursing, the recording of work done, and the clearing up after herself... not leaving the 'fag' work for younger nurses or Probationers." The superintendent believed that her nurses were special but not superior. She did not want to create private duty nurses who would leave dressings, poultice dishes, bathrooms, and bathtubs for servants to clean.

As central players in one of the world's most advanced hospitals, the students were immersed in the state of the art. The diary of a member of the class of 1897 reveals an astonishing array of experiences. Over the course of two years, she witnessed operations for the removal of ovarian cysts and fibroid tumors and for the repair of torn tendons and strangulated hernias. She later assisted in the operating room, scrubbing instruments, fixing catgut sutures, and preparing ether cones and cotton balls. On the wards, she administered dozens of hypodermics, made plaster splints, viewed intubations, prepared solutions according to the metric system, filtered salt solutions, made iodoform gauze, started sterilizers, and performed bladder irrigations and intrauterine douches. She also gained experience in the accident ward, the nursery, the children's ward, the women's medical ward, the dispensary, in post-op, on special duty, with infectious disease cases at North Brothers Island, and on night duty.

And she did all this under Maxwell's critical eye. "For her there was just one right way of making a bed, or of bathing a patient, or of doing anything which a nurse had to do," reported Rev. Coffin.

Miss Maxwell showed the way and expected her pupils to follow without deviation. This was not, as some self-styled progressive educators foolishly suppose, to ruin initiative. The graduates of this school are conclusive evidence that their originality and ingenuity have not been suppressed...

The girl who could not meet Miss Maxwell's exacting standards found the school an uncomfortable place, and her stay in it was usually brief. The stupid, the inattentive, the lackadaisical, the scatter-brained, the lazy, the careless, the rebel against rules, met with no mercy. She could be satirical if she thought a probationer thick-skinned or obtuse. A reprimand from her was an event not likely to be forgotten by its unhappy recipient. Her severity was due to her standards for her profession and her insistence that the sick deserve only the most skilful and painstaking care...

Miss Maxwell demanded not only brains which worked with concentration, precision and unflagging alertness; she went deeper and required in nurses a rigidly disciplined personality. It is a mistake to fancy that she was not a woman of strong and warm sentiment—witness her patriotism, her devotion to this school and its graduates, her lifelong passion for the honor of her profession, the steadfastness of her friendships—but she abhorred sentimentality. She proceeded to knock any traces of it out of her pupils. Feelings, temper, tongue, nerves, muscles were to be under strict control. The military ideal at its loftiest dominated and was embodied in her.

Maxwell inspired all sorts of reactions in her pupils, from awe to fear to respect. One alumna remembered the superintendent, an above-average five feet, eight inches in height, as a "tall, dignified figure guiding us through what seemed to us then the interminable mazes of the old hospital. She could outwalk us all. As we scurried after her, breathless, she would suddenly stop, turn and with a twinkle in her eye, say: 'Nurses must learn to walk fast.'"

"How well I remember the first time I walked up that long corridor with you and how you gave me a demonstration of my carriage and walk, which was not at all that flattering," recalled Edith Ambrose '94 in a letter to Maxwell. "How I practised to hold myself and walk like you, in my bedroom when no one was looking."

A member of the class of 1915 remembered: "Once she put the question: 'What are the little things in nursing?' A squirming, uncertain, anxious-to-please probationer hemmed and hawed and tried to make up a list of 'little things.' It was impressed upon us that 'there are no little things in nursing.'"

"Every student has a fund of memories whose center is a certain tall figure in white who suddenly confronted one 'with the goods,'" recalled another alumna.

Some never-to-be-forgotten lesson was sure to be learned at such moments. They may have dealt with the fashion of one's hair or the length of one's skirt, or with far more weighty matters of professional etiquette or treatment of patients. Be that as it may, by that presence an awe akin to fear was inspired, commanding the promptest obedience. It usually wore off, that worse stage of quaking, but that prompt response to suggestion—never!... Surely none of us feel, after quitting the field of our training, that we are meant to rest on those laurels and let it go at that. Rather she makes us feel the progress still to be made—with the fight always on for a world of health and sanity.

Few students were foolish enough to complain about conditions to Maxwell, whose stoicism was legendary. One evening, as the story goes, Maxwell and her usual retinue of house officers (whom she recruited as escorts to the opera or theater) hopped in a cab back to the Hospital. After a block or so, Maxwell calmly asked if they could stop for a moment so she could get her finger out of the door.

"There was a majesty about Miss Maxwell and an imperious quality in her will that secured obedience," added Helen Young '12. Unfortunately, it also evoked fear and suppressed the valid expression of emotions. "Miss Maxwell had sharply criticized my work — and justifiably," recalled a member of the class of 1915. "I did not tell her why my mind was not wholly in my loved and chosen work. I was taught not to make excuses." The student kept silent even though her brother had been hospitalized on Ward's Island for threatening to commit suicide. A week later he did. When Maxwell found out, she summoned the student to her office. The alumna remembered, "I stood stone still for a moment. She said: 'You have been expecting this?' I said: 'Yes, he has made several attempts.'... To my astonishment, she then said: 'My child, why didn't you tell me this?' Then gathering me into her motherly arms, her stiff dignity gone (for the moment), I wept. Then, practical as always, she said: 'What are you going to do now?'"

"Many considered her autocratic and stern," observed Albert Lamb.

Possibly she was, in carrying on the ordinary routine of her position but when any of her nurses were in trouble no one could have been more sympathetic and gentle, sparing no amount of time and trouble in helping the situation.

I remember well the time when one of her students was found dead in her room one morning... The coroner insisted upon an autopsy, refused to do it at the hospital and said it must be done at Bellevue. Miss Maxwell not only went down there but spent the whole day until the matter was settled. She wanted the family to know that the girl had not been left alone even after her death. She did not send someone else which a really cold person would have done. She went herself.

Maxwell only appeared to be unemotional. As Lamb added, "[her] proud but albeit sensitive spirit seldom allowed her to show her real feelings to the outside world." At the same time, she craved companionship, keeping a busy after-hours schedule. Many an evening were spent at the theater, the opera, the Cosmopolitan Club, and the Woman's City Club. "She loved people," noted the *American Journal of Nursing*, "enjoyed social intercourse, and because of her physical strength she was able to indulge her pleasure in social things. It is said of her that after a strenuous day—and what day was not strenuous—Miss Maxwell would go out in the evening, would return about midnight, work for awhile, throw herself on the bed, and be up again ready for another day at five-thirty the next morning."

In order to complete Maxwell's two-year trial by fire, students had to pass a series of tests and quizzes, culminating in a day's worth of oral examinations in medicine, surgery, and materia medica (given by a physician and a surgeon) and practical examinations on the wards (given by Maxwell). The diary of a student from the class of 1897 indicates that she was asked by Maxwell to describe the number and position of the lobes in the lung and to demonstrate the preparation and application of an ice poultice.

Each year the final exams were used to select the top six students, who were awarded the honor of exhibiting their newfound skills to the public. With the aid of convalescent patients, the "first six" demonstrated how to treat rheumatism, apply bandages and poultices, change mattresses, prepare and serve food, and dress and bathe a baby. The pioneering demonstrations originated with the first graduating class, presumably to show Presbyterian's managers that their money was being well spent. Impressed, the president requested a repeat performance for outside parties, including the city's leading nurses and physicians. One year, a special series of demonstrations was presented to a class of fifteen students from Cornell University Medical College. In time, the lay public was invited, too, and the demonstrations became a widely accepted educational tool. The *New York Herald* covered the event in 1901. In an article entitled, "Graduating Nurses Show Their Skill," the newspaper reported, "The infant seemed to enjoy the process as much as the spectators did."

Presbyterian Hospital authorities were thrilled with the positive press coverage. As W. Gilman Thompson of the Medical Board recalled,

> One of the most important of the immediate benefits conferred by the establishment of the Training School was that it put a stop to the tirades of abuse which certain daily papers (they were not called yellow in those days, being merely of a plain mud color) were accustomed to bestow upon the hospital whenever news was otherwise dull. I quote from the scare lines of such a paper published in the year before the school was opened. "Shocking

cruelty charged against the Presbyterian Hospital Nurses." ... "Sick and dying alleged to have been beaten and cursed." ... [I]t was found that this [latter headline] emanated from an enterprising young man who, drinking not wisely but too well, woke up to find himself on one of the hospitals wards where being deprived of his customary alcohol and opium, he dictated a pipe dream which he sold to the newspaper for ten dollars ... [S]ometimes reporters would feign illness so as to be admitted to the wards and write them up from the bedside.

On May 15, 1894, the Presbyterian Hospital Training School for Nurses graduated its first class, twenty-one pioneers in nursing. After a musical interlude by the Mendelssohn Quartette, the commencement address was given by William H. Draper, M.D., president of the Medical Board. "It is hard to exaggerate the importance of this auspicious event in the history of the Presbyterian Hospital ... " he proclaimed. "Without the intelligent, well-trained, and faithful nurse these noble buildings, with their admirable equipment and staff of skilled physicians and surgeons, would not constitute a hospital; there would still be lacking the one essential element which gives life and order and efficiency to the work of mercy that is done within these walls."

Then, quite laudably, Draper expressed his preference for the nurse steeped in science over one steeped in sentimentality:

> The presence of the Sister of Charity, in her sombre garb, accentuates the function of the priest in the sick room rather than that of the doctor. The immortal soul of the patient seems to be a greater concern than his helpless and bruised body ... Science has ... demonstrated that disease and accident are commonly the result of ignorance or the reckless violation of natural laws, or of conditions and circumstances beyond our control. Hence we are not in need of encouragement to pious resignation and penitential endurance when disease and injury afflict us as we are of a more exact knowledge of the causes of disease and of enlightenment as to the means of preventing as well as of repairing the ills to which our flesh is heir.

Enchanted as he was about the capabilities of the well-trained nurse, Draper did not bring himself to question health care's arbitrary pecking order, and he proceeded to turn history on its head to reaffirm the need for the physician to remain in charge. "The trained nurse has been naturally evolved out of the progress that has been made in the science of disease and the art of healing," he said, blissfully unaware that it was Nightingale's principles of nursing that gave rise to hospitals, which in turn gave rise, in parallel and in concert, to organized medicine and organized nursing. While nursing gained from scientific advances in medicine, medicine gained from nursing's creation of an orderly practice environment. That scarcely mattered to Draper, who portrayed the physician as the ultimate, if fallible, authority. "Your relations to the doctor are those of a subordinate..." he told the graduates.

> Doctors are often responsible for the faults of the nurses, sometimes through their failure to give explicit directions, more often from the careless habit of leaving too much to the discretion of the nurse. It is natural under these circumstances that the nurse, especially if she be vain of her knowledge and experience, should assume responsibility which does not belong to her... You have the right to exact specific instructions from the doctor. It is not unlikely that you will sometimes be able to improve upon his suggestions, but you must be careful to do this without giving offence, and always maintain the attitude of respectful submission to his approval.

Ten of the twenty-one graduates found steady employment in private duty nursing in New York City; eight joined the staff of Presbyterian Hospital, five as head nurses; two graduates returned home, probably to marry or to assume family responsibilities; and one died shortly after graduation. This pattern of employment continued in the ensuing years, except that several of the graduates became superintendents at other institutions while others went abroad to pursue missionary work and establish training schools. One of those brave souls was Katherine Stephanova Tsilka '98, who journeyed to Kortcha, Albania. In 1901 she wrote to her friends at the School, "I have opened an abscess in the breast, and was very successful, so much so that the doctors... have reported me to the Government, but the Government, instead of stopping me, asked me to become a Government nurse." A few years later she started a school of nursing.

While a few other training schools could boast a similar record, most sent their graduates out to an uncertain freelance future. The rank and file had little chance of earning a staff position, which went only to the choicest graduates. And they did not possess the knowledge or initiative to start their own programs or the confidence to work abroad.

To assist alumnae in obtaining employment and the public in finding skilled nurses, the School established a registry of its graduates in 1894. The registry was an instant and unexpected success. Families were more than willing to pay the fee of a Presbyterian nurse, which ranged from twenty-one to twenty-eight dollars a week. In 1899, for example, the registry received 780 requests for service; 598 were filled by Presbyterian nurses, the rest by qualified graduates of other training schools.

It was soon apparent the alumnae needs went well beyond the means or purview of the Training School. The School's registry was welcome, but it was not enough. In 1897 graduates banded together to open a residential club house at 54 West 83rd Street in Manhattan. Harriet Gibson '94 was appointed the first directress. Within a year the venture was self-supporting and applicants had to be turned away. The group's activities were formalized the following year with the formation of the Alumnae Association of the Presbyterian Hospital Training School. Under its first two presidents, Frances A. Stone '94 and Amy E. Pope '94, the association drafted a constitution and by-laws, selected a motto ("Labore et Scientia"), and designed a membership pin (a Maltese cross of white enamel with a blue center bearing the letters P.H., surrounded by a wreath of laurel).

The alumnae had more immediate goals, including the establishment of funds for graduates who needed emergency loans, who had taken ill, or who were sick or retired. Just before the turn of the century, the association staged a series of demonstrations in elementary nursing, raising a grand total of $27.55, the embryo of a health-benefit and loan fund. From this modest beginning emerged a consummate fundraising team. By 1908 they had collected $50,000, half of that from Hospital President John Kennedy. Tens of thousands more were raised for a pension fund, including $20,000 from the Andrew Carnegie family and $25,000 from William Sloane, a later president of Presbyterian.

The campaign for the endowment fund got off to a slower start. Not until 1919 did the alumnae make a concerted effort to establish a fund that would give the School more independence, aiming for a lofty goal of $5 million. The delay was understandable since there was a more immediate need to provide for graduates who fell ill or ran into a streak of bad luck. Anna Maxwell, the association's first honorary member, helped the association accrue funds by donating seed money for two money-making ventures: an Alumnae Shop on the Hospital's main floor, which sold books, candies, cigarettes, and gifts, and a radio rental service for patients. Little support came from the School's usual benefactors within the Hospital community. Maxwell was incensed. In 1902 she wrote:

> Almost daily one hears of generous endowments for the investigation of scientific subjects, of great gifts to schools and laboratories, that the men who have chosen the medical profession shall be perfectly equipped for their important work. But one hears almost nothing of a concerted effort for the preparation of the one who stands next the doctor; who often has to face most alarming conditions, calling for the highest intelligence and judgment; the one who is the connecting link between the doctor and the patient, often in

the most important crisis of life; the one who must carry out orders with fidelity and knowledge. In order to put training school instruction upon an educational basis by teaching the theory as a preparation for practical work, as is already done in all other educational lines, we need increased living accommodations and an Endowment Fund for the Preparatory Course.

The association's goals were not all inwardly directed. At the beginning, the group expressed an intent to "promote a common fellowship among graduate nurses" and advance their interests "in every way." So in 1899, when the Nurses' Associated Alumnae of United States and Canada (later, the American Nurses' Association) announced a new publishing venture, the *American Journal of Nursing*, the association immediately purchased two hundred-dollar shares, and individual members solicited one hundred subscriptions. In subsequent years the alumnae funded several of the School's studies and raised great sums of money for student scholarships. Fundraising gave alumnae a shared purpose, but it was the association's magazine, the *Quarterly*, which first appeared in 1906, that truly forged a "common fellowship" of nurses, particularly among the School's far-flung graduates. Issue after issue contained letters posted by alumnae from all over the globe, detailing their exploits, from the exotic to the mundane. Readers grew accustomed to stories of classmates who met kings and queens, who founded training schools in Lebanon or Turkey, who witnessed revolutions, or who simply settled down and started families; to news of innovative nursing programs at Presbyterian and around the country; and to calls to rally around this or that political, social, or health care issue—all for one dollar a year (a price that held firm until 1948).

By any measure—except Anna Maxwell's—the School was off to an auspicious start. In what is perhaps the most understated annual report in history, she wrote in 1895 that "there is little to be said that is especially new or interesting."

5

Dressed to Heal

A seeming loss of individuality may be one of the clouds
which you will experience as you see yourself mirrored
in the sea of blue uniforms. The uniform equalizes all
and will make you dependent on personal resources to
create an individual identity. It is only in doing so that
you can attain personal satisfaction through the nursing profession.

Suzanne Festersen '60
(Student Handbook, 1959)

TURN-OF-THE-CENTURY NURSING LEADERS had to be expert clinicians, educators, *and* image-makers. If the field were to advance everything about
nurses in the public eye had to be beyond reproach, better yet, the embodiment of an ideal, for the masses still looked askance at young women who
dedicated their lives to the sick and injured and not exclusively to husbands and children. Astutely, nursing's pioneers, with historical roots in
religious and military orders, recognized the symbolic power of a uniform.

The first nursing uniforms—with their charming frills and laces, long-
boned corsets, floor-length bell-shaped skirts, layers of starched petti-
coats, high choking collars, and leg-of-mutton sleeves—accentuated the
female silhouette and fostered the romantic image of the nurse. Elabo-
rately costumed, nurses stood no chance of being mistaken for hospital
scrubwomen or for domestic servants while on private duty. As a reporter
for *Munsey's Magazine* observed, St. Luke's graduates (wearing an Anna
Maxwell design) were "all that the most inveterate reader of sentimental
war stories could desire."

If the early uniforms were attractive, they also were impractical and
nonhygienic. "A nurse taking care of a patient with an infection could not

be on duty more than a half hour without getting her sleeves contaminated..." note Kalisch and Kalisch in *The Advance of American Nursing*. "Nurses who rolled them up were severely criticized since their appearance was thought to be 'unladylike,' suggesting the image of a laundress or scrubwoman."

The cap was more practical. It dated to medieval times, when a woman's obedience and humility were signified by the wearing of a bridal veil. While the cap symbolized the nurse's service to humanity, it also covered the fashionably long and complicated hairstyles of the day. The washing of long hair was tedious and not to be undertaken too often.

Bellevue was the first school to adopt a uniform, though not without protest. Some students perceived a uniform to be the mark of the servant class — at least until they caught a glimpse of the charming prototype designed by a fellow pupil, Euphemia Van Rensselaer, from society's upper crust. Other schools followed suit, each seeking its own mark of distinction.

Graduate nurses generally wore the uniforms of their alma mater wherever they worked: as head nurses in other institutions, in private duty, even overseas. The uniform thus became a wearable resume. According to Jamieson et al in *Trends in Nursing History,* "patient and doctor learned the particular virtues concealed beneath each school costume. Pride in individual achievement lost itself in school pride which gradually assumed an intense form. Inevitably, the barrier raised grew higher and symbolized itself in devotion to a school uniform which assumed a fixity that made any future modification very difficult."

Not surprisingly, unscrupulous educators exploited the uniform's symbolic power. In the early decades of the twentieth century, disreputable correspondence schools of nursing lured prospective pupils with the promise of certificates, caps, school pins, and uniforms. "This paraphernalia paralleled that supplied to students in hospital programs, and in the public's mind gave the graduates of these diploma mills the same status accorded hospital school graduates," notes Jo Ann Ashley in *Hospitals, Paternalism, and the Role of the Nurse*.

Anna Maxwell went to great lengths to ensure that her students were, figuratively and literally, nurses of a different stripe. Seeking something different from the checks and plaids and stripes adopted by other schools, Maxwell patterned the Presbyterian Hospital uniform after a blue-and-white-striped taffeta dress she had observed in a London museum. Sparing no expense, she imported the finest gingham from Glasgow. "I want a uniform which my nurses will be proud to wear always, and which they need not be ashamed of when they go out into the home to do private duty nursing," she said.

Students were no doubt proud, yet they probably blanched at the cost. A receipt belonging to Amy Chamberlain '94 indicates that she spent $16.46 —almost two months' stipend—for the complete school uniform, including gingham for the dress, muslin for the apron, as well as collars, studs, bibs, belts, buttons, and caps.

The Presbyterian cap, patterned after the Puritan maiden's cap, was designed with gathers to be worn over the contemporary pompadour and top-knot hairstyle. When soiled, the handsewn organdy cap was replaced, never laundered. (For reasons unknown, Maxwell never wore a cap herself, only a white linen uniform typical of head nurses.)

Reflecting nursing's military and religious heritage, the School used its uniform to mark one's rank. The stripes were awarded only to those who successfully completed the probationary period. Until then, students wore an undistinguished gray chambray uniform (although other colors were reportedly used in the early years; Emily Clatworthy '98, for instance, remembered that hers was pink). The probie uniform put the pupil in her place, but it also warned staff members and patients that the wearer was a novice. It "protected the students while they were working in the clinical area...and it protected the patients," says Helen Pettit '36. Successful probies were awarded the stripes and the cap, but they still were required to wear the black stockings and shoes. White stocking and shoes were distributed on graduation day, when the new alumnae were awarded the privilege of wearing the full plumage of the graduate Presbyterian nurse.

So important was the uniform to Maxwell that she devoted some of her remarks at the 1899 meeting of the Associated Alumnae of Trained Nurses to the topic. "Why is the uniform necessary for those undertaking the work of nursing?" she asked. "Is it not because, being made of light washable material, it is comfortable to work in, easily cleaned, quickly adjusted, agreeable to the eye, and, being so distinctively associated with the profession, inspires confidence in patients and friends invaluable to the wearer? ... The rightminded women connected with our profession throughout the land are proud to wear the uniform of their school unchanged, as the soldier is proud to wear the distinctive mark of his company or regiment."

In her textbook Maxwell intoned that "nurses should always be immaculately clean, trim and tidy. An untidy appearance gives the impression of carelessness, and carelessness is a characteristic that is not tolerated in a nurse...The nurse's uniform is, as it were, her passport to scenes and places from which other people are excluded and in which an impersonal, professional, dignified bearing is essential."

It was perhaps inevitable that Maxwell's passion for the School uniform would become the subject of a practical joke. "One seldom saw Miss Maxwell nonplused," remembered Albert Lamb. "One morning she was amazed and quite discomfited when several members of the house staff appeared in shirts and ties made of the same [blue-and-white-striped] material. She never did find out how this came about."

Students looked forward to the time when they could wear the School's "stripes," even if they were uncomfortable and restricting. "The day I got my uniform, I was on the roof [an open-air ward] where the temperature was perhaps 150 degrees," recalls Alice Bliss Smith '19, more than seven decades after the fact. "I didn't feel the heat at all. I was so proud of my uniform."

"The worst thing about nursing school was getting dressed when you overslept," said Pamela Heydon '60. "There were so many buttons. But as much as we hated buttoning those sleeves in the morning and unbuttoning them to do certain procedures, we were still proud of the uniform. No one had one like ours."

Joanne Yodice Heide '65 fondly remembered the "weekly delivery of elongated brown cartons full of stiff uniforms that had to be tamed and pegged onto our bodies, and the ritual drippings of white organdy into murky bottles of Elastic Starch." She also recalled that "expert ironers" in her class were able to pick up extra money "finishing caps for those of us less skilled who nevertheless wished to look presentable."

With her distinctive uniform and cap, there was no mistaking the Presbyterian nurse. "It seems that I'm the only one in this hospital...who doesn't wear a plain white dress," wrote a 1926 alumna who was practicing in another state. "Many people have told me how pretty the uniform is ... Tonight a man walked up to me and said, 'As I live and breathe, Presbyterian Hospital, New York City. Won't you come work for me? Your very uniform gives me confidence, and I alone can keep you more than busy.'"

Presbyterian Hospital graduates were also distinguished by a special pin, emblazoned with the motto "Salus Generis Humani" (Health of Humanity) on the front and "Neighbors" on the back. The first pins were a gift of Frederick Sturges, longtime member of the Training School Committee, who "gave his mind and heart to the concerns of nurses," noted the *Quarterly*. At a special pin presentation ceremony in 1896 for the first three classes, he said, "You came to us to be trained for the profession of nursing, and when you graduated we gave you a diploma stating that you were possessed of a certain practical knowledge. Is that all you learned … I know it is not. You are none of you the same women that you were. You have had an experience of life and its tragedies, vouchsafed to but a few, and that must have awakened you to a new birth … You have learned that you have the power to fill a large space, and the practical knowledge to make it available."

Sturges acknowledged that many of the graduates would leave or had already left nursing to raise families or to pursue other endeavors, such as missionary or charity work, but he hoped they would not dissolve their ties to Presbyterian or to the profession. Believing that neither the diploma nor the pin were enough to represent this principle, he added, "We have resolved then to institute for you in our Hospital the 'Order of Neighbors' … If you will always bear in mind that you can be a *neighbor* in every sphere of life, you will recognize the value of the training you have received here, and will give to us the happiness of feeling that in your hands our work is going forward with ever increasing results."

6

What Should We Have Done Without You?

We must all deprecate war and its horrors, and women
will ever wish for eternal peace... When war does come
and our brave men go forward to fight, they can never
go alone — the hearts of and helpful activities of American women must go with them.

Red Cross Report (1898)

BEFORE THE NINETEENTH CENTURY would run its course, another war would
figure prominently in the history of American nursing. This time it was a
conflict between the United States and Spain over Cuban sovereignty. Fortunately, it was a little war (though not so "splendid"), for the U.S. Army was
woefully unprepared, both to do battle and to care for casualties. The lessons of the Crimea, reaffirmed in the Civil War, had become a historical
footnote to this generation's politicians and generals. Once again, thousands more lives would have to be expended to demonstrate the value of basic
sanitation and a well-organized medical corps.

Despite its unpreparedness, the Army was initially reluctant to involve
female nurses on a large scale. Surgeon General George M. Sternberg
believed women to be "out of place" in the military. Why women, in the guise
of nurses, could survive twelve-hour days in civilian hospitals steeped in
death and disease and misery and suffering but could not tolerate the same
in military hospitals was never explained. The Army, however, held out as
long as possible, and even resorted to the use of untrained infantrymen as
medical corpsmen. But chauvinism was a luxury it could ill afford. Few men
volunteered for hospital duty. No wonder — it brought little reward (i.e.,
money or status) and much danger. This was a war not of bullets but of
microbes. While hundreds of American soldiers died in battle, behind the

lines thousands died of disease, mostly typhoid, contracted in squalid domestic military camps. Yellow fever, malaria, measles, dysentery, and diarrhea further thinned the ranks. Thirty percent of the American forces fell ill during the five-month war. As Victor Robinson writes in *White Caps,* "The soldiers had rushed to the colors, thinking they were going to fight the Spaniards and liberate the Cubans; no one told them they could die in America of fecal matter." Finally, after a serious outbreak of typhoid at Camp Thomas, a Georgia training center for 50,000 men, Sternberg relented, opening a new era for the military and for nursing.

Organized nursing, led by Isabel Hampton Robb, was quick to offer its services to the nation. Two days after the war erupted, the newly formed Nurses' Associated Alumnae (NAA) of the United States and Canada petitioned the government to involve trained nurses in the military. When Sternberg finally relented, he turned to a physician and Washington insider, Anita Newcomb McGee, M.D., of the Daughters of the American Revolution. McGee and nursing's leaders shared some concerns—namely an interest in liberating women's energies for social good—but not others. In selecting Army nurses from a list of 5,000 applicants, McGee judged all training school diplomas to be of equal value, hired untrained nurses, and dispatched nurses individually to military base hospitals, where they fell under the jurisdiction of unwelcoming medical men—all of which flew in the face of organized nursing's desire for hospitals staffed by high-quality graduate nurses under the command of the profession's elite. In total, the Army contracted the services of about 1,200 nurses from 200 different diploma programs. Each received thirty dollars a month plus board and transportation.

As the summer progressed and typhoid ascended, Robb and her NAA associates pressed on, striving for the same standards they had successfully instituted in civilian hospitals. In alliance with the Red Cross Society for the Maintenance of Trained Nurses of New York City, also known as Auxiliary No. 3, they petitioned the Army to expand organized nursing's involvement in the war. The auxiliary's leaders, a trio of wealthy social reformers, were dispatched to the White House to meet with President William McKinley and Surgeon General Sternberg. The result was historic: for the first time, organized groups of nurses, under their own command, would be allowed to work in military field hospitals.

The auxiliary looked to Anna Maxwell, who had written several personal appeals to the surgeon general on the Red Cross' behalf, to direct its recruitment effort. Operating out of her Presbyterian Hospital office, she motivated, by example or by persuasion, some 200 graduate nurses to enlist.

"When early in August, 1898, I read in the Boston papers that Miss Maxwell had sent out a call for nurses for Chickamauga Park...I immediately offered my services," said nurse Jane F. Riley. A number of Presbyterian alumnae also answered her call, serving in the South, in Puerto Rico, on the hospital ship *Relief,* and at Montauk Point, Long Island, a quarantine station for returning troops.

Maxwell and several other New York City superintendents were invited to the camps to lead the battle against the microbes. Though almost fifty, she readily accepted this hazardous assignment. She knew that the stakes were high, that nursing was on public trial. According to Kalisch and Kalisch, she "constantly reminded the nurses that their work...would forever speak for or against the women of America."

On August 7 Maxwell and her assistant, Frances A. Stone '94 (who were granted leaves of absence by Presbyterian's Board of Managers) and a contingent of forty nurses set off for Camp Thomas in Chickamauga Park, Ga. They were assigned to establish a nursing service at the new Sternberg Field Hospital, which would eventually expand into a network of 200 tents and rough wooden huts, staffed by 160 nurses. They arrived on the twelfth, the very day Spain and the United States signed the armistice. Peace, however, had no bearing on the nurses, who had traveled, it seemed, back in time to the scene of a medieval plague. As Maxwell recalled, "It was certainly a most harrowing sight to see the long narrow cots filled with what had been strong, splendid men, hollow-eyed, emaciated, muttering in the delirium of fever, sores in which dead flies were encrusted filled their mouths, making swallowing almost impossible. Their bones protruding through skin and bed sores several inches deep were not uncommonly found on hips, back, elbows, often on the head and ears and it was here that the energies and resources of the trained nurse were called forth in making the lives of these men less wretched and in restoring them to health."

That first day was a nightmare. "In all the long years of experience among the sick," commented Maxwell, "my eyes have rested on no sadder more pitiable sight ... We were helpless to pay the sick soldiers the necessary attention." The nurses arrived to find 136 new patients, an unfinished hospital, unpacked supplies, and uncooperative military workers. The commissary commander explained that work would be suspended at 6 p.m. and that the utensils couldn't be used until they were inventoried, per Army regulations. "The imbecility of the situation was too much for Miss Maxwell, and she informed the authorities she would open the [train] cars by force unless she received the supplies immediately: her wrath cut the red tape," recounts Robinson.

"Even before they had their suit cases unpacked they were at work," recalled the hospital's acting steward, Edwin B. McDaniel, a second-year medical student. "I can see the sad, determined face of Miss Maxwell as she controlled herself and made the best of it ... But our able general was in command and did the impossible that day and in the strenuous days to come. She was up seemingly day and night. I know for I saw her."

The pace never let up. Each day during their one-month tour of duty, the nurses toiled from sunup to sundown, with twenty minutes off for lunch and again for supper. Some days more than 200 new casualties arrived. According to Maxwell,

> In many instances they were brought long distances, driven through a broiling sun at midday, and had to lie in the ambulance from two to three hours, before they could be moved to their beds. When you consider that often as many as four men were crowded into one ambulance, suffering from thirst and heat, scarcely able to move in the cramped and narrow space allotted to them it is no wonder that many suffered from shock, exhaustion and convulsions...
>
> The course of our work was often impeded and made difficult by such stumbling blocks as sanitation of the most primitive kind, insufficient disinfections, water supply and accommodations for washing utensils, ... lack of medicine, milk, ice and other supplies ... Add to this the heat, the dust, the moisture and the flies and you have the picture complete.

"Late in the summer," Robinson adds, "when the regiments departed, the commanding officer deprived Miss Maxwell of her orderlies, \though hundreds of sick remained behind ... She was willing to overwork her nurses in an emergency but not kill them. She announced that if she did not get the orderlies at once, she would withdraw her nurses within twenty-four hours. Before the expiration of her ultimatum, the orderlies suddenly appeared in camp."

During Maxwell's one-month stay, the nurses attended to 900 sick and wounded soldiers. Only sixty-seven died.

Sternberg Hospital must have been quite an eyeful, with its endless rows of tents and stretchers, dotted by scores of nurses in uniforms of every cut and design imaginable. Since the military made no provision for standard dress, the nurses wore their own uniforms, the marks of their respective schools: stripes and checks and plaids in blues and whites and pinks in endless combinations.

The colors and patterns did not mask the fact that camp life was grim and hard, however. There were three toilets for the entire nursing staff. The only laundry was miles away. Typhoid fever afflicted many a nurse and felled at least one. Most of the nurses returned home with a chronic gastrointestinal illness. Maxwell, true to form, claimed that they had "not only the necessities but many of the luxuries of life," referring to the Red Cross–supplied dormitories, bathhouse, store rooms, kitchen, dining room, housekeeper, and servants. Despite her unwavering stoicism, she won the respect of everyone. "Sane, cool headed, sympathetic, commanding, she inspired confidence in all around her," wrote McDaniel, the steward. "She won cooperation by the sheer force of her personality."

Isabel Hampton Robb contended that it "was through this Auxiliary that the best nursing [in the war] was done." Taking notice of the Red Cross' success and the military's pitiful preparation, President McKinley appointed the Dodge Commission to investigate the conduct of the Army Medical Department. The commission recommended, among other things, the creation of a reserve corps of trained women nurses.

Characteristically, the military balked and even accused the nurses of "coddling" soldiers during the war. Nursing leaders (Maxwell included) and other social reformers recognized that it would take an act of Congress to institutionalize Army nursing. Through their efforts the War Department was forced to support a bill that led to the creation of the Army Nurse Corps.

Maxwell was also instrumental in creating a reserve of military nurses, the Red Cross Nursing Service. She became one of the first members, even though she was technically too old to enroll. In an early recruitment meeting, Mary E. Gladwin (who closed down Sternberg Hospital after Maxwell's departure) asked, "Miss Maxwell, why don't you enroll?" With a laugh, she answered, "Nonsense, I am too old. The Red Cross wouldn't have me." To which Gladwin responded, "Your nurses will never enroll in sufficient numbers unless you set them an example and they see you wearing the pin. Suppose you, Miss [Jane] Delano, and I fill in blanks and send them to Washington without mentioning our ages." They did, and they were promptly accepted.

Back at Presbyterian Hospital the dispensary (clinic) building was transformed into a forty-bed military ward. The soldiers made for fascinating medicine (they were "200 of the most interesting cases of typhoid and malignant malaria fever which it has been ever been my privilege to study," reported physician W. Gilman Thompson), but they were a severe strain on a hospital burdened by the city's own typhoid epidemic as well as by a crippling heat wave. According to Hospital Superintendent C. Irving Fisher, the "nurses voluntarily gave up rest and recreation hours to service," dutifully administering ice baths every four hours, which were required to keep the fevered patients from slipping into shock.

The not-so-splendid little war of 1898 was a turning point in United States history. It launched the political career of Theodore Roosevelt, the famed Rough Rider of San Juan Hill, who came to personify interventionist America, and it announced the arrival of a new naval power. The United States was now strategically supreme in the Caribbean and a new force in the Far East (where a small part of the war was fought). It was the beginning of the American century.

It was also the beginning of a new era of nursing. The government finally acknowledged the indispensability of organized nursing in wartime. This was no small accomplishment. One of the most regimented and chauvinistic segments of American society had been convinced that professional women should be taken seriously.

The military's change of heart was best expressed by Camp Thomas' chief field surgeon, Colonel John Van Rensselaer Hoff. To Anna Maxwell he said: "When you arrived we did not know what we should do with a contingent of women in the camp; now we are wondering what we should have done without you."

7

Rooms of Their Own

> [Florence Nightingale] Hall is fully equipped with
> every possible necessity … and is not only a haven of rest
> and recreation for the nurses, but is looked upon as a
> potent factor in their education.
>
> *Anna Maxwell (1904)*

SHORTLY AFTER the Presbyterian Hospital Training School opened, Anna
Maxwell realized that her nurses needed rooms of their own. Living over
the "shop" might be appropriate for bakers and grocers, but not for nurses.
"Our greatest present need is a nurses' home apart from the hospital
building," she wrote in 1894. "It seems essential, both from a hygienic and
rational point of view, that the nurses of a hospital should have complete
change, fresh air, and the atmosphere of home surroundings when off duty.
The lack of these comforts is sorely felt after a fatiguing day in a hospital
ward."

The Board of Managers agreed, partly because the move would free space
for one hundred badly needed beds. The Hospital, they reported, "is
crowded to its utmost capacity and many patients must necessarily be turned
away." However, it would be another decade before the nurses would vacate
their cubicles on the top floor of the ward pavilion.

By 1898 the highest of the hurdles to a new residence had been cleared
—or so it seemed. The managers had selected a site (the corner of 71st Street
and Park Avenue), chosen an architect (James A. Baker), and secured
financing (an anonymous gift of $410,000). Ground was already broken
when a lawsuit brought construction to a halt. Nearby residents, led by one
John Moller, feared that the proposed residence would upset the character
of this area, which since the Hosptal's founding had evolved into an afflu-
ent residential community. The proposed building, he contended, would
violate covenants in the property's deed that prohibited the construction

of railroad stations, slaughterhouses, forges, livery stables, tallow chandleries, brass foundries, opera houses, breweries, and other enterprises that "may in any way be noxious or offensive to the neighboring inhabitants." Moller had a point: The new building would be eight stories tall, twice as high as any surrounding structure, and contain its own heating, electrical and refrigeration plants. But a nursing school was hardly a slaughterhouse. Nonetheless, in 1901 he won a temporary injunction restraining Presbyterian Hospital from construction.

An editorialist for the *World* made a mockery of the suit:

> Justice Freedman of the New York Supreme Court is struggling with the questions whether a "nurses' home" is an offensive business such as would justify an injunction against its erection near the property of a plaintiff.
>
> The average layman could settle that question quickly. He would merely ascertain whether the nurses are of the kind that beat insane patients, boil idiots in too hot bath water, get drunk on pay-day and knock out each others' teeth. A "happy home" of such nurses would be a nuisance within half a mile and disgrace anywhere in the city.
>
> But if the nurses are the kind that wear neat white caps and speak in low treble or contralto, that have the still tread, the soft touch and the gentle manner that many a sick-room knows, why, nurses of that kind are an ornament to an neighborhood. Their presence ought to be worth a premium to a real estate owner.
>
> If the nurses in this case are young women, and if the learned Justice has had experience of illness, the plaintiff's chances are worthy—but it is highly improper to discuss judicial decisions before they are made.

While the Moller suit wound its way through the legal system, two long-time Hospital benefactors stepped forward to give the nurses a respite from city life. In 1901 the J. Kennedy Tods generously offered the School weekend use of their estate, Innis Arden, in Sound Beach (now Old Greenwich), Conn. Innis Arden, a scenic strip of land jutting into Long Island Sound, served as a retreat from the summer heat for almost four decades. The Tods' generosity did not end there. After Mrs. Tods' death, the property passed to the Hospital, which sold it and used the proceeds to finance additions to the nurses' residence.

Although the court eventually ruled in Presbyterian's favor, the decision did not matter. The managers had already decided to build the residence on unrestricted parcels of land just to the east. Ironically, Moller succeeded only in turning the original building site into a large green pool that befouled the neighborhood for more than a year. "The stagnant pool lies in the heart of one of the best districts of the residential portions of the city and looks more like a New Jersey swamp than a building lot in New

York," read a newspaper account.

Finally, in July 1904 Maxwell and her nurses moved into their long-awaited home-away-from-hospital, a splendid structure featuring a roof garden, gymnasium, assembly room, parlor, dining room, domestic science kitchen, laundry, and underground tunnel to the ward building.

Presbyterian's president, John S. Kennedy, the not-so-anonymous donor, was given the honor of naming the new red brick and limestone residence. Graciously declining requests to name it after himself, he christened it Florence Nightingale Hall. The name, he said, "would as nearly as possible express the character of the building and the purpose to which it was to be devoted."

Maxwell, thrilled with the new residence, exclaimed that it marked "a new era in the life of the school." And she added, "Here, it is hoped, can be corrected some of the faults arising from the serious lack of home training so apparent in the young women of today. Already the general health of the students is improved, although small change has been made in the articles of diet provided. The fact of improved conditions for cooking and serving has made a marked change for the better, and the luxury of a single room for each student means everything to her."

Still sensitive to Moller's suit, Maxwell made sure that her nurses did not appear out of place in the ritzy East-Side community. "We wore hat and gloves while walking to and from the hospital ... so as to be treated kindly by our wealthy neighbors," remembered Margaret Wells '29.

In only five years, the School outgrew its new home, forcing the Hospital to convert the gymnasium into eight dormitory rooms and to rent a residence annex for probies at 5 East 73rd Street.

Florence Nightingale Hall preceded by a decade or two a rush to improve accommodations for student nurses around the country. Sickness among students was legion because of overcrowded and unhygienic conditions. As the competition for applicants intensified in the first quarter of the century, a time of unprecedented hospital and nursing school expansion, administrators began to clean house. When a European hospital administrator visited a nursing residence in New York in the 1920s, he was moved to remark that when he died he hoped to be reincarnated as an American nurse.

Unfortunately, this was the least important and most successful of the reforms sought by nursing leaders in the early 1900s. The battles for upgraded and standardized curricula, for nurse registration, and for educational and clinical autonomy were yet to be won. Nursing remained a nineteenth century phenomenon well into the twentieth century.

8

The Unfinished Business of the Hospital

> In the hospital where modern appliances and supplies
> are abundant, there is very little scope for originality; in
> the homes where there is practically nothing, [the stu-
> dent nurse] must of necessity improvise and economize
> and this is generally done with good results. Going into
> the homes of the destitute people and seeing and know-
> ing them as they really are, teaches her adaptability and
> resourcefulness and develops humanitarian instincts.
>
> *Margaret Bewley '02 (1908)*

THE ORGANIZATION OF HOSPITALS in the final stages of the nineteenth century was nothing short of remarkable, a shining example of American
compassion and ingenuity. But the work of the country's social reformers
was far from over. People had already started to complain that hospitals were
intimidatingly bureaucratic and impersonal and that physicians were overly
specialized, treating "diseases" instead of whole patients who are part of a
family and a community.

There were even deeper concerns. As medical science flourished, so did
medical technology. Although new devices and techniques unquestionably improved the delivery of health care, they also inflated the cost of doing
business. As budgets tightened, private voluntary hospitals strayed from
their charitable origins, growing less and less tolerant of nonpaying cus-
tomers. The wealthy came first, the poor last, and the middle class did not
come at all, unwilling as they were to submit to ward care but unable to
afford a private room. It was estimated that only one in ten people who
needed care actually sought the services of a hospital.

With uncontrolled industrialization and immigration, the task of satisfying the health care needs of the lower and middle classes grew
immeasurably harder. New York City in particular was overwhelmed by

the influx of immigrants, who in the early 1900s accounted for more than 40 percent of the population of 3.5 million. Southern Europeans, for the first time, added to the cultural mix in appreciable numbers. With these new nationalities came new social, economic, and health problems. Immigrants old and new were crowded into sweatshops by day and unsanitary tenements by night. They were routinely victimized by their landlords and by each other. Contagious disease was rampant. The streets were crowded and filthy. Parks were few, and the countryside, with its clean air and water, was inaccessible. This was no promised land.

In this time of great social flux, the reformers recognized that hospitals had to become more flexible. "Both economics and humanity," historian Charles Rosenberg explains, "underlined the need for regional planning, for improving and even expanding outpatient facilities, for better convalescent and long-term care, for the provision of socially appropriate yet economically viable facilities for middle-income patients... The responsibility of the hospital did not stop with perceived sickness, [the reformers] contended, nor were its boundaries defined by admission and discharge."

As one Presbyterian physician commented, someone was needed to look after the "unfinished business of the hospital."

On New York's Lower East Side, at 265 Henry Street, the reformers discovered a humane and affordable answer to urban America's crushing public health care woes: the visiting nurse.* Henry Street was home to nurse Lillian Wald's Settlement House (established on another site in 1893), an independent, privately funded organization that sent nurses out to the homes of the poor, offering both nursing care and health instruction, in that order of priority.

The concept of visiting, or district, nursing was not new to Anna Maxwell. Years before, in Boston, she had participated in an early, if failed, attempt to extend hospital nursing out into the community. Encouraged by Wald's success, she wrote in 1894, "We have a hope of district work in some form in the future, possibly in the care of those who can partially pay for the service rendered, and who yet cannot afford the higher price accorded the graduate nurse. There must be a large class of self-respecting people, too proud to ask for charity, and entitled to skilled care and attention when ill, who would avail themselves of this plan." Unfortunately, Maxwell's plan fell victim to Presbyterian's shortsighted policymakers. Preventive care did not carry much weight in medicine's increasingly diseased-focused

*The current term, public health nurse, was coined in 1912 with the formation of the National Organization of Public Health Nursing.

philosophy. The decision would come back to haunt them. Nine years later the Hospital complained that it was "crowded to its utmost capacity and many patients must necessarily be turned away." Short of cash, the managers could not afford to convert the nurses' quarters back into functional, income-generating, wards.

Well aware of the Hospital's predicament, Maxwell submitted a second proposal for visiting nursing, this time emphasizing its potential for relieving hospital overcrowding. Nurses, under the direction of a physician, would be sent out to the homes of individuals who were too "healthy" to be hospitalized but too sick to be left alone (e.g., the elderly and chronically ill); who had been discharged from the hospital but needed followup care; and who needed care but would not go to the hospital. In the home the nurse would feed and clean a patient, change a surgical dressing, monitor a patient's progress, or teach a young mother the basics of health, nutrition, and hygiene. Maxwell envisioned visiting nursing as part of a continuum of care, beginning with what is now called discharge planning for ward and dispensary patients.

Presbyterian's managers could no longer ignore the potential contributions of the visiting nurse. Finally, in 1904 they established the Department of Visiting Nursing and Social Service. As Charles Rosenberg notes, "Even in the world of academic medicine, the reductionist view of disease had not swept all before it; work diet, stress, individual habits, and dwelling places all might play a role in predisposing to illness."

No doubt, the managers were swayed by a gift of $5,000 from Mrs. William K. Vanderbilt, Sr., wife of the wealthy industrialist, covering the plan's startup costs. From countless visits to the surgical corridor, where her sister-in-law, Mrs. J. Borden Harriman, was hospitalized, Vanderbilt took great interest in the life of the Hospital. The two befriended several nurses, including Maxwell, and "decided that in no way could their time, money and effort be more profitably spent than by helping provide a nursing service in the homes of the poor," according to Eleanor Lee '20, the School's first historian. As members of the Hospital's governing committee for visiting nursing, they toured tenements to learn firsthand the conditions they were trying to ameliorate. (Vanderbilt generously supported the department for another two decades.)

Not surprisingly, physicians were slow to embrace the new department.* "Our first effort," said Maxwell, "was to interest the doctors and

---

* Only after the Sheppard-Towner Act of 1921, which spurred the enormous success of community-oriented preventive health services, dominated by nurses and social workers, did physicians seriously embrace the concept of preventive care. Fearful of losing ground, organized medicine con-

persuade them to refer the patients to our social service department... [I]t took the best part of the year before the doctors spontaneously asked for such services." When infant care services were offered to Vanderbilt Clinic, Maxwell was told, rather coldly, "Well, the June crop of babies are dead, a few may be saved in July and August; yes, you may try the experiment for two months."

Patients, too, were hesitant. "The connection between the homes and the nurse was almost as difficult to establish," Maxwell noted. "This was due to a distrust of anything that seemed to interfere with private life."

Nevertheless, the department flourished. In 1905 alone the nurses, sporting dresses of blue gingham and coats and hats of Cambridge gray, made 12,284 visits to 4,109 patients in a large swath of New York City, from the Battery to the Bronx, but primarily on the East Side between 79th and 100th streets—an astonishing caseload for a handful of graduate and student nurses. The department was largely tied to Presbyterian's Vanderbilt Clinic (notably, Walter B. James' tuberculosis clinic and Samuel Lambert's medical clinic), yet it also handled patients from the Cornell Dispensary and the Society for Improving the Condition of the Poor. In addition, the visiting nurses were assigned by the Health Department to manage all tuberculosis cases between 63rd and 79th Streets and Fifth Avenue and the East River.

In keeping with the Hospital's mission, the service was provided free of charge to the poor. All others were assessed a modest fee of ten to twenty-five cents, which supported the purchase of food, fuel, flowers, linens, and nursing supplies for the less fortunate.

Visiting nursing quickly lived up to its promise. According to department head Margaret Bewley '02, a veteran of six weeks' training at Henry Street, the visiting nurse was instrumental in stemming the spread of deadly contagious diseases. "For instance," she wrote, "she sees in an early stage a case of measles, which is promptly investigated and reported to the Board of Health, thus saving an epidemic in the community, and keeping a larger number of children from [missing] school." Moreover, the nurse helped to dispel the popular notion of hospitals as places of "gloom and death," which kept many from seeking care. "In the days before this plan came into use," she added, "many [cases] would go along from bad to worse, and finally

vinced federal authorities that private physicians should be the sole stewards of health matters. Sheppard-Towner programs were subsequently closed and private physician practices expanded. "The private doctor's take-over of public health services was a social, not a medical phenomenon," writes Sheila Rothman in *Woman's Proper Place*. "It reflected, as its timing makes clear, a medical response to a political innovation."

be compelled to enter a hospital ward, with resulting great loss of time, general inconvenience and family upset."

Four years after visiting nursing began, Maxwell wrote, "It seems permissible to suggest that in the work of the department the 'art of healing' has taken on a new phase that might well be termed the 'art of prevention' ... The presence of the nurse in the clinic establishes greater confidence between the physician, the patient and the nurse, and enables her better to enforce prophylactic measures in the home." She later observed, "Our patients return less and less frequently for hospital and dispensary care, because they learn to economize their earnings to secure better food and to preserve health."

Since Vanderbilt's gift was the department's primary source of funding, the department had to make do with a student-dominated staff. Though it could have accomplished more with fully trained graduates, the service prospered—and so did the students. The experience was priceless. "To a great extent she is thrown on her own responsibility, and must adapt herself to the home conditions of each family; to face exigencies met with in private nursing, and she is expected to use her own head in emergencies, instead of appealing to someone in authority," reported Bewley, the School's first instructor in visiting nursing, to the 1908 Convention of the Nurses' Associated Alumnae in San Francisco. "She also learns to think of each patient as an individual as well as a case of illness, for under care at home his progress is often dependent on the financial and social condition of the family. The nurse is called upon to keep all this in mind and frequently to make decisions in cases to be reported to the instructor, for immediate relief, medical advice, removal to hospitals, etc."

Maxwell wisely offered visiting nursing as a two-month, senior-year elective, allowing students to self-select for this particularly challenging branch of work. They entered, as Eleanor Lee noted, "with the right spirit, carrying a new atmosphere into the homes they visited." That spirit was exemplified by Alice E. Burbidge '07, who wrote,

> There is undoubtedly a stimulating effect on the mind in doing a work so entirely different from the routine work of the hospital. This experience comes generally well on in the third year when we have come to the point that makes us wonder if the course is not necessarily long. We are too tired to study, we know the routine work, and are restlessly longing to get out of harness...
>
> The chance to study human nature with all the barriers down...is one for which every nurse should feel grateful... Patients in the wards are very much alike, or, if they show any marked eccentricities, they are generally of a most

trying nature. But in their homes, where they are not obliged to conform to any rules, they are their natural selves, whether pleasant or the reverse.

Margaret Gillis '07 also exhibited the special spirit of the visiting nurse. "The nurse enters the tenement home; the little baby is sick and there are three, four, seven or more other little ones," she wrote.

> The mother looks tired and weary; she is untidy and very often dirty, the children are unkempt and dirty, the home is poor — very poor. The windows are closed tight because the weary mother thinks the cool air will hurt the sick baby ... Here is the opportunity for the nurse. My own method is ... to win if possible the mother's love, at any rate, to try to make her see that I am indeed her friend, and that I am going to help her, not only with the sick baby, but also with the whole family...
>
> Then I find out the other children's names, how many go to school, and how many help the mother, how many are able to wash their own faces and hands and make themselves look pretty, and, while I bathe the sick baby, I ask the mother to sit down and talk ... teaching her how to take care of the baby ... [T]hey love to tell you all about themselves and their husbands and their lives, and you can advise and counsel, and sometimes you will see the weary look displaced by a bright smile and a look of happiness that you wish you could always be there...
>
> The mother is shown how to prepare the feeding for the baby. In doing this, there is opportunity of teaching her order and neatness in the kitchen ... [I]t has more than once surprised me how much there is to these women; how quickly they respond to kindness, and how willing and eager they are to learn ... You will find the mother watching for your coming the next morning, her home will be cleaner and neater, the children will be clean, and she herself much improved in appearance through the use of soap and water.

Of course, not every household visit was so rewarding. Edna Whitelaw '01, attached to Vanderbilt Clinic's Department of Applied Therapeutics, told of a encounter with "Mr. A," seriously ill with tuberculosis:

> I try to be charitable and think that the disease has warped his naturally sunny(?) disposition. I was greeted with "Why didn't you come yesterday, I told you to and why are you so late today?" Then he began complaining that no one ever did what was right toward him. The Charity Organization didn't give him enough money ... the doctor didn't come often enough, and the medicine was no good anyway. This man had been sent home from St. Joseph's, the Metropolitan and Riverside Hospitals for fault-finding. His version was that the places were run by cranks who didn't know anything. I rubbed his back and fixed his bed and tried to give him a more normal view of things, but it was just as bad the next day. His wife had been in various stages of drunk for a week and the filth of those two rooms was beyond description. I had to stand over her and make her clean up, for a self-respecting

pig could not have stayed there. Of course the woman never in all her life had touched any liquor, she was ready to swear that to me! Her nerves were unstrung from worry and grief about her dear husband! At that, the "dear husband" pulled himself up in bed and threatened to throw a flat iron at her. I calmed them both down, told the man I would report him for forcible removal (which he dreaded); told the woman I would have her locked up for neglecting a dying man, and departed with the promise to come to-morrow. They lived in Hell's Kitchen!

All in all, it was no surprise that Bewley found that students showed "a more eager interest and marked improvement in their general work upon resuming their duties in the Hospital wards."

Visiting nursing was rewarding, but it also was exhausting and dangerous. As Burbidge recounted,

> The stairs, of course, are the bug-bear of our existence and we sometimes wonder if the risk we run in nursing patients with pulmonary tuberculosis is not very great, even when every precaution is taken. We climb up four or five flights of stairs, then gasp, rather than breathe, in the infected air in our patients' room…
>
> Sometimes it seems to us that all our patients live as near the sky as possible and the dark, narrow, evil-smelling stairs are certainly a sore trial, though not so much as the almost inevitable tenement cat! It is always wise to poke an inquisitive toe into the darkest corner of the darkest flight of stairs and often one is rewarded by an ear-splitting "meouw." This however is better than a prolonged song-cycle when one steps carelessly and forcibly on poor puss!

Though Burbidge's sense of humor may have protected her from the psychological hazards of the tenement home, it offered no immunity to the physical hazards. Hospital wards were dangerous enough, but at least the environment was controlled, sanitized to the greatest extent possible. Tenements were another story altogether, at least until the nurse had her way. On average 80 percent of student nurses in general hospitals harbored the tuberculosis bacillus by the time they were graduated.

Ill students at Presbyterian always had access to a staff physician, but according to Albert Lamb, "there were no continuing records and numerous girls were admitted to the School with no adequate knowledge of their physical condition other than a letter from the family physician that they were in good condition. Not infrequently did this turn out to be true and girls had to be dropped who should not have been admitted in the first place."

Pressed by Maxwell, the Board of Managers in 1910 appointed a salaried physician (Lamb) to the Training School to deliver acute care, conduct regular examinations, and assess prospective students. The following year the class of 1912 agreed to volunteer for tests of a typhoid vaccination (although a few students were excused when their parents' objected). "For succeeding classes it was made compulsory," recalled Lamb. "I believe our nurses were the first as a group [outside of the army] to have typhoid immunization. Other prophylactic measures were instituted as they came along." Dental care was added in 1922.

The work of the nurses was greatly eased in 1916 with the gift of a motor car and chauffeur from the managers. "It has been invaluable," wrote Maxwell, "in saving the time and strength of the nurses, in multiplying home visits, in carrying sick patients to and from the hospital, in taking convalescents to railway stations, and in bringing pleasure to some of our 'shut-ins' by taking them with the nurses on their rounds."

"Our nation is at last awake to the alarming condition of public health and the immediate need of providing a remedy," Maxwell wrote around 1918. That year every student was required to attend a lecture on public health and then accompany social workers into the community.

Not long after, the School collaborated with Henry Street and Teachers College to give students public health nursing experience. The result was an intensive four-month elective that each week included seven hours of lectures and conferences at the college and thirty-three hours of field work and case-report writing under the supervision of a Henry Street nurse. This replaced the elective with the Department of Visiting Nursing and Social Service, partly because the department had begun to emphasize social service and partly because it could not offer students sufficient attention. (A few years later the department dropped "Visiting Nursing" from its title.)

Maxwell actually preferred that public health nurses receive postgraduate training, not a cursory diploma-level introduction to the subject. In a 1923 speech to the Albany Guild for Public Health Nursing she argued that advanced education was essential for the nurse "to establish a social conscience, to understand civic conditions, to gain a knowledge of infant welfare, child hygiene, the conduct of clinics and health centers, school nursing, or industrial welfare work, rural nursing, etc., etc." Public health measures, she insisted, are the "best investment a nation can make."

The nurses and students of Presbyterian Hospital were involved in other vital public health measures, most notably the Katie Geitz Milk Kitchen. Again a former patient and a Vanderbilt played central roles. During a year-long stay in the Hospital, Geitz grew interested in the plight of the city's poor. When she recovered in 1905, she offered the Hospital the use of her ground-floor apartment on East 85th Street as a site for distributing free or low-cost milk and other foods to undernourished infants and children. Many of these "milk kitchens," as they came to be called, evolved into preventive health centers.

According to Elsie Patterson '01, the School's second instructor in visiting nursing, the idea for Presbyterian's milk kitchen originated with a graduate of the Training School. Upon visiting the Walker-Gordon Farm in Plainsboro, N.J., a producer of specialty milk products, this alumna observed that the company was discarding up to forty quarts of still-useful milk "wastes" each day. The company was persuaded to donate the byproducts to Presbyterian, which turned it into baby food for distribution through Geitz's milk kitchen.

In time donations poured in from private philanthropists, permitting Geitz to move to larger quarters in the new East River Homes on 77th Street, an innovative subsidized housing project for tubercular patients and their families that was bankrolled by Mrs. Vanderbilt. The kitchen's services gradually expanded to include a wider variety of foods and patients. In later years meals were supplied to "open-air" classes for tubercular schoolchildren held on the roofs of the Homes and the nearby public school. By 1913 the kitchen had dispensed 35,700 quarts of milk, 840 dozen eggs, and 9,000 portions of soup, stew, and other edibles. Geitz retired in 1925. Shortly after, when the Hospital moved to a new neighborhood, the kitchen closed.

Presbyterian's Department of Visiting Nursing and Social Service was also involved with two day camps for tubercular children, one on the *Middletown*, an old Staten Island Ferry boat anchored at East 91st Street; the other, called Hill Top, on the grounds of the summer home of Herbert Carter, M.D., in Hawthorne, N.Y.

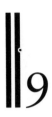

9

Not Quite a Profession

It is...co-operation of brain and hand which distinguishes the artist from the artisan and the practitioner
of a profession from the worker at a trade.

Theodore C. Janeway, M.D.
(Commencement exercises, 1914)

IN ONLY A MATTER OF YEARS Anna Maxwell had established one of the finest training schools in the nation. But her work was unfinished, her goal of
raising nursing "to the level of a profession" unrealized. With this goal in
mind she became a founding member of the American Society of Superintendents of Training Schools for Nurses (1893) (forerunner to the National
League for Nursing), the Nurses' Associated Alumni of the United States
and Canada (1897) (forerunner to the American Nurses' Association), the
International Council of Nurses (1899), the New York Counties Registered Nurses' Association (1904), and, later, the Eastern Council of Nursing Education (1921). The minutes of these organizations are dotted with
her name as chairperson or member of countless committees and boards.

Despite these organizations' efforts, nurses could not lay claim to
professional status, even by the most lax standards. Unlike medicine,
nursing had yet to gain control over its own destiny, assemble a unique base
of knowledge, devise a system for advancing or evaluating its skills and
theories, or set standards for education and practice. Census figures from
1900 indicate that there were 109,000 untrained nurses and midwives but
only 12,000 trained nurses, many of whom were products of marginal
schools. Thirteen dollars and a few months of home study could earn anyone an impressive-looking diploma and all the necessary nursing
accoutrements from the National Correspondence School of Health and
Hygiene in Detroit. Women of all backgrounds were streaming into nurs-

ing's wide-open back door, diluting the potential for professionalism.

Accordingly, nursing leaders fought vigorously to close that door. One tactic was to define legislatively, state by state, what it meant to be nurse, a task that consumed several decades. Ironically, the registration movement faced some of its stiffest opposition from within, from the many lesser-trained nurses who feared the consequences of restrictive standards and who saw registration as a narrow concern of the education-minded elite. Lofty ideals didn't put food on the tables or clothes on the backs of working nurses. The movement also encountered opposition from physicians and administrators from the poorer hospitals, who thought nurses were already overeducated.

As the undisputed capital of nursing in the United States, New York was the most influential state in the registration movement. Anna Maxwell and other prominent nurses, under the umbrella of the New York State Nurses' Association (NYSNA), the country's first state nursing society, won passage of the era's most restrictive legislation, the 1903 Nurse Practice Act. Under the act, a Board of Nurse Examiners set basic educational standards for schools of nursing. The standards were relatively low, far below those of Presbyterian, St. Luke's, and other acclaimed schools. Nevertheless, just nineteen of New York's ninety-eight incorporated training programs could qualify without substantive changes, such as the addition of obstetrics and maternity wards in their hospitals. Under the act only graduates of approved programs could sit for state examinations and (if they passed) call themselves "registered nurses."

Lamentably, the realities of health care politics dulled the act's potential. Since women did not yet have the vote and many rank and file nurses opposed registration, NYSNA was forced to turn to influential physicians and hospital administrators for help in winning the act's passage. While some fought it bitterly, others gladly obliged—for their own reasons. Registration, to the medical men, was a way to secure a more reliable supply of nurses, to deliver a crushing blow to their competitors (small private hospitals with inferior and possibly unsalvageable training schools), and, most important, to ensure them a continued role in shaping nursing's destiny. Nursing relinquished further control by surrendering the act's administration to the Board of Regents, an old and respected state agency that oversaw higher education. This strengthened the authority of the legislation, but because of the Board's strong ties to organized medicine, it also weakened nursing's influence and the act's standards.

Even more frustrating, the final version of the act called only for *voluntary* compliance. In other words a woman could call herself an "R.N." only if she met certain standards, but she did not have to be registered in order to practice. This did not seem to bother the public, inexperienced as it was in the health care marketplace, so unregistered private duty nurses found the act no barrier to employment.

The unparalleled scientific advances of late 1800s heralded a new age of health care, an age that cried out for deeper nurse involvement and better-trained practitioners — at least nurses thought so. Nursing's vanguard pressed for a standardized three-year curriculum with more scientific content, as well as for reduced ward hours, improved physical conditions, and postgraduate training. (Actually two years was plenty, though not within the prevailing apprenticeship system, which was not about to be overturned, at least not industry-wide. Student nurses still had to earn their keep, which required long hours at the bedside.) Mixing service and science, it was hoped, would help reverse the genderization of nursing, which had long stymied professional advancement.

Physicians vociferously opposed any expansion in the intellectual aspect of nurse training. To great applause William Alexander Dorland, M.D., a prominent member of the University of Pennsylvania medical faculty, stated, "If a little knowledge is a dangerous thing in most avenues of employment, in nursing it is more dangerous — it is fatal ... I believe that a superficial knowledge of physiology and anatomy, together with a thorough acquaintance with hygiene, will answer every purpose." He added that "a nurse may be over-educated; she can never be over-trained."

The same argument was heard closer to home. In a letter to the Training School, Samuel W. Lambert, M.D., the new dean of Columbia University's College of Physicians & Surgeons (P&S), wrote, "The argument that ... theoretical studies do no harm, even if no immediate good results, is fallacious, for it is far from harmless to distract a tired woman from her important and useful work with details even of elementary science which can be of no use to her."

Presbyterian's own W. Gilman Thompson, one of the School's founders, similarly proclaimed, "The work of a nurse is an honorable calling or vocation, and nothing further. It implies the exercise of acquired proficiency in certain more or less mechanical duties, and is not primarily designed to contribute to the sum of human knowledge or the advancement of science ... The function of the nurse [is] to make an ill person comfortable in bed [and] ... to observe and record certain data of the patient's condition." Thompson conveniently ignored that nursing's glacially slow professional evolution was due in no small part to physicians. In the typical training school, one without an enlightened administration or the countering influence of an Anna Maxwell or an Isabel Hampton Robb, medical men restricted the scope of nurse training to the acquisition of domestic skills.

Taking another tack, an editorialist for the *Journal of the American Medical Association* contended in 1904 that "conditions of incomplete development of the genital organs in women are much more frequent than used to be the case. It would seem as though the intense mental application so freely encouraged by our modern educational system may very well serve to divert nature's purpose of developing the sexual side of the being."

Of what were physicians and administrators so frightened? Loss of power and money. Nurses of greater skill, education, and autonomy posed a real threat to the medical men's control of the clinical setting and of a highly profitable pool of workers (student nurses). The new century saw the creation of hundreds of new specialty hospitals in which nursing generated the bulk of the revenue. Without this income, historian Jo Ann Ashley argues, "it is doubtful that so many small hospitals could have been established or stayed in business. Medicine was scarcely developed to the point of having many services to offer."

Moreover, nursing was far ahead of medicine in the use of the hospital as an educational laboratory, and curriculum reform threatened to widen that gap. Until the early 1900s medical schools were primarily commercial ventures, unattached to hospitals and universities; they placed little emphasis on the use of patients as living textbooks. Not so coincidentally when nursing started clamoring for more theoretical and clinical training, medicine initiated a drive for equal educational access to patients and against nursing educational reform.

Nurses were not without their physician supporters, however. To the class of 1914, Theodore C. Janeway, M.D., a visiting physician at Presbyterian Hospital and Bard Professor of the Practice of Medicine at P&S, proclaimed:

> In spite of protracted search, I have never met [the overtrained nurse], and I am coming to regard her as a mythological personage. The conceited nurse … the lazy nurse … the slipshod nurse … I know … But the overtrained nurse, a nurse who actually and absolutely knows too much, is to me as an absurd idea as an over-educated physician. Sometimes I half wonder whether, if there were more over-educated physicians, there might not be less so-called overtrained nurses …
>
> Scientific knowledge and technical skill are … the basis of successful practice of either profession, and the object of all professional education is to impart these fundamentals in proper proportion …

> [T]he glorification of the technical skill has its dangers, no less than the magnification of learning. Mere dexterity in the performance of even complicated tasks is not enough to qualify a good nurse. She must have trained powers of observation, must know how to detect every change in a patient's condition, and how to interpret what she observes. She must recognize the danger signals that call for action, and discriminate between them and the seemingly alarming ... She must appreciate the limitations of her knowledge and know when to mistrust her judgment, yet never lose her calm and poise. She must be resourceful in an emergency, applying old principles in new ways.

Despite physician opposition, curriculum improvement did occur. History was on nursing's side. By the turn of the century the United States was well into the progressive era, a time when middle-class city dwellers rose up to protest the evils and abuses of unbridled urbanization and industrialization. Women entered the workplace in record numbers in response to loosened religious, economic, and social constraints, including liberalized divorce laws. In nursing, young women found a somewhat respectable means of escaping to the big city and away from family and societal pressure to marry.

It was in this enlightened atmosphere that Maxwell lobbied for an expanded curriculum at Presbyterian Hospital, seeking to broaden the students' experience beyond the traditional branches of nursing (medicine, surgery, obstetrics, gynecology) into the burgeoning specialties of "contagion, orthopedics, eye and ear, rest cure, mental nursing, alcohol and allied habits, care of children, and scientific preparation of infant formula and other foods." A revised, three-year curriculum was implemented in 1898 (thus no class was graduated in 1900).

Some nursing historians contend that expanded programs merely subjected students to another year of "hard labor." At Presbyterian the new curriculum covered virtually the same ground as the original, though presumably in greater depth — no detailed description of the early courses has survived, so it is impossible to tell. New lectures were added in "The Ethics of Private Nursing" and "Opium and Allied Habits." The extra year, Maxwell claimed, afforded students more experience with "executive" tasks. "In broadening the work," she wrote, "the third-year pupil gains valuable experience in extended time in the care of private patients, or acting head nurse of wards, as third assistant in the office, or in substituting for the night superintendent, thus gaining an insight into the management and discipline of the School and Registry that tends greatly to increase her usefulness and efficiency in whatever branch of the profession she may select after graduation."

Around this time, as a member of the American Society of Superintendents of Training Schools for Nurses, Maxwell helped to bring about the country's first true postgraduate course in nursing. Finding it difficult to locate qualified assistants and head nurses, superintendents around the country collaborated in 1899 to institute a year-long program in hospital economics at the newly formed Teachers College of Columbia University. Through courses on such topics as psychology, history of education, organization and administration, hygiene, food production, household chemistry, and dietetics, the program prepared graduate nurses to become teachers in training schools and superintendents of nursing in hospitals. The educators' underlying aim was to bring uniformity to training school curricula.

Though the Teachers College program was influential, spurring nursing's advance, the nurse-training industry was expanding uncontrollably; quality control was almost nonexistent. Nursing was not quite a profession.

Discontented with Presbyterian's curriculum, even after the recent program overhaul, Maxwell renewed her quest for professional-level nursing education. In 1901 she called for more intensive clinical and theoretical instruction and, more importantly, for a considerable change in, if not an end to, the apprenticeship system. "At the present time," she explained, "the demands made upon 'the Nurse' are as complex and varied as they were formerly simple and uniform, and a revolution in education methods is demanded." Nurses, she pointed out, needed preparation for a staggering variety of roles — nursing school principals and instructors, hospital superintendents, sanitary inspectors, public school nurses, army nurses, settlement workers, seaside and floating hospital nurses, and resident nurses in colleges and schools, hotels, and department stores.

"We must ... look forward to having a definite curriculum with paid instructors; the pupils should be asked to help in the payment of the instructors," she added. Mindful that some students needed the School's meager monthly stipend, she proposed scholarships for "the few who are not financially well placed." She was also aware that the Board of Managers would look first to the question of dollars and cents and pointed out that the new system would "save a neat sum to the hospital," as much as $2,000 annually, or 20 percent of the Training School budget, even with a substantial increase in enrollment, which then stood at seventy-six.

Two years later Maxwell and her assistant, Frances Stone, submitted a new curriculum to a special committee of the Medical Board. They recommended that course work be concentrated in the first two years, leaving the senior year for "branch work and for lectures upon liberal subjects, intended as an offset and balance to the purely technical and as broadening the nurse's point of view." They also proposed that the probationary period be extended to six months and that pupils not be permitted on the wards until receiving elementary training, including daily lessons in anatomy, physiology, and nursing and household economics and daily practical demonstrations in cooking and housekeeping. Probies would be closely watched and frequently evaluated, with an eye toward weeding out as many unsuitable pupils as possible.

Apparently, Maxwell's vision of nursing came alarmingly close to the realm of medicine. A few years later W. Gilman Thompson, then a lecturer in the Training School on "Nursing in Typhoid Fever," was moved to complain that nursing studies "in many instances belong to the first or even second year of a medical college course." He preferred the old two-year curriculum—under physician control—and perhaps a year or more postgraduate specialty training for a select group of nurses. Not only that, he proposed that some students be graduated after only six months. These workers would be called "trained attendants." Thompson reasoned, "What an elderly patient requires with paralysis lasting several months is not an overtrained nurse who can talk about 'coloperineoplasty' or write a thesis or [interpret a] urinalysis and give her views on Bright's disease ... but someone who can feed her, adjust her pillows, and report any sudden change in her condition to the physician."

Paradoxically, Thompson also criticized nursing schools that tended "to dwell upon inflexible, unthinking routine, and advanced pedagogic methods, to the exclusion and cultivation of the nurses's individual judgment, tact and common sense." His schizophrenic stance mirrored the medical establishment's mixed reaction to the advance of the American nursing. While it prized the well-trained nurse, it feared her as well.

There were, to be sure, sympathetic people in influential circles. For instance, Henry Fairfield Osborn, a professor of zoology at Columbia University and director of the American Museum of Natural History, openly accepted nursing's quest for knowledge in his commencement address to the class of 1907. "As the ideal well rounded man in any profession, not alone that of medicine, should have his knowledge tempered by a deep and sincere love of humanity, so the ideal woman should have her natural sympathies, her compassion, her tenderness, and above all her spirit of self-sacrifice tempered and directed by knowledge ... " he said. "Knowledge and love, or science and sentiment, should be twins, they should go hand in hand in every department of human activity. Unfortunately they do not."

And eight years later commencement speaker James R. Sheffield, a member of the Board of Managers, astutely recognized nursing's growing role. "I believe that your profession will be used, more and more, for a better understanding of disease," he speculated.

> The laboratory will still determine the nature of the bug, the learned doctor will diagnose the disease or injury by name and prescribe for it by rule; but the hourly vigil by night and day, watching every change in color, pulse and temperature, will teach the well-trained nurse some truths about the patient and the disease which are not recorded on the chart, or written in the bedside notes.
>
> Alive to your opportunity, you can add much to the store of knowledge upon even the commoner forms of illness, and, blest with your womanly sympathies, in addition to your professional skill, you may make your work not alone a benefit to the patient, but an enduring contribution to the science of medicine.

In this ambivalent atmosphere the Board of Managers approved Maxwell's proposed curriculum in 1904, but with specific "suggestions" — a laundry list of limitations. The board wanted all instruction in medicine, surgery, and pathology to be arranged and supervised by one of its own in conjunction with the head of the Training School. Courses in bacteriology, urinalysis, and chemistry were to be limited to practical instruction. Chemistry, for example, was to be taught only in relation to the principles of diet and cooking. Similarly, the study of materia medica was to be restricted to practical instruction in poisons, antiseptics, and the preparation of solutions. The board accepted at least the need for broader clinical experience and graduate-level study.

Exactly how much Maxwell acceded to the board's suggestions is hard to discern. The preliminary course in "Bacteriology," for instance, appears to be more than cursory, judging by a brief description in the School's 1906 bulletin. Probies learned the principles of sterilization, preparation of culture media, common species of bacteria, effect of heat and chemicals on the growth of bacteria, isolation of bacteria from common sources, bacterial diseases, and sources of contamination. In "Anatomy and Physiology," they studied the "general anatomy and physiology of the human body, the composition and properties of the tissues, the circulation of the blood, and the elaboration of the food into blood."

Final exams for the class of 1906 also suggest that the curriculum was substantial and challenging. Some of the questions were:

> What care would the nurse give a pneumonia patient?

How does the white of an egg differ from the yolk of an egg? Which of the three constituents predominates—proteins, carbohydrates, or fats?

What are the abdominal symptoms in typhoid, with special reference to pain, tympanites, and the presence of blood-mucus and undigested foods in the stools?

Describe the post-operative treatment of a case after tracheotomy for oedema of the glottis?

How would you give a high enteroclysis [injection into the abdominal cavity] in a private house?

[Demonstrate how to] Prepare and hold a child for intubation.

[Demonstrate] Artificial respiration for suspended respiration.

[Demonstrate how to] Apply tourniquet for abdominal hemorrhage.

Though Maxwell's plea for a tuition charge, which would support the hiring of additional instructors to relieve the head nurses, was ignored, the Hospital itself supplied the needed funds. With this new bounty the superintendent assembled a faculty with expertise in the theory of nursing; bandaging; preparation of supplies; dietetics; demonstration of materia medica; reading and voice training; district and visiting nursing; gymnastics; anatomy and physiology; surgery; medicine; bacteriology and urinalysis; massage; and ethics. The new staff included, among others, six Presbyterian graduates (one, a former superintendent at New York Eye and Ear Infirmary), a graduate of Teachers College Hospital Economics program, and two physicians.

The new curriculum consisted of four stages: a six-month probationary term, followed by a six-month junior term, a year-long intermediate term, and a year-long senior term. Though more emphasis was given to academics, life in nursing school remained hard. A typical day for a probationer consisted of five hours of practical work on the wards and in Florence Nightingale Hall, two-and-a-half hours of classes and demonstrations, one-and-a-quarter hours of study, and two hours of recreation. On Saturdays she worked and studied until one in the afternoon, on Sundays until three. Each student was allowed four weeks of vacation in the summer, but any time lost "through illness, or any other reason," had to be made up. Free medical care was provided.

All in all, the reform movement of the early 1900s failed to bring nursing to the level of a profession. Many states passed nurse practice acts and many schools upgraded their curricula. Yet students continued to learn as apprentices and the mix of "science and sentiment" never quite jelled, disrupted by the addition of a new ingredient into the practice of nursing. After Henry Ford's wildly successful experiment with automobile mass-production, "efficiency" became *the* answer to society's woes. According to nursing historian Susan Reverby,

> Efficiency in this era had both a moral and managerial function. It signified a hardworking, disciplined, unemotional person, willing to break with traditions to become an effective "expert." As promulgated by "scientific managers," efficiency required the systematic breakdown, analysis, and timing of the steps in a work process; the search for standards and the "best way" to perform each task; the separation of mental from manual labor; and, ultimately, managerial control over the planning and execution of their work.
>
> Accepting these ideas of capitalist rationality was not perceived as antithetical to nursing's historical commitment to service and duty. Efficiency was to be the link between service and science, the bridge over which nursing traveled to be accepted as a profession.

A further complication was that nursing's and medicine's idea of efficiency did not always overlap. "While an Isabel Stewart might worry about the best way to insert an intravenous needle," Reverby explains, "in most hospitals, nursing and hospital administrators were concerned with how quickly student nurses could perform the task. But once the methods and tools of the efficiency experts were introduced they could be used, not to upgrade nursing, but to subdivide and increase the work." Efficiency was a worthy goal, but it was no bridge to science.

Reformers in nursing, some historians argue, failed in a larger sense. Jo Ann Ashley, for example, faults nursing's vanguard for the narrowness of its approach. "The basis of the problems confronting nurses was the relationship between men and women at the turn of the century," she argues.

> Underestimating this, perhaps because of their fears or because of their self-image as reformers, many leaders did not go far enough in examining the repressive atmosphere with which they had to contend in an effort to change the political, social, and economic status of women entering nursing...Had nurses identified the problem correctly, and early enough, they might truly have become "social reformers" in the new century. Instead, their concentration on limited educational issues over which they had no control did little in the way of solving their problems or in elevating their own status or the general status of women. They did have educational problems, but a far more important problem was the social order in which women were dominated by men.

Perhaps the nursing reformers did not go far enough, yet they unquestionably contributed to social reform and most surely opened many eyes to the potentialities of women. The larger travails of women in American society were often discussed within the School's community, and it is hard to imagine that Presbyterian was alone among leading programs in this regard. In 1914 the *Quarterly* published a scathing and sometimes sarcastic three-part series on women's suffrage, addressing both sides of the issue. "We have ... a large number of opponents to woman suffrage because 'women are too sacred to descend into the muddy pool of politics,'" wrote one Frances G. Ecob, whose connection to Presbyterian is unclear. "Isn't that a beautiful sentiment? If politics are dirty, no one can blame women for it ... Suffragists don't hold forth about purifying politics, but we don't think we'd make them any worse."

Ecob's bold words apparently ruffled some *Quarterly* readers. Yet the editors continued the series "because it seemed right that a readable magazine for professional women ... should contain information about the principles that control our living and working conditions. Political education is strongly advised by Miss Maxwell ... [T]he time has gone by when the self-supporting woman can afford to be ignorant upon public and political questions."

The fair-minded editors allowed anti-suffragette Margaret Doane Gardiner equal space. "To woman belongs by nature the creative, individual work of the world," she wrote. "To man belongs by his nature the administrative and corrective side of life. Not that each cannot do the other's job, but that each does best what is natural to them, and that neither can do both well. The best surgeon would be but a poor nurse, and the perfect nurse a fifth-rate surgeon."

Intriguingly, Anna Maxwell also opposed the suffragettes. According to her close friend, nursing pioneer Isabel M. Stewart, the superintendent "was very much anti-suffragist and thought it was a terrible thing for nurses to behave so badly ... [I]t never caused her to break with any of them. She just thought that they had gone astray." That, of course, is not to say that Maxwell was not a social reformer. Nurse training, especially that of high quality, gave women "access to skilled work that was a powerful hedge against the economic dependence that helps to maintain women's subordination," notes historian Barbara Melosh. "Few other institutions in the twentieth century could provide young women with a comparable experience of female autonomy. Seldom explicitly feminist in their ideology, the schools nonetheless empowered young nurses as women by expecting much of them, and by denying the cultural contradiction between femininity and commitment to work."

Maxwell and her peers achieved reform from within, generally obeying the rules of social politics—and for good reason. As Jo Ann Ashley explains, "Acutely aware of their dependency on the good-will of the managers, medical directors, and boards of trustees in private ownership, leaders had no intentions of antagonizing these groups at the very outset of their work. Trained nurses had prestige, recognition, and visibility; therefore the necessity for radical public action seemed unwarranted to the majority. Although they would in less than a decade, nurses had not yet thought of moving away from privately owned schools to collegiate education for their profession."

In Maxwell's realm, a woman could get things accomplished without the vote, something she proved on countless occasions. When she spoke, men listened. "One had to be very sure of one's ground in opposing any of her ideas," noted Albert Lamb, her personal physician. "Even then she never gave up without a good fight." Helen Young added, "She had not the slightest fear of any man, be he dean or president of the board or a Vanderbilt...A quick tongue and a ready wit softened the way."

Raised to respect lines of authority, Maxwell worked successfully within the system, using whatever means were at her disposal—the force of her personality, the weight of her record, the influence of her friends—to win more rights for nurses and better care for patients.

One of Maxwell's biggest disappointments was her failure to secure a sizable endowment for the School in order to free nursing education from the *economic* needs of the Hospital. Because she won so much support from the managers over the years, she did not see an overwhelming need for *administrative* independence. "Never in her conversations with me did she speak of the school being incorporated independent of the Hospital but always as an integral part of the responsibilities of the Board," recalled Young.

Had Maxwell adopted more rebellious or more forceful tactics, the nursing and women's reform movements might have progressed more rapidly. Then again, she might have been suppressed, and her career might have warranted but a footnote in the history of nursing.

In 1908, at the age of fifty-seven, Anna Maxwell contemplated retirement. Evidently, she had learned well the pleasures of rest and relaxation during a recent six-month sabbatical in the old world. It was a retirement undoubtedly deserved. Her accomplishments of recent years — the revised three-year curriculum, the opening of the visiting nursing service, the establishment of military nursing, the creation of several nursing organizations—were a fitting end to an unusually long and fruitful career in a field where practitioners generally retired after only a few years, usually to raise a family.

She also was a best-selling author. With Amy Pope '94, she wrote *Practical Nursing*, published by G.P. Putnam's Sons in 1907. It was one of the first texts for working nurses as well as students. The reason for this oversight, an *American Journal of Nursing* reviewer noted,

> has undoubtedly been, that many text-books of nursing have been written by men, who were not so well posted in practical nursing as in anatomy, physiology... The present volume differs widely from this class... Practical experience speaks from every page of the book — this gives it at once its greatest value and charm. With all due regard to other schools of nursing throughout the country it must be acknowledged that many are unable for one reason or another to attain the high standard which the Presbyterian Hospital School of New York has set, and it is a matter for congratulation that those who have made the success of the school are so generous in sharing the result of their experience and labor. Not an idle word—not a shred of padding is to be found between these two covers.

The book, which went through four editions and was translated into Danish, Spanish, Chinese, and Korean, was widely used by nurses and lay people for a quarter-century. Approximately 250,000 copies were sold. "The appearance of this work ... marks a turning point in nursing literature," wrote the *AJN* reviewer.

But at the insistence of the Board of Managers, Maxwell did not resign. There was so much more to be done—for the Training School, for nursing in general, for the country, and beyond. Before long the world would feel the rumblings of war. Men would be injured. Nurses would be needed.

10

The Hamlet of the Setting Sun

And so again, while men fight and maim and kill—the
women, as always, bind up the wounds, nurse the sick
and comfort the dying.

James R. Sheffield
(Commencement exercises, 1915)

IN JUNE OF 1914 Archduke Francis Ferdinand, heir to the throne of Austria-
Hungary, fell victim to an assassin's bullet, precipitating a war of unima-
ginable proportions. Over the next four years ten million soldiers and twenty
million civilians perished—all for an uneasy and short-lived peace.

The United States remained (officially) neutral until the latter stages of
the hostilities, when President Woodrow Wilson reluctantly declared war
on Germany "to make the world safe for democracy." The public was generally disinclined to war, too, not yet ready to assume the role of the world's
policeman. "That there was no spontaneous urge to fight was suggested by
the strong measures taken: a draft of young men, an elaborate propaganda campaign throughout the country, and harsh punishment for those
who refused to get in line," notes Howard Zinn in *A People's History of the
United States.*

Nurses were among the first to "get in line," though for reasons that had
nothing to do government propaganda or threats. Indeed, the participation of nurses, individually and collectively, preceded Wilson's declara-
tion. With a sizable American military commitment likely, nursing leaders
were not about to stand idly by and watch history repeat itself. Still fresh
in memory was the Spanish-American War, when young men in uniform
suffered horribly in the absence of an organized nursing corps. The Army
and Navy Nurse Corps were born of that debacle, but they were inadequate to the demands of a global conflict.

In 1916, unbeknownst to the president, who was then still hostile to any preparedness planning, the American Red Cross, the Medical Department of the Army, and prominent physicians and nurses quietly collaborated to establish base-hospital units at the country's most prominent medical centers. Each unit would have enough supplies and personnel to field a 1,000-bed hospital that could be mobilized in a matter of days.

The first of fifty such units was organized at Presbyterian under the direction of George E. Brewer, the Hospital's chief surgeon, and Anna Maxwell. Together they recruited twenty-five physicians and sixty-five nurses and raised $25,000 for supplies. U.S. Base Hospital No. 2, as the unit became known, was ready to serve by the start of 1917.

The leadership of the unit's nurses fell to Maxwell's capable assistant, Janet B. Christie '98. Though healthy and active, Maxwell at age sixty-four was too old for official overseas service (the Red Cross cut-off was thirty-five). Nonetheless, in the summer of 1916 she accompanied Irene Givenwilson on a Red Cross-sponsored tour of Europe to evaluate the status of volunteer nursing. In about one month's time they visited sixty-seven hospitals in France, England, and Belgium as well as a number of aid stations near the Western Front. (It was the first of two trips that Maxwell would make to the war-torn continent.) Maxwell also edited Givenwilson's influential report to the Red Cross.

It is likely that the superintendent encountered a number of her former pupils during the tour. Before the war Presbyterian alumnae could be found all over the globe—in Alaska, Albania, Cuba, China, Egypt, France, Japan, Korea, the Philippines, Puerto Rico, Russia, South Africa, Turkey, and elsewhere—serving as nurses and teachers and administrators and missionaries. Now, as volunteers, numerous alumnae were individually assisting the war effort overseas. Two of them, with the rank of captain in the Canadian Army Medical Corps, were directors of nursing at English military hospitals.

Glenna Bigelow Tyler '01 was the first Presbyterian nurse, and probably the first American nurse, engaged in the war. In the summer of 1914 Tyler was caring for a prominent Belgian in his chateau in Liege when the Germans attacked. Instead of retreating, she stayed on for months to nurse wounded and burned Belgian soldiers before escaping to safety and returning to the United States. A few years later Tyler joined the Army Nurse Corps and served in European base and mobile hospital units. She documented her early war experiences in *Liege on the Line of March* (1918).

Edith T. Hegan '07 was one of the first Canadian nurses to serve overseas, in England, France, and Russia. As a member of the Anglo-Russian

Hospital Corps in Petrograd, she witnessed some of the bloodiest battles of the Bolshevik Revolution from Prince Dimitri's palace (which had been converted into a hospital), blocks away from the Winter Palace. "As nurses, enlisted in the service of our country," she wrote in *Harper's Monthly*, "our first duty is to relieve suffering, and attend to the wants of our patients. But one does not often see a republic in the making, and so we watched the progress as much as we could from our second-story window... Our patients ask us for news, but beg us not to remain at the windows, as already bullets have struck inside the hospital... One hummed through the window directly between our heads... But we go ahead and do our work—for the daily tasks of a nation must be done, even if thrones totter and fall and kingdoms are ground to dust beneath our feet."

Helen Young '12, an up-and-coming faculty member, took a leave of absence from the School to work at the American Hospital in Juilly, France, in 1915. In a letter to Maxwell, she wrote that many patients "have developed the most horrible wounds from infections... [They] gradually become emaciated men and... eventually lose an arm, a leg or a life." Humorously, she added, "Miss [Gertrude] Drake ['08] keeps telling us 'I never worked so hard in my life. Not a minute off duty.' We told her she must not forget when she was 'in training.'"

Before the first American soldier set foot on European soil, Maxwell's nurses had already gathered wartime honors. Three alumnae, Edith Campbell '07, Mary Boulter '08, and Catherine Scoble '12, were decorated with England's Royal Red Cross for distinguished nursing service by King George V. In Kiev Helen Linderman '10 was personally congratulated by Czar Nicholas. Clasping her hand and looking directly in her eye, he said, "I thank you so much for coming over to help care for my soldiers." Word of Presbyterian's reputation spread to the Queens of Bulgaria and Greece, who requested places in the School for several of their countrywomen. It seemed as if all the royalty of Europe had come to appreciate Maxwell's nurses. Soon the young men of Europe, the soldiers of misfortune, would come to appreciate them, too.

Letters from alumnae depicting the horrors of war were routinely published in the School's *Quarterly*. Unfortunately, they did not get wider circulation, for the horrible tales they told might have helped shatter the romantic myth of wartime nursing held by thousands of inexperienced young women, including well-educated socialites, who clamored at the gates of the Red Cross. Many people, even in the military and in nursing, believed that volunteers with a big heart and a little preparation could contribute to the war effort as health care workers. Most nursing leaders disagreed, fearing a dilution of their hard-won standards. According to nursing historian Susan Reverby, "By the eve of the First World War, the idea that high-quality nursing care depended on more than a nurse with practical skills, a kind heart, a well-developed sense of duty to the patient, and deference to the physician was just beginning to gain acceptance. When the United States entered the war ... the demand for nurses in both civilian and military hospitals almost shattered that fragile understanding."

A panicked Clara D. Noyes, director of the new Red Cross Bureau of Nursing, wrote to Adelaide Nutting at Teachers College, "the most vital thing in the life of our profession is the protection of the use of the word *nurse.*" Noyes, Nutting, and other prominent nurses wanted to support the war effort, of course, but they believed that recruitment goals could be met by different means: by stepping up recruitment at existing schools of nursing, creating accelerated programs for college-educated women, and establishing a school of nursing within the military.

In the end the nursing establishment won, convincing the military to accept only graduates of training schools with sound theoretic and practical courses (although standards were gradually loosened) and to open the diploma-level Army School of Nursing.

Patriotically, the Presbyterian Hospital School of Nursing quickly shifted its attention to the war effort. (The timing was unfortunate since New York City, with nurses and social workers in the lead, was just beginning to respond to the dismal state of public health.) The turnabout was certainly disruptive, though hardly paralyzing. The School had never been content to confine its ministrations within the walls of Presbyterian Hospital. Anna Maxwell routinely dispatched student and graduate nurses to affiliated hospitals, public schools, private homes, milk kitchens, rural communities, and military field hospitals. In short, nurses were sent where nurses were needed. Now, with war raging overseas, the School's "community" was not all that different, just a bit wider. And the School's goal was the same—to produce as many quality nurses as possible—although now it had to do so without dozens of staff nurses who were away serving the war effort. As a countermeasure the School trained 154 Volunteer Nurses' Aids for ward duty. They were helpful, but not a substitute for the real thing.

Three weeks after the United States declared war, six base hospitals were summoned for duty and assigned to take over general hospitals of the British Expeditionary Force in France (later units operated Red Cross and U.S. Army Hospitals in France and England). Presbyterian's unit was the third to depart, on May 14, 1917, aboard the steamer *S.S. St. Louis*. Hastily and excitedly, the nurses gathered at the Hospital for meetings and vaccinations and uniform fittings, told only that they were going "somewhere in France." To complicate matters, Chief Nurse Christie was bedridden with a bad reaction to paratyphoid vaccine the final two days ashore.

"During those feverishly busy days, with a multitude of tasks to be attended to, [Maxwell] found time to talk to us, to inspire us afresh with the magnitude and seriousness of the work before us," recalled a member of the class of 1915. "She knew that we might not all come back. One of us did not."

"It was bewildering," wrote Anne K. Williams '15 in her unpublished memoirs of the unit, "The First Six Hundred." "It was difficult to believe we were actually at war. Familiar internes suddenly bloomed out as important looking majors, captains, and lieutenants. We found it difficult to take them or ourselves seriously. It all seemed unreal."

Just before the unit departed, Noyes wrote to Maxwell and the unit's nurses: "The eyes of the world are upon you—there will be double necessity for discreet conduct, and professional lines must be carefully drawn." Whether Noyes' words had any effect is hard to tell, but the nurses did soon "realize that entering military service was a solemn business," wrote Williams. "We were required to sign an oath of allegiance to our officers, and it had been impressed upon us that we were, like all soldiers, subject to court-martial."

Maxwell, of course, needed no such reminder from Noyes. A veteran of many nursing campaigns, military and civilian, she recognized the importance of outward behaviors and appearances. Which is one reason she pushed so hard to have her nurses—and all other nurses—properly attired for wartime service. According to the *American Journal of Nursing,* "When she heard that the nurses were to be ready to sail in ten days with no provision made for an outdoor uniform, she was greatly concerned ... Should the American nurses go overseas in civilian clothes, she said, it could never be understood by those already in uniform. She felt keenly that the American nurses in the theater of war needed to have the protection of a uniform."

Maxwell brought her concerns to Jane Delano, head of the American Red Cross Nursing Service, who appointed her chairwoman of a new uniform committee. With a little help from her friends and a diligent clothing manufacturer, Maxwell designed and produced 300 uniforms in six days, enough for Unit No. 2 and the two units that had already departed. Her design, somewhat modified, became the regular Army nurse uniform.

Yet another of Maxwell's contributions to military nursing involved the fight to secure rank for Army nurses. Like Spanish-American War nurses, World War I nurses generally received little respect from medical officers and, especially, hospital corpsmen. The War Department had declared that Army nurses have "authority in matters pertaining to their professional duties (the care and of the sick and wounded)." However, the vaguely worded regulation left authority over important ward matters (e.g., ventilation, sanitation, light, temperature) open to interpretation, which seriously eroded the nurses' control.

Later, as the military battle in Europe wound down, a political battle at home heated up. The first salvo was fired in 1917 by militant suffragists, who enlisted the aid of several prominent nurses, including Maxwell (not a suffragist but a veteran advocate for nurses' rights). The nurses quickly took the lead and realistically lowered their sights to the goal of *relative* rank, which would give nurses the title of officers and authority over nursing matters, but not the commissions, pay, or benefits of regular officers. In the face of significant opposition from various congressmen and officials (including the secretary of war and two successive surgeon generals who had opposed rank of any form), it was the reasonable thing to do. Relative rank was finally awarded to Army nurses in 1920.

"To [Maxwell's] service on our finance committee, whose chairmanship no other would accept, we are indebted to a freedom from anxiety as to funds without which we could not well have gone forward," wrote Helen Hoy Greeley, counsel to the National Committee to Secure Military Rank for Army Nurses, in a letter of appreciation to the School and its alumnae. "Of the total sum raised and expended for rank, almost a third was obtained by your dearly beloved Anna C. Maxwell of New York." Greeley also praised the School's alumnae, who diligently responded to calls in the *Quarterly* to petition their congressmen for relative rank and to ask their physician, soldier, and woman friends to do the same.

It must have been quite the eyeful that clear blue afternoon in May 1917 when out of New York harbor slipped the *St. Louis,* its deck teeming with nurses in navy serge dresses and topcoats, matching felt hats, and dark tan gloves. They were the first Army nurses to wear an official outdoor uniform — not a momentous occasion, but nonetheless a symbolic step toward recognition of nursing's place in the military. It did not seem to matter then that the uniform was too hot; they were later replaced with a lightweight shirtwaist and navy-colored suit.

The *St. Louis* sailed alone for one week, with only seven naval guns for protection, virtually defenseless against the German U-boats that prowled the Atlantic. (Among the few civilian passengers was Lillian Gish, star of D.W. Griffith's movie, *Birth of a Nation*.) The days were occupied with safety drills and instructions, a constant reminder of the subterranean dangers. Daily, the doctors and nurses practiced donning their Everwarm safety suits, which purportedly could keep one alive in the water as long as four days, with the aid of a special food and supply pouch. "We laughingly visualized ourselves bobbing serenely upon the surface of the ocean, courteously exchanging the civilities of chocolate and brandy flasks, and intermittently playing tunes on the tin whistles provided for signaling!" wrote Williams. But the safety measures were no joke. On another ship, the unit later learned, one nurse was killed and two others injured when a defective shell exploded on deck during gun practice.

Unit No. 2's crossing was uneventful, save for a blustery storm and a scary bump in the night. A whale? A dead mine? "No official information was forthcoming," recounted Williams, "but it made everyone realize the tension which we were unconsciously living." The *St. Louis* was met off the coast of Ireland by two U.S. destroyers for an escort through the dangerous passage to Liverpool. "During the last two nights," reads Christie's diary, "we were ordered to remain on deck fully dressed and to carry with us our life belts and nonsinkables, and whatever else we felt was a precious possession."

Once ashore, the nurses began to sense the tremendous social impact of the war. "Girls were driving buses, girls were carrying plumbers' kits, sacks of coal, girls were serving as mail-carriers, in fact doing everything there was to be done," wrote Williams. "It was a novel and touching sight." Overseas the war had severely strained society's neat division of labor along the lines of gender. If women could be plumbers and coal carriers, they could be most anything else. No wonder Williams and her compatriots were exhilarated by the sights. (Back home the lines remained well demarcated, which was reflected in the commencement address of James R. Sheffield, a member of the Board of Managers, to the class of 1915. "The first thing that appeals to me about this splendid career you have chosen is that it is so essentially women's work," he said. "No man can do it. It is your destiny and privilege.")

Next on Unit No. 2's itinerary was London, peopled with convalescent soldiers from every corner of the British empire. "Hundreds of private homes, and buildings of every description, had been converted into hospitals. It seemed at moments as if all London were one vast hospital," Williams observed. After a week in the English capital, which included afternoon tea with the American ambassador and Lady Randolph Churchill, the unit crossed the Channel (nicknamed "Death Alley") aboard the hospital ship *Panama*. The immediate destination was the French city of Le Havre. Despite an escort of submarine chasers and hydroplanes, the Germans mounted a minor attack, skimming a torpedo perilously close to the snip. Finally, on May 31, they arrived at the mystery destination, Etretat, a small village on the Normandy Coast, which would be their home for the next eighteen months.

Base Hospital No. 2 could not have found a more charming spot than Etretat, known as "the hamlet of the setting sun." Each year, in peacetime, as the damp, cold, and dismal Normandy winter faded into memory, artists and writers and vacationing French and English families descended upon this small fishing village, lured to its half-moon beach and majestic cliffs, beautifully depicted in a series of paintings by Monet.

The war changed all that, but not the village's hospitality. Alerted by the town crier ringing his bell on every street corner, most of the townsfolk came out, flags awaving, to greet the doctors and nurses of Unit No. 2. A British honor guard and military band added to the fanfare; nobody in the unit much cared that they played Sousa's "Stars and Stripes" thinking it was Key's national anthem.

The celebrations soon ended, quieted by the realities of war: meager food; damp, cold, bug-infested living quarters; mud and more mud; military discipline; and travel restrictions. Flu periodically enfeebled the staff, and now and then bombs dropped from the skies. Worst of all was the endless stream of wounded young men, victims of the latest technologies of combat. Far from romantic, World War I nursing was a grisly lesson in the repair of bodies ripped apart by fragmentation shells, high-explosive blasts and steel-jacketed bullets, in the treatment of eyes, skin and lungs scarred by chlorine and mustard gas, in the continuous cleansing of wounds infected with the myriad pathogens of Europe's well-manured soils. Operating theaters were high-speed butcheries, where buckets overflowed with severed limbs. This was a time for expert nurses, not civilian angels of mercy.

Late in the war, while serving at the front with a mobile hospital, Williams wrote, "Our sense of humor was tickled ... by the appearance in camp of a *Cosmopolitan* magazine, having as its cover the picture of a dainty, immaculate 'Red Cross nurse.' The contrast between the picture and our own appearance was too funny. Between heat and dust and the natural ravages of the day's work we were not dainty. Doubtless the picture of the nurse at the front as she actually appeared ... would hardly appeal to the artistic eye of the public. Her clothes were spattered with blood, and streaked with dust, her face grimy with perspiration, her hands anything but immaculate."

"The first morning after our arrival [in Etretat]," wrote Williams, "we were awakened by a terrific clatter and thought surely the Prussians must have arrived. Peering down from our garret window into the street, we were assured by the sight of a couple dozen French children in sabots, clumping over the stones. They made an excellent alarm clock."

Over the next few weeks, the Americans gradually assumed control of the British hospital. Although improvised out of a local casino, several hotels, and a private villa, the hospital was exquisitely organized—as it had to be to handle up to 1,700 patients at a time. The operating room, a former tea parlor, had a glorious view of passing fishing sailboats and convoys and their destroyer, dirigible, and hydroplane escorts. There was even a well-equipped pathology laboratory for routine tests and the study of problems peculiar to military medicine, such as trench fever and trench nephritis.

On June 7 came the first trainload of wounded, conveying hundreds of soldiers of various nationalities, including German prisoners of war. Most were seriously injured. "Imagine having 418 patients brought to you in an hour or two," reads the diary of Elspeth Gould '09, the unit's assistant chief nurse. "We began to realize what war really meant."

Unit No. 2, like other base hospitals, was the penultimate stop in a highly efficient medical evacuation system established by the British. The wounded were hurried from the front to a field dressing station, to a casualty clearing station, to a base hospital, and, finally, to a convalescent hospital in England; special cases were whisked from the front to England within twenty-four hours.

At Presbyterian's unit the average stay was about fourteen days. First the wounded men were quickly triaged; emergency cases went to the operating theater, all others to the wards for delousing and treatment. According to Williams, "Within a very few hours after the arrival of a train, every man had been fed, cared for, cleansed, and assigned a clean, comfortable bed. To them it seemed heaven after the misery of the trenches, with the perpetual cold, rain, mud, vermin, and the awful nervous strain...To us with our ideas of what a modern hospital should be, the arrangements seemed very crude and simple."

"This was the first place," added Christie, "where the wounded found even simple conditions of restfulness and cleanliness such as would give them a chance to recuperate from their injuries and from the horrors of the battlefield ... The fortitude displayed by the wounded, always grateful and appreciative, even when their suffering appeared unbearable, was to the nurse a constant inspiration." The nurses needed that inspiration. Once a week, for months on end, the hospital trains would roll in, disgorging one shattered body after another. Things got so hectic the nurses were allowed only one afternoon off every seven days.

The fighting occasionally quieted, permitting the staff to wander about the cliffs and countryside, arrange a dance, stage a musical ("Hello, Etretat"), or visit Paris—anything to try to forget why they were over there. A few of the doctors and nurses contributed their free time to a neglected local orphanage, run by a "retired" octogenarian physician.

In July of 1917 Christie cabled Maxwell to send more nurses. Thirty-one were immediately equipped, only to remain idle for six weeks at a military staging area on Ellis Island while awaiting orders. They did not arrive in Etretat until October.

Though the unit was short-handed, it was asked to send two surgical teams to casualty clearing stations at the front in support of the great British offensive in Western Belgium. Each team consisted of a surgeon, an anesthetist, an operating room nurse, and an orderly. At least five different teams, and possibly as many as eight, were assembled from the unit.

The teams were on call around the clock and generally worked sixteen-hour days for six weeks at a time. Sometimes as many as 200 wounded men would arrive at once, keeping seven operating tables continuously occupied. "The pre-operation tent defies description after a drive, the most ghastly and pathetic spectacle I ever hope to see, and not a murmur from one [soldier]," wrote Louise Marsh *'08*. "In the theatre, amputation after amputation, many double; lads of nineteen and twenty; abdominal wounds with cavity full of free fluid and rapidly spreading peritonitis ... We are provided with gas masks in case we get 'gassed,' with metal helmets in case we get shelled and trenches ready to get into."

One of the new roles women assumed during the war was that of anesthetist. When Presbyterian's second surgical team arrived at the front without a male anesthetist, a British colonel cried, "But where is your anesthetist?" Major William Darrach, the team's surgeon, motioned toward Anne Penland *'12*. "But often there are eight or ten patients at once, big chaps, and they struggle," the colonel protested, adding a few colorful terms, and insisted that a medical man take her place, per army regulations. Darrach (a future dean of P&S) explained that Penland had more experience than any officer in the unit. "Wait and see," he replied, with a confident grin. "Wait and see."

The wait was not long. That night, over 1,200 casualties, many of them victims of Germany's first mustard gas attacks, poured in from the front. There was little time to debate women's proper place. As recounted in *White Caps*: "It happened that on a table lay a big Britisher who, not content with fighting the enemy, was now fighting the ether. He did not relish the idea of losing consciousness, and his broad shoulders heaved ominously. At the proper moment, Anne Penland murmured: 'There, dear, it won't hurt you a bit—there—there.' Tommy's eyes opened in surprise—that feminine voice, the low tones, the Southern touch—it was something new in his young life. He was hypnotized before he was anesthetized. Soothed, comfortable, confident, he smiled sheepishly, and went under like a lamb."

During a lull in the action the British colonel went to Darrach and said, "She always seems to draw the quiet, peaceful chaps." Try as he might, the Britisher could not bring himself to praise a woman anesthetist.

Nevertheless, Penland's impressive performance did inspire the British to train their own nurse anesthetists, who eventually relieved over one hundred physicians for medical and surgical duty. Several hospitals became anesthesia training centers, among them Base Hospital No. 2, with Penland as instructor.

In late August 1917, out of desperation or sheer inhumanity, the Germans began to bomb the casualty clearing stations, which were plainly identifiable day or night. One veteran of these attacks, Jane Rignel '13 (who, only two years out of nursing school, had pioneered a workmen's compensation health aid station at the Western Electric's New York City plant), wrote:

> I feel certain that we can never take the same interest in beautiful clear moonlight nights again—they will mean only one thing to us, an air raid and bombing. Night before last we were trying to operate on a patient when Fritz came over, and three times in the next hour we fell flat on our abdomens, with steel helmets on our heads, and held our breath while our operating theatre was shaken with the vibrations of eight huge bombs dropping uncomfortably close... We always wish we had been better boys and girls about the time the big crash rattles so close. And yet we can remember the days when we were neutral [about the war]. It would be a splendid thing for W. J. Bryant and La Follette to be as uncomfortably close to the big noise as we are—and they might change their attitude.

Nonetheless, Rignel added, "I am so glad I came to France—how miserable I should have been at home, utterly miserable. The satisfaction of knowing that we are doing our bit is compensation for any trying circumstance. I have yet to hear any Tommy, no matter how seriously injured, complain."

During one raid Beatrice MacDonald, a nurse with Presbyterian's first surgical team, leaned from her cot to retrieve her helmet when a shrapnel fragment tore through her cheek and eye, destroying it. A few months later, after being fitted with an artificial eye in Paris, she bravely returned to the front. "Imagine deliberately bombing a camp of wounded," wrote Penland, "and I don't mean one camp but as many as they could locate... Think of Miss MacDonald having to sacrifice an eye for such outrages as these." MacDonald was among the first four American women to receive the U.S. Distinguished Service Cross for bravery under fire. She also received Britain's Royal Red Cross and a personal letter of commendation from General George Pershing.

A few months later, another tragedy. In the relative safety of Etretat, Amabel Scharf Roberts '16, less than two years out of nursing school, died from virulent septicemia, acquired through an abscessed tooth. "It was a great shock to us all," remembered Anne Williams. "On Sunday, she had appeared in her place at the mess. On Wednesday, she was dead." Hundreds of physicians, nurses, soldiers, and villagers, even wounded patients hobbling along on crutches, attended her funeral. Roberts was buried in the local cemetery among the soldiers she had served. "Far off in one corner of the cemetery lay a German, a prisoner of war and one felt that in the great democracy of death all war had been forgotten," read an account of that gloomy day in *Dooins,* a weekly newspaper published by the Base Hospital.

Roberts was one of 296 American nurses who died during World War I. Remarkably, she was the only fatality among the Presbyterian nurses. The library of L'Ecole Florence Nightingale in Bordeaux (a nursing school established by three American nursing organizations—with significant help from Maxwell—as a memorial to the country's nurses) was subsequently named in her memory.

Inconceivably, the ordeal of Etretat intensified. Morale reached a new low during the ebb of winter, 1918, when Germany launched its last great offensive. Ceaselessly, the hospital trains rolled in. Because the clearing stations had suffered terrible bombardment, the wounded arrived in unspeakable condition. Funerals became an every-day affair. Refugees poured into the region. "The tender, enchanting beauty of springtime was darkened by the tragedy about us," wrote Williams.

The nurses were constantly amazed at the soldiers' spirit and recuperative powers. But even this could be depressing. "To see patients recover

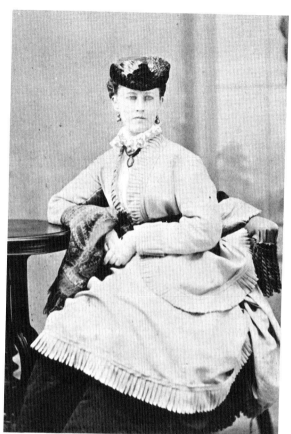

Jane Woolsey, 1870

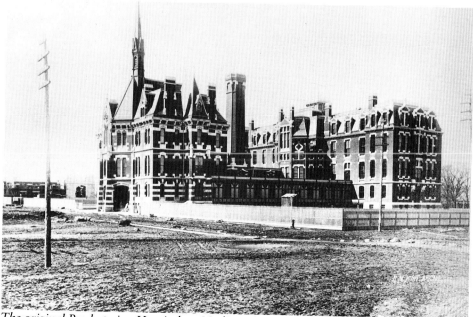

The original Presbyterian Hospital, at Madison Avenue and 70th Street, circa 1880

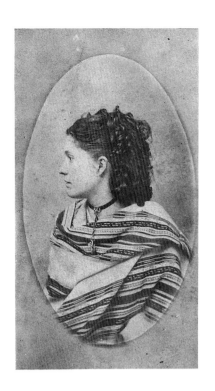

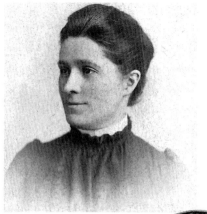

*Anna Caroline
Maxwell, age 15,
in 1868 (left) and
in 1883 (above);
Maxwell's school
pin (right)*

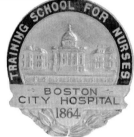

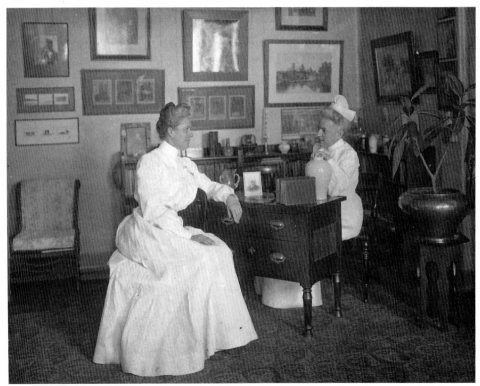

Maxwell (left) and assistant Frances Stone '94 in Training School sitting room, 1910

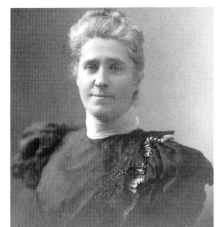

1898

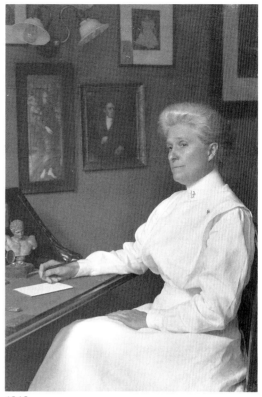

1910

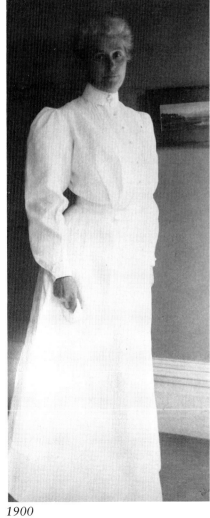

1900

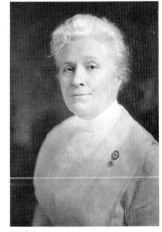

1920

Right: *Students of class of 1897: (back row, left to right) Frances R. White, Charlotte Cowdrey, Constance B. Rose, (middle) Amy A. Chamberlain, Jeanette Bonner, (front) Mary Magoun Brown*

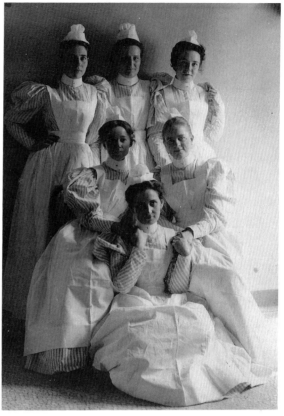

Below: *Sarah Key Davis '94*

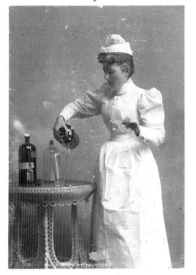

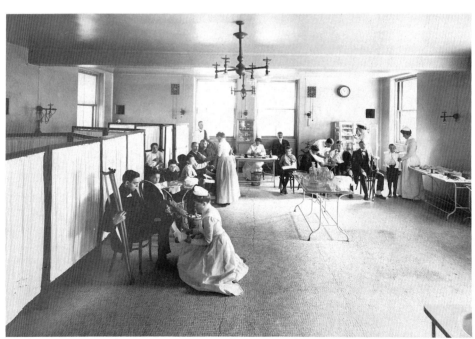

Presbyterian Hospital emergency room or clinic, circa 1900

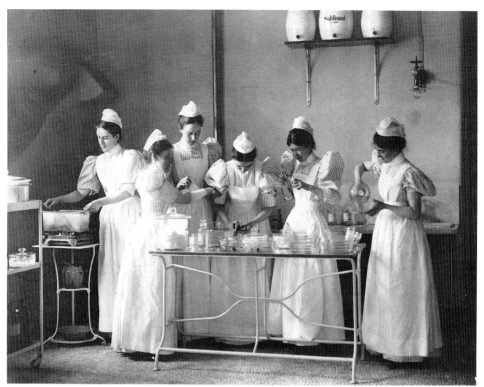

Students of the class of 1897

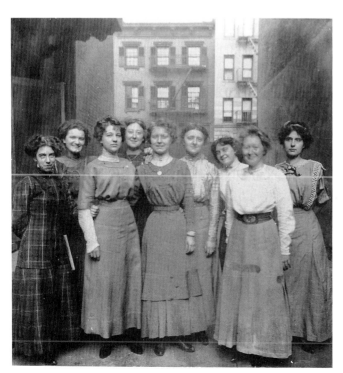

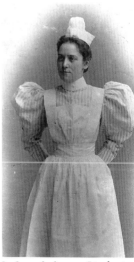

Left and above: *Students, circa 1895*

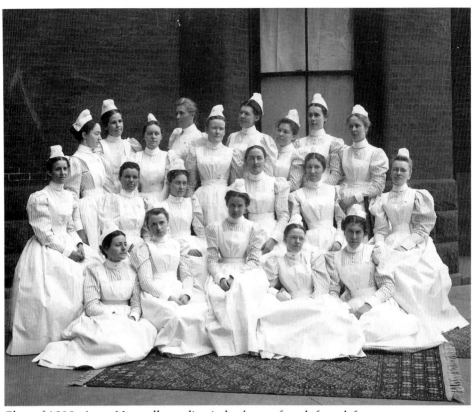

Class of 1898; Anna Maxwell standing in back row, fourth from left

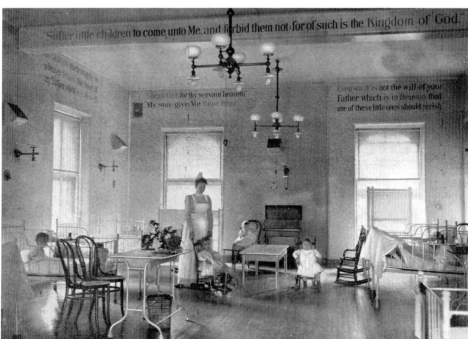

Children's ward, 1899

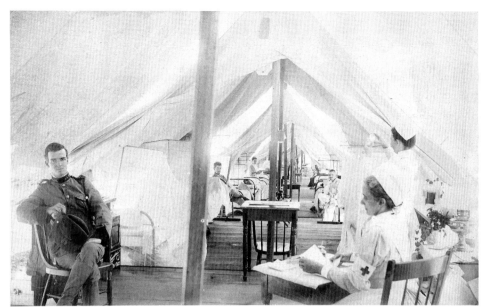

Convalescent tent, Sternberg Field Hospital, Chickamauga Park, Ga., during the Spanish-American War, August 1898; at right, Mariel R. White '97, pouring medicine

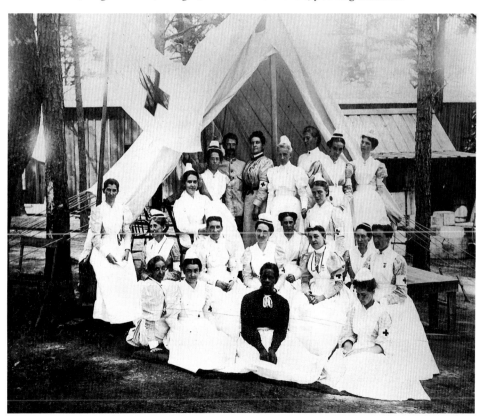

Anna Maxwell (back row, third from right), Frances Stone '94 (in front of tent pole) and the nurses of Red Cross Auxiliary No. 3, Sternberg Field Hospital, 1898

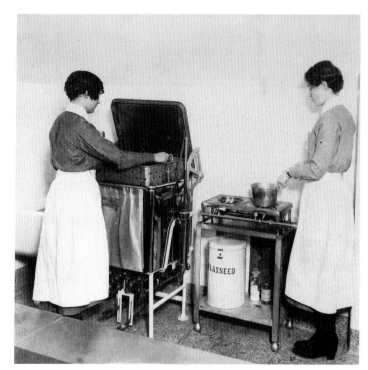

Right: *Probationers, circa 1910*

Below: *Readying typhoid patient for a bath, 1902*

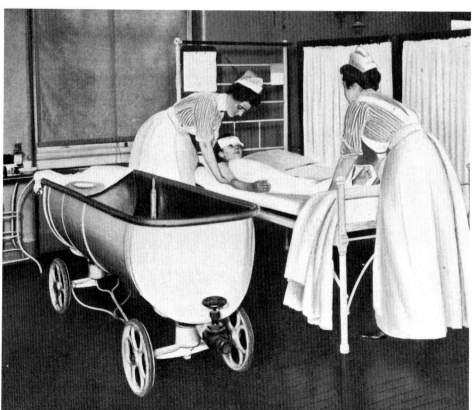

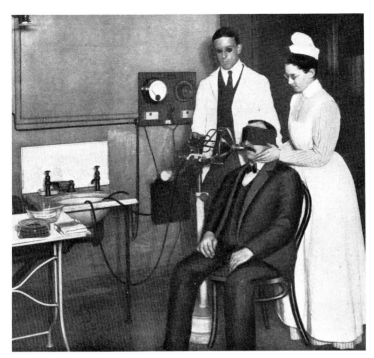

Left: *Assisting with application of Finsen light, a treatment for skin disease, 1902*

Below: *Operating room nurses at the ready: Anna Maxwell (far right), Sarah Strain '01 (middle), Sylvia Davis '04 (far left), 1903*

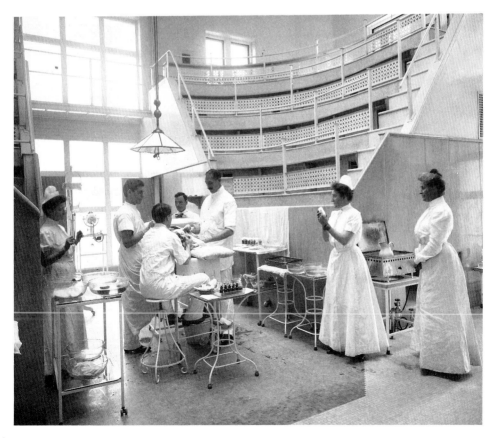

Right: *Applying an ice coil, circa 1900*

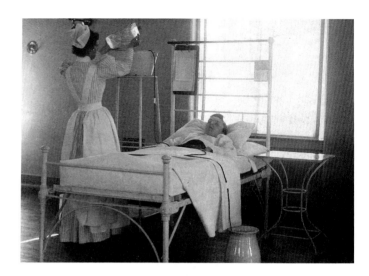

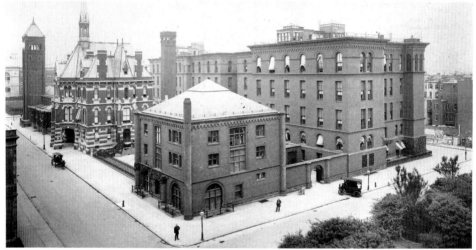

Above: *Presbyterian Hospital and Florence Nightingale Hall (at right), 1904*

Right: *Hospital dispensary, ready to receive patients, 1903*

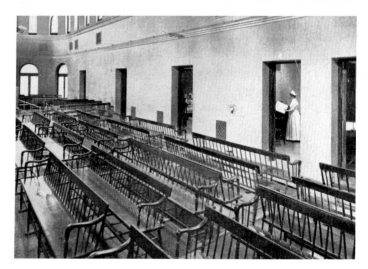

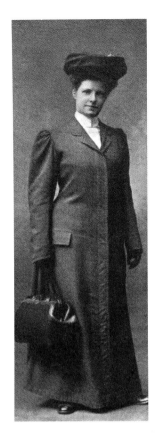

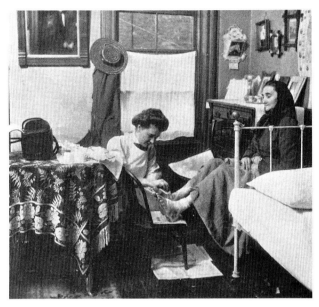

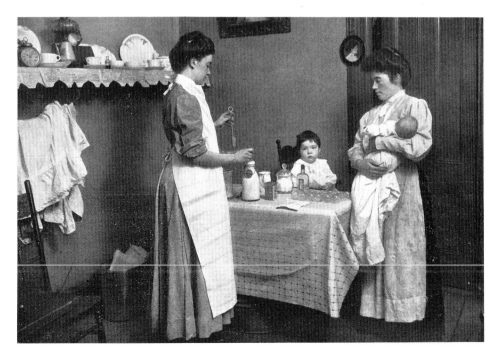

Right: *Frederick Sturges in the dispensary, prepared for commencement exercises, 1904*

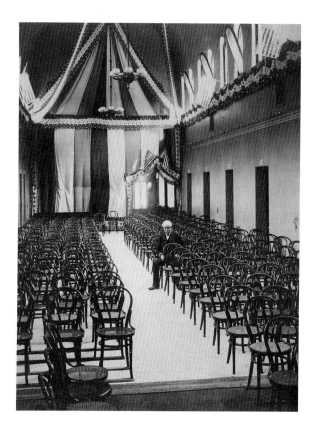

Below: *Anna Maxwell teaching in the assembly room of Florence Nightingale Hall, circa 1904*

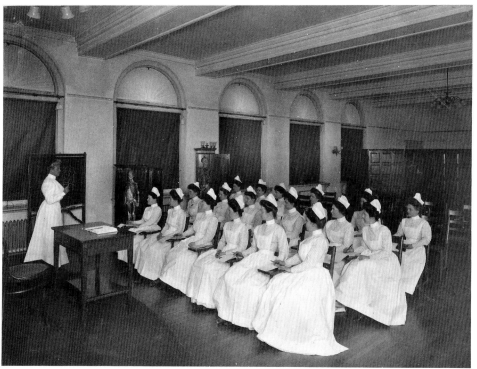

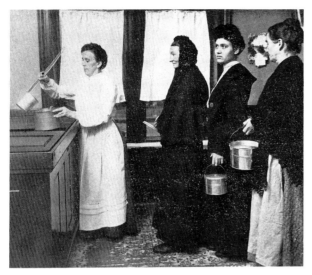

Left: *Katie Geitz Milk Kitchen,*
1908

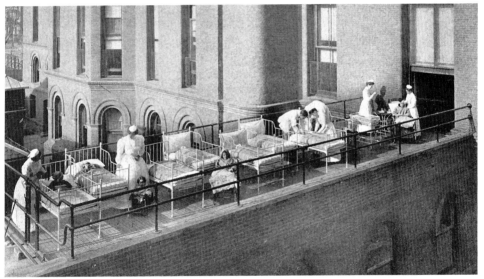

Above: *Open-air children's*
ward, 1906

Left: *Class in domestic*
science, 1905

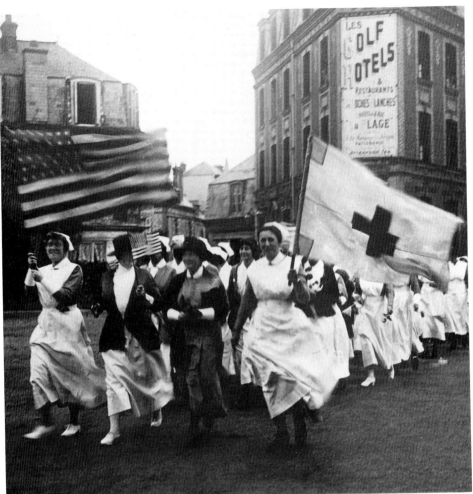

Nurses of Base Hospital No. 2 in farewell parade for Anna Maxwell during World War I, Etretat, France, 1918; Red Cross flag is from Maxwell's Spanish-American War unit

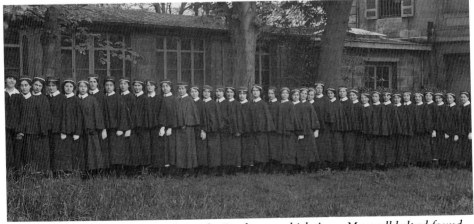

Students of L'Ecole Florence Nightingale, Bordeaux, which Anna Maxwell helped found as a memorial to World War I nurses who died in service, circa 1920

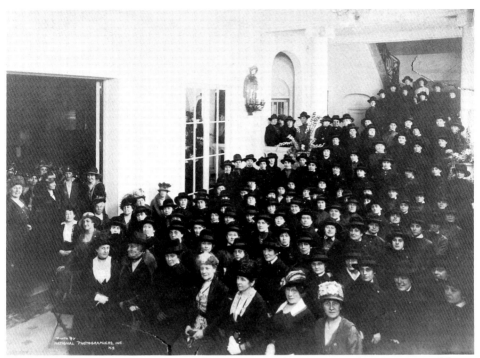

Above: *Nurses of Base Hospital No. 2 prepared for departure, May 1917*

Below: *Base Hospital No. 2 arriving in Etretat, 1917*

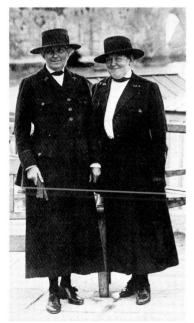

Above: *Anna Maxwell (left) and Janet Christie in Etretat, 1918*

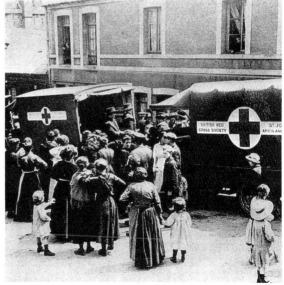

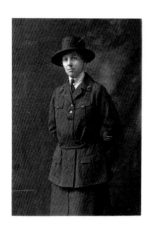

Left: *Anne Penland '12, 1917*

Below: *Nurses of Base Hospital No. 2 bidding farewell to Anna Maxwell, Etretat, 1918*

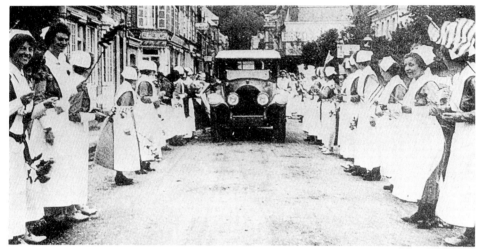

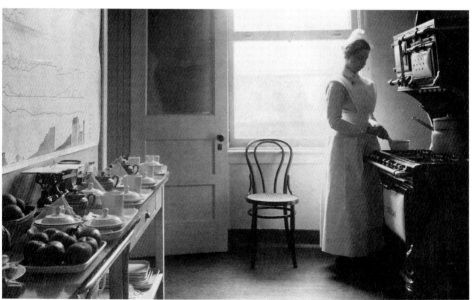

Student in diet kitchen, Presbyterian Hospital, 1916

quickly was only to face the thought that for them it meant further fighting, another wound, probably death," Williams noted. "The only happy ones were those too seriously wounded to fight again ... Even for those one could not predict a safe journey. Who could say that their brief journey across the channel would not be balked by a torpedo."

Among the injured were German prisoners of war, who were segregated from the rest of the patients. Anna Maxwell had told her nurses, "If you have any wounded Germans to care for I shall expect you to do it as though they were British, or French, or American." According to Williams, the nurses did: "[The prisoners] had medical treatment, comfortable beds, the same food as the other patients, and were shown every consideration, denied nothing but freedom ... It was difficult to associate these quiet, kindly men and boys with the cruelties and hideous practices of the Prussian army in the field ... The humility of these men was very touching and genuine."

In May, the first anniversary of the unit's arrival, the Germans were repelled. "We breathed more easily and relaxed a little," Williams wrote. "Work lightened; we spent an occasional afternoon basking in the sunny beauty of the Normandy springtime."

In mid-1918 the U.S. Army belatedly introduced mobile surgical hospitals in the military health-care chain—a response to the rapidly shifting front lines, which often put too much distance between the wounded and the stationary field hospitals. A year earlier the French had recommended the use of Ambulance Chirugicale Automobiles, or Autochirs, sturdy vehicles that could house and quickly transport a bare-bones surgical hospital. Mortality rates among the seriously wounded, they had found, could be lowered as much as 40 percent.

Twenty-two nurses, ten physicians, and a handful of ancillary personnel were siphoned from the Presbyterian unit to form one of the first such rolling hospitals, U.S. Mobile Hospital No. 2. In eight hours their fifty-truck convoy could be transformed into a 250-bed hospital, replete with operating rooms, staff quarters, and kitchen. Over the next six months the staff would become experts in its assembly and disassembly, moving from open fields to forests to abandoned chateaus to trenches, just steps behind the troops and always within range of the enemy's mammoth guns.

Led by Captain Fordyce St. John and his future wife, Jane Rignel, the mobile hospital left in June for preliminary training at a Red Cross hospital at Auteuil, the famous race track on the outskirts of Paris. Some of the nurses went directly to the capital, where they met Anna Maxwell at the outset of a summer-long inspection tour of dressing stations and evacuation hospitals at the front. ("Gallant and inspiring as always, her few words made us realize the great opportunity before us, and we were close to tears as we piled into the staff cars provided for the first lap of the journey," remembered Anne Williams. "She was the last to see us on our way, as she was the first to greet us on our return," recalled another alumna. Maxwell's itinerary included a brief visit to Etretat and another stopover in Paris for the July Fourth parade of American nurses down the Champs Elysees. The superintendent arrived home on September 19, the *Quarterly* reported, "looking as if she had been on a delightful vacation, and not just arrived from a long and tiresome sea voyage.")

In a matter of weeks the mobile unit found itself encamped at Bussy, in the thick of war. The story is best told by eyewitnesses.

"We were awakened by the most terrific barrage..." recalled one nurse. "This was followed by the gas alarm, when we all groped wildly for our gas masks...Shells were bursting everywhere; the hut next door was blown to atoms."

"Stretcher after stretcher was brought in until it seemed as if there were no more beds to hold them," Williams recounted. "They came in filth and grime — torn, weak, exhausted masses of tortured flesh and broken bones, their faces pale and ghastly with the agony of their terrible ordeal. Some died before they could be placed in bed. Many were missing a leg or arm. None of the wounds had been dressed. No sooner had we ministered to one than another was at hand... It was a scene to the make the brain reel, blood and horror, terrible suffering and death."

Manelva Wylie Keller '10 reported: "Patients were pouring in, shells were shrieking about our heads furiously; our hearts were torn between our longing to do the work that so sadly needed to be done and our powerlessness to do it."

"The nurses of Mobile Hospital No. 2 showed remarkable heroism during the bombardment at Bussy," wrote one Major Conkling in *Iodine and Gasoline* (the title of which refers to wound-cleansing solutions used in the war). "They were advised at the beginning of the bombardment to take cover, but refused to leave the patients."

"The next day, July 15, orders came to move the wounded out of shell range," added Emily Clatworthy '98. "The hospital was partly demolished. The Germans were being driven back, and, before noon, Mobile No. 2 was taking up the work again about twenty kilometers farther back—and so began our life at the front."

"So you see my life is being filled with excitement, thrills, and heartaches!" remarked one nurse. "At last I am beginning to do my bit over here, and oh, what a privilege it is. I wouldn't change places with anyone on earth."

Nothing quite matched the bedlam of that night at Bussy. But there were further challenges, minor and major, humorous and horrifying. Wherever they camped flies and wasps filled the mess, fires and floods wrecked the tents, disease weakened the staff, and bombs rained from the sky. "We were fated to be beset by the seven plagues that summer," joked Williams. At one site the unit tended to a platoon of Algerians, whose "savage instincts cropped out most unexpectedly," Williams wrote. "They had a gruesome habit of bringing enemy ears into the hospitals in their knapsacks, and objected strongly to parting with them."

Later, the mobile unit participated in the long Argonne campaign, at once the saddest and happiest chapter of its peripatetic life. Two thousand soldiers, all severely wounded, passed through its hands every week for seven weeks; 400 were buried in a nearby cemetery. "It was a dark time, lightened only by the news which filtered through from time to time that our troops were slowly but surely gaining ground," penned Williams.

It was in the Argonne Forest in November that the unit learned of the signing of the Armistice. Around then a German plane appeared. "Everyone ducked for cover," Williams recalled. "It passed over, no bombs dropped, and we wondered. Next morning was found a pamphlet, dropped from the plane, which was an appeal from the Kaiser to the American soldiers of German parentage to desert 'the traitor Wilson' and 'come to the arms of the Fatherland.'"

The mobile unit did go to Germany, as part of the occupying forces in Treves. After weeks of idleness and anticipation the unit slowly made its way back to Etretat, by then virtually emptied of patients, but full of their grateful Normandy hosts, who staged a joyous sendoff. All of Unit No. 2 reassembled in the port of St. Nazaire on the Bay of Biscay, where still more weeks of waiting followed. Finally, on January 26, 1919, it sailed for home aboard the small fruit boat *Matapan*.

"Long would be remembered the lovely, delicate beauty of Normandy: the rich fertile glory of the Marne Valley, which not even an invading army could entirely destroy; the glorious vineyard country to the east," Williams reminisced. "We breathed a prayer that the soil of France might never be trodden by the feet of its enemies."

Two weeks later the Presbyterian unit arrived at Hoboken, N.J. In a stream of ambulances the physicians and nurses were whisked up Fifth Avenue to Polyclinic Hospital for physical examinations and delousing, then on to Hotel Albert for a few days of demobilization. (The unit was soon disbanded, yet kept intact on paper as a potential Red Cross disaster response team.) The ensuing days were filled with parties and celebrations. Maxwell presented each of the nurses with a special blue-and-white enamel pin, adorned with "'17-'19" on the front and "Service" on the back.

(The folks back home never forgot the men and women overseas. One holiday season the students collected gifts and food for the wounded. Another, the seniors canceled their Halloween dance and used the savings to send Christmas boxes to the unit. In appreciation, the Board of Managers hired an orchestra for the students, so they had their party after all. In the spring of 1918, the School and other members of the Hospital community got together to stage a benefit circus for the Red Cross, replete with clowns, "wild men" from Fiji, and fat ladies. Dressed as "the Spirit of the Red Cross," from the famous Harrison Fisher poster, was Anna Maxwell. The usually composed and dignified superintendent was known to let down her guard now and then. Annie Goodrich, the renowned nursing educator, once told of a Cosmopolitan Club pageant in which Maxwell, at age seventy or so, played the role of a different sort of pioneer, Christopher Columbus.)

Lives slowly returned to normal, or as normal as they could be after witnessing a war. Janet Christie and Elspeth Gould resumed their duties at the School. Anne Penland returned to her post as chief anesthetist, which she held for almost four decades. Nearly one hundred graduate nurses mastered the intricacies of anesthesia at her hands.

"The Army of the United States is under deep obligation to the nurses who served so gallantly and faithfully," remarked Secretary of War Newton D. Baker when presenting the Distinguished Service Cross to Beatrice MacDonald. "That our losses were so slight, relatively, is undoubtedly due to the fidelity, self-sacrifice and heroism of the women of the nurse corps who ministered to our men at the very front." Similar words of appreciation were expressed by Merritte W. Ireland, the Army surgeon general.

Wartime honors were bestowed upon many other Presbyterian nurses. Britain's Royal Red Cross was awarded to Anna Balen '13, Mary Boulter, Edith Campbell, Silla Marguerite Carr-Harris '07, Janet Christie, Elspeth Gould, Hilda Havergal MacDonald '13, Harriet Meiklejohn '06, Naomi Meiklejohn '12, Mildred Parkins '10, Jane Rignel, Edith Tilley Hegan '07, Elizabeth Russell '97, and Catherine Scoble. France's Croix de Guerre went to Ruth Hovey '14, Rignel, Alice Smith '15, Phoebe Taylor '13, and Agnes Warner '01.

In addition, Madelon Battle '05* received the Order of the Croix from King Albert of Belgium. "I was a proud woman when King Albert pinned the Order of the Croix on my chest … " she told Maxwell, "but it wasn't a patch on how said chest swelled when I got your letter this morning … I've got four Belgian orders, an English, with another one on the way in a few weeks, and the Presbyterian pin—almost too much good luck for one poor 'tar heel,' isn't it?"

Lastly, France's Medaille d'Honneur de l'Hygiene Publique went to Anna Maxwell. A gold medal and special illuminated parchment were presented to Maxwell in 1927 at her sickbed in Presbyterian Hospital.

In all, about 200 Presbyterian alumnae served overseas during the war —more than a third of all the nurses who had ever been graduated from the School.

After the war a group of eight alumnae joined the American Commission for Relief in the Near East, working in such places as Armenia and Syria. Another outfit of seven alumnae went with the Red Cross to Siberia, and still others joined relief efforts in France, Serbia, and Turkey.

"It was over," Williams wrote upon her return. "Our army career was ended … [I]t would be safe to say that despite all the hardships and dangers, not one would exchange for anything in the world the comradeship, the deep experience, and all the memories, grave and gay, of our two years stay in the sister republic … To us, France would always mean something more than a resort for tourists. It would be our second home."

* Battle dropped out before completing her studies and thus did not actually graduate with the class of 1905. She was awarded a pin and diploma at the war's end.

11

No Stone Left Unturned

We have long claimed Miss Maxwell for our own, but
we have come to realize that she belongs, not to the
Presbyterian Hospital, but to the world.

C. Irving Fisher, M.D. (1922)

WORLD WAR I PROVED, once again, that war is good for business — and for
nursing. As an indispensable contributor to the war, organized nursing
accrued political clout, which it used in the partially successful struggle for
military rank. Official rank, as the leaders had hoped, did give nurses greater
authority in the armed forces and boost nursing's overall public image. But
the profession had far more serious problems. Its weakness, in any setting,
military or civilian, had little to do with formal titles and much to do with
formal education. Graduate nurses in general were products of an inferior
educational process and were respected accordingly. Even worse, half of
the nation's 300,000 nurses had had no training at all. Nursing desperately needed a sounder academic foundation.

The war delivered a piece of that foundation by sparking new ties with
academia. During the conflict roughly 20,000 nurses — most highly trained
— were sent overseas, seriously depleting the domestic supply. The profession did gain new recruits as a result of the romantic image of military
nursing, which was greatly overplayed by the media in the name of patriotism. It lost countless others, however, to the truer and far less attractive
image of civilian nursing that seeped through the cracks in the propaganda campaigns. Potential students learned that the typical nurse, either
in hospitals or on private duty, led a life of drudgery and was denied a living wage.

Ironically, many would-be nurses were thwarted by the war they were
trying to support. For example, Gladys Thivierge, a high school student in
Rouses Point, N.Y., dreamed of studying under Anna Maxwell, but when

her two brothers volunteered for duty, she was left in charge of the household and a young niece, leaving little time to study. To make matters worse, her local school had closed for long stretches because of the flu epidemic. Undaunted — and unprepared — she applied to Presbyterian in 1918; Maxwell had no choice but to reject her. At the superintendent's urging, Thivierge returned to school and then enrolled at nearby Champlain Valley Hospital. It was a great disappointment. "I felt I was doing just right by going to a nearby hospital," she wrote Maxwell more than two years later. "But my eyes are open, my mistake shall be rectified if you will consider my application ... I feel the various types of diseases limited and the educational training weak [at Champlain Valley]." Satisfied with Thivierge's new credentials, Maxwell accepted the determined woman into the class of 1924.

As the wartime nursing shortage intensified, nursing educators recognized that traditional recruitment methods were sorely dated. In the early months of the conflict the Committee on Nursing (a group of prominent nurses attached to the General Medical Board of the United States Council of National Defense) launched a highly successful nationwide campaign to recruit high school graduates, which ultimately increased enrollments by 25 percent. Boldly, the committee aimed even higher, at better-educated women, who were needed throughout nursing. Top schools had been attracting college women for many years, though not in any organized fashion. To attract these women into the field the committee asked nursing schools to offer a shortened program to college graduates with strong backgrounds in science.

Not all schools were convinced that graduates deserved special treatment or would make better nurses, but Presbyterian quickly agreed to the plan "in the belief that the college woman, having developed powers of observation by means of good scientific training, and having acquired a certain amount of technical skill in the handling of laboratory materials, in the study of art, or in practical procedures, such as cookery, etc. may be able, in a shorter space of time than the average individual, to master the technical processes demanded in nursing, and, as a further result of mental training, to concentrate on essentials, assimilate more readily the theoretical instruction, and single out elements of value in the practical experience." One year of college work in biology, chemistry, sociology, and psychology (or in related fields) was required for admission into the shortened course. (High school graduates were still accepted into the traditional three-year program.)

Within six months of the program's June 1917 announcement, the School received over 1,900 inquiries from would-be nurses, roughly three times normal. Flush with an unusually large number of qualified applicants, the School added an extra section of probies to the class of 1920, twenty-two of whom were housed in the homes of benefactors until a house could be let at 825 Madison Avenue. Of the class' seventy-eight members, over half had college experience (twenty-two had degrees). Total enrollment was 174, a 30 percent increase over previous years.

To make sure the faculty was up to the task of educating these elite students, Maxwell hired instructor Alice Francis Bell, a new baccalaureate graduate of Teachers College.

The Committee on Nursing's experiment escalated the following year with a special summer-long nursing preparatory course for college graduates at Vassar College, Poughkeepsie, N.Y. The novel program (originally conceived as a glorified nurse's aide course) attracted over 400 women, who went on to thirty-three of the finest nursing schools in the nation. Twenty-one of them enrolled at Presbyterian in the fall of 1918, including Priscilla Barrows '20, who had immediately responded to the call to duty. "I walked home ... and told my Mother in faltering tones (for I knew she wouldn't like it and she didn't) that I was going to attend a Training Camp for Nurses ... " she recounted. "There was an almost electric atmosphere about the Camp that summer. Everyone was on their toes, eager to learn, eager to make strides toward that date in September when she would enter the real battlefield of disease and be done with books." Other participants in this experimental class were two future directors of the School, Eleanor Lee '20 and Margaret Conrad '20 (who later became dean of the World War II incarnation of the Vassar school at Bryn Mawr), and Gertrude Banfield '20, who became director of enrollment and recruitment of the American National Red Cross during the Second World War. Much of nursing's leadership over the next generation arose from the brief Vassar experiment.

Despite the signing of the Armistice that fall, the overwhelming majority of the Vassar graduates completed their studies. Many other nursing students did not. Thousands came to nursing because of the wartime glamour and left when it faded, seeking better prospects in marriage. As the *Quarterly* noted, "A sudden influx in 'Father's Bank Account' has undoubtedly turned many a prospective nurse to a life less strenuous, and since the armistice the attraction of a dashing, overseas surgical career has vanished ... Our much lauded vocation of abnegation has become an avocation." The war also legitimized a few other forms of occupation for women; they no longer had to answer a "calling," such as nursing, to gain respectability in the workplace. Presbyterian was not immune to this phenomena: twenty-seven students resigned in the wake of the war. Thus, the conflagration had ended, but the nursing shortage did not.

Resources were further strained by the influenza epidemic of 1918-20, spread around the globe by the continual movement of troops. Over a half-million Americans died during one ten-month period, five times the number of U.S. military deaths in the war. Hospitals were overwhelmed, and nurses were needed more than ever.

Presbyterian Hospital added forty cots to the medical service, which was devoted entirely to influenza patients. More than 850 flu patients were treated during one four-month stretch. Most surgery was curtailed and only emergency cases were admitted. Since there were no preventive or curative medicines, the staff wore masks and gowns and scrubbed their hands with great care. But quarantine measures failed to prevent the epidemic from incapacitating ninety student nurses, two of whom died, in the first winter of the epidemic. Classes and demonstrations were canceled during the flu's peak. Somehow the staff prevailed, with help from several married (i.e., retired) alumnae who returned to duty. "We had to rely entirely upon symptomatic treatment and good nursing care," wrote Presbyterian historian Albert Lamb. The flu returned the following winter in a less virulent form.

By 1920 the country was short an estimated 65,000 nurses. Tens of thousands of excess deaths were attributed to inadequate staffing. In May of that year the School of Nursing graduated fifty-eight students, its largest class ever but not large enough. Hospitals and agencies submitted requests for three times as many graduates. One Southern state alone asked for ten graduates to cover its entire territory as public health supervisors. Many positions in "industrial nursing" went begging, prompting Maxwell to suggest that hospitals should establish a six-month course in this specialty for graduate nurses. "Corporations would no doubt aid in allowing classes to visit the plants, and, if approached, might be liberal in subsidizing the schools for such a course in order to provide nurses for their own plants," she said.

With so many job offers and relatively few graduates, Maxwell decided to add another section of probies. She placed paid notices in leading magazines and newspapers and pleaded to alumnae for recruitment assistance. Astonishingly, no one applied. That even a top school could fail to attract students was undeniable proof of nursing's dismal image. Several of the School's college-educated students gave talks at women's colleges, including Smith, Vassar, and Wellesley, in the hope of future returns, but Maxwell knew it would not be enough. "Extensive publicity will be necessary in the immediate future," she wrote. "The standard schools [those adopting the National League of Nursing Education's 1917 curriculum standards] will have to take part in this campaign or the 300,000 patients occupying beds, which are said to be provided for the sick in America, will not be properly cared for."

To make up for the shortage of students at Presbyterian, "ward helpers" were engaged in 1921, relieving the nurses of some noneducational duties, including wheeling patients to and from examining rooms and clinics, carrying specimens to laboratories, transferring and discharging patients, and retrieving supplies. (This was apparently modeled on the experience of a few years earlier, when the Hospital found it advantageous to hire clerical workers in the outpatient department to assist the overburdened nurses. The positions were filled with women who had taken first aid courses at Presbyterian.) Two years later the Hospital added floor clerks, who from a desk positioned at the entrance of each ward received visitors, answered the phone, and took messages. These measures helped as well as hindered, since they were charged to the School's existing budget.

In another move to boost staff levels, the School recruited graduate nurses for a new three-month "Added Experience" course. Thirty nurses from fourteen countries signed up, at a salary of sixty dollars a month. Unfortunately, many of them spoke little English.

The post-war experience was telling proof that nursing education was in dire need of an overhaul. The product was faulty—students weren't buying and patients and physicians were complaining. To rally public support for reform, nursing leaders initiated the high-profile Goldmark study of nursing, but its results would not be published for several years (see Chapter 12). Something had to be done immediately. One obvious remedy was to shorten the students' marathon workdays (often twelve-hours long), which were long enough scare off even the most fervent applicants. In 1918 the National League of Nursing Education asked schools of nursing to institute a fifty-two-hour work week. Presbyterian consented, but delayed the new plan until late 1919 because of the influenza epidemic and the many Armistice-related student resignations. Some students did not mind the long ward hours. Alice Bliss Smith '19, for instance, remembers, "I loved it, every single minute," she said. "I just hated to get off duty. My heart was in it."

(Earlier, Maxwell had spoken out against twenty-four hour shifts for special duty nurses, showing a concern for rank and file nurses often lacking in "elite" academicians. At the 1916 New York State Nurses' Association annual meeting, she remarked,

> In many cases, for example after a major heart operation has been performed, the necessity of watching for hemorrhage is almost constant. Can a nurse who has had a strenuous day be relied upon for such service? She may be able to catch a few hours of broken sleep provided the patient does not require constant waiting upon, but she bears the responsibility if anything goes wrong and a human life may be at stake...
> In many states stringent laws are in force, regulating the hours of railway employees, so that the "man at the switch" may not, by falling asleep, endanger the lives of the public. Is it not of as vital importance that the hours of a nurse shall be as reasonable, so the life of her patient may be safe in her hands?)

Actually, the students' hours were at a historical low. For the first time they had an off-duty life to speak of. Like the rest of the working class, they had little experience with the concept of "leisure time" and fell into some disturbing habits. There was particular concern over the rising abuse of late and overnight passes, the "predilection for owning library books," and improper conduct during prayers. They also put their free time to good use. Emboldened perhaps by the women's suffrage movement and nursing's political battle for military rank, students at a few nursing schools dabbled in self-government. At Presbyterian they convened a meeting in April of 1920 to discuss ways of addressing pressing nonacademic matters, including rules barring women from the Hospital tennis court. Consequently, they voted to establish a Student Association, replete with a constitution, rules and regulations, officers, and a host of committees. (*P.H.*, a brief student quarterly, was launched a few years later.) Maxwell, a member of the association's advisory council, told the students, "Do not attempt too much at one time, but see to the finish what you undertake to accomplish."

Judging by an early set of rules and regulations — which incorporated many existing policies — the students undertook a great deal, addressing virtually all aspects of student life. All off-duty students who missed an association meeting faced a fine of ten cents. Students were required to observe "quiet hours" in the residence hall from 9 a.m. to 4 p.m. and 10 p.m. to 7 a.m., which was enforced by student proctors. Only with a late pass could students stay out past 10 p.m., but not beyond midnight, unless they had an unimpeachable excuse and notified the School by telephone or telegraph. Special overnight passes could be obtained, providing a destination address and phone number were supplied. Except for night nurses, students were required to report for 6:45 a.m. breakfast and prayers. Three missed breakfasts in a week triggered a report to the advisory council. Rooms were inspected each week by a student proctor, who made sure that dresser and table tops were free of "unnecessary material" and that beds were stripped and windows raised while one was on duty. Use of the kitchenettes and library was strictly controlled. Uniforms could not be worn on the street, except by those who resided outside Florence Nightingale Hall; they had to wear a coat and hat. In keeping with the almost religious belief in the recuperative powers of fresh air, students were allowed to sleep on the roof, so long as they did not use white bedding.

On the back of a pocket-sized pamphlet of rules and regulations were the following suggestions:

> Don't be afraid to be yourself; be ashamed not to be.
>
> Have a large circle of acquaintances but go slowly in forming intimate friendships. You have three years in which to form friendships, and all your life to keep them.
>
> Don't be ashamed to study.
>
> Don't cut classes—or friends—or breakfasts.
>
> Remember you have a representative government. If things aren't going the way you want, it's your own fault.
>
> Be thoughtful of those who are studying. Remember, busy signs should mean locked doors even to friends.

Aided by Maxwell, the student government won the right to use the Hospital tennis court, which had been restricted to men. "No harm so far has come from this unprecedented break in technique save an endemic infection of tennis in the school," reported the *Quarterly*.

Student government gave the pupils some voice in their own affairs, though it did relatively little to lighten their load. In 1923 a student identified only as "A.B.S." submitted a poem entitled, "The Trained Nurse," to the *Quarterly*. One of the stanzas read:

> *For social life she has no use,*
> *Nor any gaiety;*
> *She likes to live as a recluse,*
> *She's but a nurse you see.*
> *The strength of Hercules she needs*
> *To stand the strenuous life she leads.*

The School of Nursing's second linkage with academia was a joint diploma-baccalaureate degree program with Teachers College, an indirect result of a tentative affiliation between Presbyterian Hospital and Columbia University. Although the 1911 agreement dealt primarily with medical education and practice, it strengthened relations between the institutions' respective nursing programs. In 1917 those relations coalesced into a three-year program for women with at least two years of college experience (including certain science prerequisites) leading to both a nursing diploma and a bachelor of science degree. Enrollees were required to complete a shortened (twenty-five-month) nursing course at Presbyterian plus thirty-two credits (one academic year) at Teachers College.

It was a highly unusual arrangement. Only sixteen colleges and universities around the nation had any schools, departments, or courses in nursing education, and even fewer had combined diploma-degree programs. "This may serve as encouragement for the advancement of admission standards in a state requiring only one year of high school as preliminary education for admission to schools of nursing," read a notice in the *Quarterly*.

At first it was recommended that students take their preliminary college courses at the college, ensuring a certain quality of candidates in the joint program. By 1921 this was made mandatory, and an extra year was added for specialty work. The program, now five years in length, consisted of two years of liberal arts instruction at Teachers College (including preclinical nursing instruction), two years of practical instruction at the Hospital, and a final year of advanced study, usually in nursing education or administration or in public health nursing at Teachers.

The new five-year program was not for everyone, partly because of the steep expenses at the college, totaling close to $1,000 a year—$250 to $300 in tuition plus $500 to $700 in living expenses. (To put these costs in perspective, a private duty nurse at Presbyterian, working twelve hours a day, five days a week, fifty weeks a year, could make only $2,000 a year, and few private practitioners were lucky—or hardy—enough to be so busy.) Presbyterian didn't charge tuition for the diploma-degree students, only a modest fifteen dollar fee for clothing, equipment, and other items. (Three years before, the Hospital had instituted its first tuition fee for regular students—seventy dollars for the entire program, which covered the cost of uniforms, books, instruments, and other essentials.)

In anticipation of the School's planned affiliation with Columbia University, both parties agreed to terminate the relationship in 1925, after some fifty women had been graduated. Their decision was more than a decade premature, since the affiliation was not realized until 1937. (See Chapter 15.)

In another cooperative arrangement between the two institutions, Presbyterian offered a five-week practical course for graduate nurses enrolled in Teachers College's 1920 summer session. The aim of the course, taught by Helen Young, was to prepare nurses to teach in schools of nursing.

Paradoxically, while the School was striving to raise educational standards, some alumnae were questioning the wisdom of overly stiff admission requirements in the midst of a nursing shortage. An unsigned article in the *Quarterly* asked, "How much education is necessary to make an intelligent, efficient nurse? Surely a B.A. or M.A. does not necessarily make a good nurse… The present standard will suffer more from the present dearth of nurses than it would by lowering entrance requirements and thus getting more nurses to do the work which at present is going undone." Even within nursing people could not agree over the value of higher education. How were nursing educators going to convince outsiders that nurses could not be overeducated?

In yet another milestone of 1917, the governors of Columbia University awarded Anna Maxwell an honorary master of arts degree "for more than thirty-five years of giving talent, knowledge and high devotion to the training of nurses for their important place in modern life [and] always holding the highest professional ideals and earnestly inculcating them in others."

Four years later Maxwell submitted a letter of resignation to the Presbyterian Hospital Board of Managers. (Simultaneously, two old Presbyterian hands, Janet Christie and Elspeth Gould also resigned. Both had worked continuously for the School since their student days.) Her modest letter read, in its entirety, "Your Board invited me—just short of thirty years ago—to undertake the establishment of the School of Nursing and to become the Director. It has been my pleasure to see the growth and enlargement of your hospital and to take some small part in this growth. The School has attained some measure of distinction through the services rendered the public by its graduates, and several gifts to the Hospital have been secured through their instrumentality."

By this time Maxwell had become somewhat isolated from day-to-day matters of the School. Her contact with students was minimal, limited to occasional lectures and disciplinary actions. A summons to the superintendent's office was met with fear and trepidation. According to Alice Bliss

Smith, Maxwell's association with students was largely confined to written notices or disciplinary meetings. "If you were sent to her," she says, "you knew the end was near. She was very severe."

Smith's classmate, Mary E. Pillsbury '19, was called into Maxwell's office a few days after graduation. "Even though I was now a graduate nurse and on duty in the hospital, being called to the office made me fearful," she remembered. "What had I done? ... I put on a clean white uniform, fastened my school pin in just the right spot and pinned on a fresh cap. I drew a long breath, knocked on the door and, when bidden to enter, stood before Miss Maxwell with my hands properly clasped behind me—the posture we always took when talking to superiors ... Miss Maxwell looked me over. We were never asked to sit unless the matter was serious, so as I remained standing I felt things weren't too bad." As it turned out, Pillsbury was summoned not for a scolding but for an assignment in Keene Valley, in New York's Adirondack mountains, where a nurse was desperately needed to help manage an outbreak of influenza.

Maxwell was not totally removed from student life. To make sure that she heard everyone's comments and concerns, she kept a mailbox on her office door and responded with little yellow, handwritten notes. "Miss Maxwell always remembered my name and expected me to know the whole earth," noted Jennie Wideman '20.

The Board regretfully accepted Maxwell's resignation and voted unanimously to continue paying her $2,500 salary for the rest of her life as well as to establish a fund that would yield an annuity of $1,500. "It is only natural ... that Miss Maxwell should have asked to be relieved of the onerous duties of her office while still able to devote her great knowledge to the science of nursing, derived from her long experience, to the advantage of the profession generally," reported William Sloane, Presbyterian's president. "Miss Maxwell will always remain a member of the Presbyterian Hospital family."

News of Maxwell's resignation reached alumnae all over the world. In May, 400 of the School's 736 graduates gathered to honor her at commencement exercises, which as usual were held in the Madison Avenue Presbyterian Church. "It was an impressive sight: the long procession of her former students among them superintendents, instructors, head nurses in white uniforms, and many other graduates once more in their blue-and-white-striped uniforms," reported Eleanor Lee. "At the appearance of Miss Maxwell, leading in the class of 1921, there was a marvelous tribute of enthusiastic applause."

President Sloane read from a special roll of parchment:

Her influence has been felt, not only in our institution, but in hospitals and training schools and in the nursing profession generally throughout the world ... Gifted with a wonderfully magnetic personality and endowed with a clear insight into the possibilities in the development of the profession, sympathetic with the successive new steps made necessary in the methods of teaching, jealous of the position of the nurse in civilian life, and ambitious for her proper recognition in military service, an inspired teacher, a helpful friend, and a superb type of womanhood, Miss Maxwell has been the glory of this institution and, more than anything else, has added lustre to its reputation for nearly a third of a century.

At the ceremony's close, the class of 1921 lined the aisle of the church and formed an arch of white diplomas, tied with blue and white ribbons, through which Maxwell passed.

The next day, at an honorary luncheon, Maxwell was given a bouquet of roses that concealed a $4,000 check "for a little spree." When the band launched into a rendition of "For She's a Jolly Good Fellow," no one could find the voice to sing. "It was the Chief herself who took the situation in hand, and tapping her foot and nodding her head, in her own imperious way, led the way out of a difficult moment," reported the *American Journal of Nursing*.

More than 800 of Maxwell's friends and admirers gathered again in February 1922 for a special tribute dinner at Manhattan's Biltmore Hotel. In one of many testimonials Haven Emerson, M.D., of Columbia University's DeLamar Institute of Public Health (later renamed the School of Public Health and Administrative Medicine), proclaimed, "Whatever Miss Maxwell's ambition for her profession, we shall know that her mind, her art, her determination will be to give her patients, whether babes or soldiers, whether tenement family, or city, or nation, something of nursing service a bit better than has been studied out before, and then to so present it and fix it in the practice of the day, that the method, the art, the technic of the service will become a part of the creed and conscience of her successors."

Annie Goodrich, who called Maxwell her "constant adviser and friend," remarked:

In this morning's news I read that Miss Maxwell was the Florence Nightingale of the United States. The Times is wrong again (I wish they would place a woman on that editorial staff). Dear Florence grew immensely stout, you'll remember, in those last years spent reforming British armies and killing English statesmen in the Cause. Not so our Anna! She is much more the great prelate type judged by her noble stature and her lofty mien ... [G]o to her for advice—it will be briefly given—yet always to the point ...

In every cause of nursing she has made an outstanding contribution: in legislation, that the sick might be ensured proper nursing care; in obtaining rank that no stone should be left unturned to further our efficiency in time of war; in the creation of the Bordeaux School that our sisters who served and fell in France should live again... Have you ever thought what it would mean to live for forty years in those great domiciles of human ills, the hospitals, their very walls reeking with pain, while Death stalks daily down the halls followed by weeping friends? To live... in this, and never to be downed; to hold fast to the joy of life; to still know it the great adventure it was meant to be. That's sportsmanship indeed! Loving and serving man, she has loved not less his art, his songs, his clever fingers twisting out his thoughts in stone, in steel, in china, or in glass. I traveled with her once in England. Castles, cathedrals, palaces and hallowed spots—she knew them all!

Anna Maxwell may have resigned from the Presbyterian Hospital School of Nursing, but she did not retire. Until the end of her life she continued to work for the School on special projects (most notably, the campaign for a new residence hall), attend professional meetings, and lecture and travel widely. Maxwell always believed in doing something extra and appealed to others to do the same. In a 1923 note to the alumnae she asked, "Is it not a privilege to accept committee work? How many of you have accepted office in state and national affairs? How many are carrying on their education in keeping up with the times? Sometimes a hint of greater things that might be accomplished is whispered. Other Alumnae have progressive programs for cultural and civic interests. What are you doing along these lines?" Maxwell herself was an active member of several women's clubs, where society's most prominent and progressive women gathered to exchange ideas and plan campaigns. The clubs were, in one sense, mutual improvement societies, where Maxwell gained the university education she was too busy to pursue formally.

The daunting task of succeeding Maxwell fell to Helen Young, a highly experienced clinician and educator, who was appointed acting director. She had one tough act to follow.

12

Infinite Courage

Seldom did [Helen Young] attempt to express the Ideal-
ism of Nursing with words or metaphors. She just practiced it as she saw it.

Franklin M. Hanger, M.D. (1967)

FREE OF THEIR WARTIME OBLIGATIONS, nursing's leaders redoubled their
campaign for professional reform, beginning with the prominent Goldmark study of nursing education and practice. They had been anticipating
such an inquiry for almost a decade—not for the results (they already knew
what was needed), but for the political fallout. Only hard data would convince a recalcitrant health care establishment, nursing superintendents
included, that nursing schools should be more selective in admitting students, separated from hospitals, linked with universities, and independently endowed.

Organized nursing was hoping for nothing less than a sequel to the
Flexner report, the devastating 1910 study of medical schools that precipitated a revolution in physician education. At that time nurses petitioned
the Carnegie Foundation, Flexner's backer, for an investigation of their own;
curiously, the foundation declined, while funding studies of dental, legal,
and teacher education.

In 1922 the Goldmark study, which was funded by the Rockefeller
Foundation, produced an indictment as scathing as Flexner's, confirming
the beliefs of nursing's vanguard. That the study analyzed better-than-
average institutions added further weight to its conclusions — or so one
would think. Remarkably, it yielded no Flexnerian change. The health care
establishment contended that nursing, in advocating more theory and less
practice, was moving in the opposite direction of medicine, which follow-

ing Flexner was awakened to the value of hands-on experience. It was a hollow argument: nursing evolved from the bedside and was naturally seeking a stronger scientific foundation. In truth, the Goldmark study (named for its secretary and primary investigator, Josephine Goldmark) stirred up old fears. Administrators were afraid of a costly disruption to student nurse staffing, while physicians were afraid of competition from highly educated nurses. The prevailing belief was that nurses were already overtrained, that technical knowledge and manual dexterity were enough; dishearteningly, many nurses agreed.

Time and again nurses were warned of the insidious, dehumanizing nature of too much scientific training, as if this were a documented phenomenon. Even at Presbyterian Hospital, an institution that cultivated and nurtured knowledgeable nurses, this message was repeated relentlessly, beginning with the first commencement exercise. To the class of 1927, Chauncey Brewster Tinker, the esteemed professor of English from Yale University, remarked, "The human soul is a fearful thing when the quality of mercy has gone out of it. Well may a patient pray to be delivered from a nurse who is so scientifically trained and so perfectly equipped as to be past all feeling." (Apparently, merciless physicians were acceptable, or perhaps physicians were immune to this phenomenon.) "Obedience, discipline, poverty, humility — they are the marks of the nursing profession still," he added. The next year the graduates were told by John Miller Turpin Finney, the acclaimed surgeon from Johns Hopkins University, "What the patient and the doctor alike want in a nurse is a thorough training and a high degree of efficiency ... But they do not want them at the expense of her womanliness and humanity." The Reverend Samuel S. Drury reminded the 1930 graduates, "You are going into an essential calling," harking back to the profession's ascientific origins. "Any fool can be efficient, but it takes a genius to be kind." And in 1931 Dean Sage, the Hospital's president, commented, "There is a danger that a professional school may become a mere machine oiled and geared to produce the trained specialist. In such a case, the individual product acquires only the rhythm of the machinery; becomes a qualified expert at the cost of a sacrifice of the priceless gift of understanding and sympathy." It was not the last time that the students would be so lectured.

The Goldmark study might have had more impact if it had surveyed all nursing schools, bringing each one's pluses and minuses to light. Flexner did just that with the nation's 155 medical schools. His study was less scientific than Goldmark's, but more specific and thus more jarring. The weakest medical schools could not survive the public scrutiny. For the weakest nursing schools, however, there was safety in numbers. Goldmark could not afford to analyze all 1,800-plus programs and was forced to settle on a slightly misrepresentative sample of twenty-three. As a result the lesser programs went unremarked and unchanged. In fact more schools were opened in the ensuing years.

The report was further weakened by Goldmark's recommendation for a subsidiary grade of nurse who would assume some of the simpler bedside and housekeeping tasks, thereby improving hospital efficiency. Goldmark, a social worker, rose to prominence studying fatigue and industrial efficiency. To the nursing leaders' taste, she was overly concerned with productivity issues. They vehemently objected to the subsidiary nurse proposal, abhorring any institutionalization of the undertrained nurse and any further obfuscation of the title "nurse." (Two years later, the National League of Nursing Education [NLNE] recommended changes in nursing nomenclature in order to improve public perception of the profession. The league preferred "nursing education" to "nursing training" on the theory that the two "do not represent identical processes and that 'training' may occur without education." Other substitutions were suggested, including school of nursing for training school, nursing practice for practical training, and director or principal for superintendent or directress. As early as 1905 Presbyterian started referring to its nursing program as the "School of Nursing," replacing "Training School for Nurses.")

The Goldmark study was not fruitless, however. It did legitimize the nurse educators' views and prompt the Rockefeller Foundation to fund various educational initiatives, notably, the first fully independent university school of nursing at Yale, established in 1924 under the direction of Maxwell's close friend and protege, Annie Goodrich.

Hopes for reform were renewed with the Committee on the Grading of Nursing Schools, another attempt to diagnose nursing's ills and write a prescription. This effort, launched in 1926, held particular promise since it was broader in scope and more widely supported than the Goldmark study, with participants from nursing, medical, and hospital associations. The committee's leader was P&S Dean William Darrach, the School's old friend.

Again, the results were an indictment of nursing education, echoing

Goldmark's recommendations for reform. More than half of the schools studied were found to have a minimum entrance requirement of one year of high school — a level of preparation, the committee noted, "less than that required for stenographers, typists, or file clerks in high grade business offices or for saleswomen in the better department stores." Most schools, it was revealed, had ill-prepared faculty (42 percent of instructors were not even high school graduates themselves), were associated with hospitals too small to offer a complete education, mandated too many hours on duty (more than most factories), and provided little coordination between theory and practice.

(To the nursing faculty at Presbyterian, the report was a confirmation of the School's relative superiority. For example, they learned that their *probationers* had better academic credentials than most other programs' *instructors*. On the other hand, the report underscored the School's need for fiscal and programmatic independence.)

And again, the health care establishment balked at the suggested remedies. Physicians contended that elite nursing educators merely wanted to eliminate the competition and that college-educated nurses were unnecessary. Hospital administrators continued to insist that they did not exploit student nurses. The facts said otherwise. A University of Minnesota study demonstrated that the nursing budget for a hospital that operated a training school and staffed its wards with students and instructors was one-half that for a hospital with an all-graduate staff.

To make matters worse, nursing superintendents were equally opposed to reform. Of 500 superintendents surveyed in one study, a staggering 76 percent preferred a student nurse service to an all-graduate nurse service. They had little incentive to change a system in which they had flourished and which they controlled.

At Presbyterian, administrators also denied that they were profiting at the students' expense. President Sage told the 1929 graduates, "It is said that many [hospitals] are operating for the purpose of providing inexpensive nursing in the wards and without due regard to the amount or quality of education provided the pupil nurse. I do not believe that the Presbyterian Hospital is subject justly to any such criticism."

The Hospital was less exploitative of students compared to most other institutions, which was evidenced by the quality of its curriculum and its graduates, almost all of whom, year in, year out, passed the New York State Board of Regents examination with scores in the eighties and nineties (in contrast, only two-thirds of all examinees in the state achieved *passing* grades). And a year earlier the Hospital had begun to hire appreciable numbers of general duty staff nurses, at a yearly salary of $1,000 plus "maintenance" (room and board). But the Sage administration was hardly guilt-free. That year, according to a School study, the average student gave the Hospital about 2,000 hours of uncompensated service, 42 percent of which had no educational value whatsoever. Assuming the remaining 58 percent had no value to the Hospital (a generous assumption), each student contributed 840 hours of service each year, at a cost to the Hospital of $208 (the School's budget, $60,000, divided by the number of students, 288), which is equivalent to an hourly wage of twenty-four cents. In contrast, a graduate nurse worked 2,700 hours a year for a total cost of about $1,200 (salary plus room and board), for an hourly wage of forty-four cents. Thus, a nursing school, even an expensive one like Presbyterian's, was a profitable enterprise.

The Grading Committee's final report, issued in 1934, capped off sixteen years of near-continuous nationwide study of nursing education—with relatively little to show for it. Strident political opposition was partly to blame, yet so was a repeated blunder. Like Goldmark, the Grading Committee could not afford to conduct a specific school-by-school analysis, which effectively negated the possibility of grassroots reform. In the wake of the two studies, many educators looked to the Depression to do their bidding for them. And indeed many of the lesser schools succumbed in the weakened economy; the number of diploma programs dropped from 2,286 in 1929 to 1,472 in 1936.

While the country's professional organizations wrestled over the future of nursing, Helen Young enriched and expanded nursing service and education at Presbyterian Hospital. Recognizing that science, not sentiment, was behind good nursing, Young supported the School's own studies of education, the results of which guided the enlargement and redesign of the curriculum and the institution of a more scientific admissions process. Recognizing that education, not service, must be a nursing school's raison d'etre, she won independence from Presbyterian Hospital and affiliation with Columbia University (see Chapter 15).

As these extraordinary events unfolded in the 1920s, Young guided the construction of the School's new home, Maxwell Hall (see Chapter 13), and helped engineer the Hospital's move to Washington Heights, where it joined with Columbia University in creating the nation's first modern medical center in 1928. At the new locale, Young retained authority over the education of student nurses as well as the delivery of nursing care. For sixteen years she deftly managed this increasingly difficult dual role, even as student enrollment doubled, the patient census tripled, and health care splintered into a slew of specialties. And for another five years after that, she continued to rule the nursing service at Presbyterian.

Remarkably, Young quickly emerged from the shadow of Anna Maxwell, who was not only the School's founder and sole leader, but also one of the profession's pioneers and a nurse of international renown. Few nursing educators had been blessed with so rich a resource and cursed with so heavy a burden. As Eleanor Lee wrote, "To succeed Miss Maxwell took infinite courage."

Like Anna Maxwell, Helen Young spent her formative years in Ontario, Canada. Young was born in 1874 in the town of Chatham to parents of Scottish origin. She was educated locally in the public schools and then at the Toronto Normal School of Pedagogy, a teacher preparatory program, finishing in 1895. The following year, she was graduated from the Toronto School of Pedagogy for high school and university instructors.

Young—tall and slim, athletic and attractive—returned home in 1896 and secured a position as a substitute teacher at the McKeough School, which allowed her to gain professional experience and fulfill family obligations. At the century's close she received tenure, securing her future in the Chatham schools. But something happened during the next decade.

In 1909 she resigned her teaching post to study nursing at Presbyterian Hospital. What brought her to nursing and to Presbyterian is unknown. It is unlikely that she was dissatisfied with teaching, for she ended up in nursing education. Conceivably, Young found in nursing what was lacking in secondary education: opportunity for advancement. Women were seldom promoted to the rank of school supervisor or principal, a disheartening reality she must have recognized after more than a decade on the job. Moreover, the teaching field was becoming glutted, limiting teachers' geographic mobility. Whatever the impetus, Young enrolled at Presbyterian just months shy of her thirty-fifth birthday, the School's cut-off age for admission. She finished in 1912, intent on a career in private duty.

Maxwell, however, was so taken with the new graduate that she persuaded her to join the Presbyterian staff as a head nurse, a position that included significant teaching and administrative responsibilities. Young assumed control of the women's surgical ward and subsequently the women's medical ward, earning a reputation as a stern yet superb organizer, teacher, and caregiver. Three years later, after the outbreak of the Great

War, Young was granted a three-month leave of absence to work at the American Hospital in Juilly, France. She further contributed to the war effort at home, mobilizing nurses for the Hospital's overseas unit.

Young returned from Europe restless to learn. To find out more about public health nursing, she skipped one of her vacations to substitute in the Hospital's visiting nursing service. A mere five years after graduation she became Maxwell's assistant (substituting for Janet Christie, who was serving overseas). Among her first assignments was to help implement the shortened course for college graduates as well as the joint diploma-baccalaureate program with Teachers College. One could always find Young in her office in the small hours of the morning, finishing all the tasks that could not be squeezed into a normal workday. Upon Christie's return in 1918, Young resumed the role of practical instructor. But it was not a demotion; she was being groomed for much more. By the time of Maxwell's retirement in 1921, Young, at age forty-seven, was a seasoned teacher, nurse, and administrator — the superintendent's logical successor. She was appointed acting director that year and permanent director in 1923.

Young was a popular choice to head the School. Her confident and dignified bearing won her instant respect and attention. Though she usually appeared stern and aloof, she could be forgiving and open. "Miss Young had a truly remarkable ability to discipline, correct, suggest new ways and yet have the individual involved feel it to be in her best interest no matter how difficult at the time," reported Dorothy Rogers '25.

Many, like Alice Bliss Smith '19, saw only the professional side of the School's second leader. "Helen Young was very much like Miss Maxwell — very severe," she remembers. "She never let down her hair at all. And she frowned the way Miss Maxwell did." But Young's demeanor was an "act." She played the ideal nurse, the woman who could handle it all, without complaint, without excuse. "I have seen her wretched with fever or pale with fatigue," noted Franklin M. Hanger, M.D., a professor of medicine at P&S, "but any notice of it on my part always produced a toss of the head and the emphatic remark, 'I am not sick.'...Everyone else with miseries...was treated with the gentleness and compassion of a woman who had an uncanny comprehension of human anxieties and physical suffering."

"The image of nursing was terribly important to her," says Helen Pettit '36. When students threatened to tarnish that image, they were immediately taken to task. She often admonished probies always to hang up their clothes and never throw them on a chair. Maria Auchincloss Look '32,never forgot the day when she and her classmates violated Young's unwritten code of behavior. "One morning at prayers when the lights were turned on in Sturges [auditorium in Maxwell Hall]," she recalled, "the large radio, which had not been turned off the night before, warmed up. Then just as Miss Young said, 'Good morning,' a loud man's voice boomed out, 'Good morning Ma!' Uncontrolled laughter — it was moments before we could settle down. Miss Young was not amused, [and said:] 'Would the girls who are responsible for this please step out of line on the way out. This has caused an unnecessary delay getting to the hospital and it is the patient who suffers when you are late.' "

With biting sarcasm Young scolded fidgeting students to put their hands behind backs. "At least you know where they are," she would bark. "Now maybe you can manage your tongue better."

But there were soft, subtle, and humorous sides to Young's personality, as Augustine Barnard Stoll '16 learned early one morning after working the late shift and returning to Florence Nightingale Hall. "I ... tubbed and was stretched out on the bed... when the phone rang," she recounted. "The dry voice of Miss Young, who was in charge of the ward where I worked, was clear: 'Miss Stoll, please come back in uniform and finish [your patient's bath]. You didn't clean under his toe nails.' ... I think there was a twinkle in her eyes as she said, 'I think you will always remember, won't you?' "

"We all remember how emphatic Miss Young was about not permitting a nurse on duty if she had any sign of a bandage. Nurses were always healthy, at least they had to look that way," said J. Margaret Ada Mutch '36. To Mutch's horror, Young once caught her on duty wearing a walking cast, the result of a skiing accident. "My heart sank," recalled Mutch. "What would she say? Imagine my surprise when she said 'I think you should take one day off to get accustomed to the cast.' "

Young's gentler side was revealed to Cecile Covell '26, who recalled:

Several of us head nurses were sent to one of the wards to make up beds for the arrival of the patients [at the new Columbia-Presbyterian Medical Center]. Never having examined the workings of a gatch bed, we were intrigued with the possibilities and experimentation soon followed. In no time we had produced beds with the most unfamiliar angles. The next step, of course, was to try them out on ourselves and on each other. Soon there was a row of bodies relaxing in positions not taught by Miss Morrison! At that moment from one of the elevators emerged Miss Young and Mr. Bush [the Hospital president]. "If you can't find anything better to do on Hospital time than this," he shouted, "I can," and left. Miss Young followed... with a controlled smile.

Ruth Nethercut Rogers '14 glimpsed a side of Young few ever did. "One day," she said, "as I dashed into a linen closet for a clean sheet, there was Miss Young, crying with her head on the pile of sheets for which I was headed. Embarrassment and concern stopped me in my tracks. Then she raised her head, wiped her eyes, smiled at me and said: 'We all have to cry some-times.' With her head held high, she returned to the ward."

Young was a stickler for nursing ethics, but largely shorn of their religious and moralistic overtones. She counseled her charges that they should not expect to change their patients' ways. "Don't think you can change this," she lectured, "even with your new found knowledge of the why and wherefores of human reactions." Marion Knox Thatcher '36 recollected, "Miss Young said she expected her girls to take a cocktail or two, if the occasion demanded—not to be prudish—but to be practical. She knew we would conduct ourselves 'in the proper fashion.' "

"Young was that rare thing, a saint with a sense of humor," added Virginia Henderson, an internationally known author and nurse-researcher. "She must have represented for me a moral force, because when she died, I was left with a sense of loss akin to that I had when Ghandi and Mr. Roosevelt and Mr. Kennedy died. It was as if a prop of the social structure had been removed."

More than a few of her nurses noted, "We worked with her and not under her"—perhaps the highest praise for a superior.

Young also won the respect and trust of the School's graduates; as treasurer of the Alumnae Association for forty years, she deftly managed and protected the graduates' sick benefit, pension, and scholarship funds. Private duty nurses, who generally had little regard for elite nursing educators, appreciated Young for her studies of private service, conducted as a member of several registry committees, including Mrs. William Church Osborne's Associated Registry Group and the Nursing Bureau of Manhattan and the Bronx.

In retrospect, Young's only weakness was that she lavished perhaps too much attention on traditional, nonacademic concerns, such as order, efficiency, appearance, and deportment. The students' clinical performance, for example, was still judged according to their enthusiasm, cheerfulness, neatness, tact, general appearance, attitude toward criticism, loyalty, courteousness, etiquette, and poise. To be fair, students were also rated for their initiative, executive ability, resourcefulness, teaching ability, appreciation of the value of social problems, and analytical powers. If Young's teachings were long on style, they were still longer on substance. In nine years, she added nearly 400 hours to the curriculum, more than doubling it. She fortified the teaching of nursing technique as well as basic science, preventive care, holistic care, and rehabilitation. "Rehab[ilitation]' was part of our vocabulary before Dr. Rusk and others had awakened the whole country to its importance," observed Margaret G. Arnstein '28, the nation's chief public health nurse in the 1950s. "At the old hospital, where the beds had posts at each side of the foot of the bed, spreads were tied to the post a good 8 inches above the bed — sheets and blankets were pleated loosely so that the patients' feet would not be flattened. Prevention of foot drop was indelibly seared into my being as an index of the importance of bodily mechanics for the patient and for the nurse." Young's pupils "learned to nurse the sick not only in body but in mind," reported *Student Prints*, a student publication. "[Her] constant thinking of us as separate individual personalities has increased our awareness of patients as individuals."

If Young was intimidated by the task of succeeding Maxwell, there was little sign of it. Immediately after assuming the superintendency she started to implement her own vision of nursing. Instructors were given their own offices, on the second floor of Florence Nightingale Hall. Guest lecturers were offered a generous, standardized pay rate of five dollars an hour. Several key personnel were hired, including an extra instructor for ward teaching (Margaret Eliot '21, a future director of the nursing service), a second assistant director for planning clinical assignments, and ward helpers to answer the phone and receive visitors (allowing more time for educational endeavors and plain old patient care). New courses in mental diseases and personal hygiene were swiftly added.

One of Young's most notable early achievements was the introduction of a new academic schedule. By the mid-twenties probies were entering in large numbers at two different times of the year, February and September, resulting in an inefficient, inflexible, and overlapping tangle of preliminary, junior, intermediate, and senior courses and clinical assignments. In this scheme students oftentimes learned the theory of a particular subject *after* the clinical experience. When the unusually large class of 1925 was graduated, the smaller succeeding classes were obliged to perform ten-hour instead of eight-hour shifts in the wards. (The students "cooperated in every way possible," Young noted, yet they hardly could have been pleased.) Outbreaks of serious illness easily destabilized the School. For instance, epidemics of scarlet fever (1925) and sore throats (1926) led to the temporary suspension of classes.

Frustrated, ninety-three members of the classes of 1926, 1927, and 1928 (two-thirds of the student body) signed a letter of protest to Helen Young, which read:

> Owing to the dissatisfaction that has prevailed in the student body for some time, and realizing the unstabilizing effect upon the general morale of the school, we have endeavored to analyze the situation and suggest a possible remedy ...
>
> 1. We request that the student nurse may be assured of her complete training during the time contracted for her hospital work.
>   (a) That she have a well balanced course covering the many branches of nursing education which the hospital affords.
>   (b) That she may have a specified period of time in each of these departments.
> 2. We request that the present call system in the operating room be abolished, and that there shall be instituted a regular night service, as in other hospitals.
> 3. We request that a system of filing applications for affiliations be established whereby the student nurse may be assured of her desired branch of work, thus obviating the possibility of a course in which there is no interest.

The solution to the scheduling dilemma, introduced in 1926, was the "block system" of instruction, which concentrated classes into definite periods: a fifteen-week preliminary term, a ten-week freshman term, and a six-week junior term. (Senior courses — specialty experiences with a little classroom theory — ran the entire academic year, independently of the blocks.) The block system had several advantages. Most importantly, it reduced course overlap and repetition, greatly stretching the reach of the School's eighteen-member faculty (nine full-time nurse instructors, eight part-time physician lecturers, and one full-time lecturer in dietetics). At any given time, only one group of students in addition to preliminary students were taking classes; the others were on full-time ward duty, usually the evening or night shift. Thus, no one on nights had to worry about attending classes the following day. Furthermore, the hours spent in class now counted toward the requisite time on duty, lessening the student's overall responsibility. "This results in better grades, better health, and fewer absences," faculty member Eleanor Lee later concluded. The block system also permitted better coordination of theory and practice and better vacation planning.

For a student who entered in the fall of 1927, the three-year academic schedule proceeded as follows: Preliminary classes ran from September through mid-December, which were followed by eight weeks of evening and night duty. The next segment, the freshman block, began in February 1928 and continued through the end of March. (Unlike probationers, freshmen attended classes and worked in the wards, spending sixteen hours in the former and thirty-four hours in the latter each week.) This led into another interval of evening and night duty, stretching all the way to November, with four weeks off for summer vacation. The short junior term, which also combined classes and ward duty, followed, ending in mid-December 1928. This was trailed by a long cycle of ward duty, including another four weeks' vacation (except for short-course students who worked straight through the second summer), ending September 1929. (This lengthy interval was not instructionless. As Lee explained in 1931 to a meeting of the NLNE, "We have ward clinics given by the doctors on the medical and surgical wards each week ... and each student writes one case study each month.") Then commenced the senior year, which consisted of several two- or three-month specialty clinical experiences and classes, ending May 1930. (The block system prevailed, with only minor revisions, through the 1940s.)

Another beneficial change for students in 1930 was a doubling of the sick day allowance (from ward duty) to thirty days, with a bonus of fifteen days off for those with a perfect attendance record.

Possibly the most consequential achievement of Young's first decade was the routinization of research. The School, which had evolved somewhat informally and haphazardly, embraced a more active and orderly search for knowledge and information. Maxwell and other pioneering nurses respected the scientific process and built their teachings around it, but they never quite adopted it as their modus vivendi. Nursing journals were largely anecdotal, and the practice of nursing was largely driven by the science of medicine.

Young supported numerous scientific endeavors, including two major studies of education in outpatient clinics; a test of the "case method" of ward instruction; the development and testing of a new method of evaluating students' ward experiences; field studies of public health, mental health, and collegiate nursing education; a survey of the alumnae; and a comprehensive analysis of clinical teaching.

The first significant research project of the Young administration was a multi-hospital study of education in outpatient nursing, funded by the NLNE. Six different hospitals in the U.S. and Canada—including Presbyterian—were analyzed in order to fashion a more rational approach to the teaching of outpatient care. The eleven-member study committee, which included Young and Marguerite Wales '20, director of the Henry Street Nursing Service and a member of the School's Curriculum Committee, concluded in 1925 that the outpatient area was a rich but underused educational resource, a site where students could gain exposure to patients and problems not found on the wards. Their report, "Pupil Nurse in the Out-Patient Department," recommended that schools hire more and better-qualified outpatient nurses who were expert teachers as well as caregivers, reduce the noneducational duties of the student nurse, increase the amount of teaching and supervision, devise more specific plans of instruction, integrate outpatient nursing into the curriculum more closely, enlist more support and cooperation from physicians, and establish advanced courses for graduate nurses interested in outpatient supervisory work.

The record is not clear, but it appears that these and other recommendations were incorporated into a three-year demonstration project in outpatient nursing education launched by Presbyterian's Dispensary Development Committee in 1928 and funded by the NLNE and the Alumnae Association. Louise Knapp, a nurse and recent Teachers College graduate, was put in charge of the project and given an appointment at the School. The project's second phase featured a one-month clinical experience in outpatient teaching and supervision for graduate nurses, which attracted practitioners from around the country.

In 1927, in the wake of Yale's successful experiment with collegiate nursing, the Alumnae Association sent Eleanor Lee, director of education, on a tour of five university programs. Two years later she was one of twenty-five nurses nationwide who received Rockefeller Foundation fellowships to observe rural nursing in Alabama, a health promotion program in Harlem, public health and mental health nursing in Rhode Island, and university nursing in New Haven. It was both a reassuring and eye-opening journey for Lee. "There is nothing better for one than to get away and to see how other people do things," she wrote. "It makes one ... realize all that is right here [at the Hospital]." Well, not all, she acknowledged, adding that the School ought to offer more instruction and experience in outpatient care and public health "in order to educate [students] to the broader meaning of nursing."

Lee spent six highly instructive weeks at Yale University, where the Rockefeller fellows attended dozens of conferences and clinical demonstrations on all aspects of undergraduate nursing. Lee was comforted to learn that Yale, the profession's pacesetter, was not that far ahead of Presbyterian. For example, Yale had adopted the "case method" of ward teaching throughout its program, a concept that Presbyterian had successfully tested and implemented on its own the previous year. (In the case method, a student was assigned to a particular patient for up to one month, learning nursing procedures as the need for them arose; a case study was written by the student about each patient. Previously, a student concentrated on a particular procedure and performed it on a variety of patients, putting too much emphasis on diseases rather than on people who have diseases. "This attitude leads to the type of remark ... 'Not an interesting thing on my ward. Just a lot of old cardiacs,' or 'Five gastric ulcers on our ward,'" wrote Mary C. Houston '32, instructor in nursing. The case method, in contrast, allowed students to "view one case each month from every angle, and make a special study of it," to "see the patient as a person or individual, with his family background, his problems, his physical symptoms and their treatment, and especially how *nursing care* can help him," and "to make for each student a small library of case studies of patients for whom she has been responsible." Each case study, preferably kept under 1,000 words, was discussed with and reviewed by the head nurse, then sent to the School office for grading.)

At the tour's close, Lee concluded: "So much more is demanded of the nurse today, she has such an important part in the prevention of disease and the maintenance of health that she is no longer merely an expert at doing technical procedures. She needs her knowledge — reasoning — and judgment. We must teach her to THINK. We must not make her a slave to hospital routine ... It was a most valuable experience for me and I feel what we need to do here is to study our own situation, our curriculum and the experience we have to offer — in other words — ARE WE MAKING THE MOST OF OUR GREAT OPPORTUNITIES?"

Another revealing study, a survey of the School's graduates, was conducted by the Alumnae Association in 1928-29, with statistical help from Ella A. Taylor of the Grading Committee. Responses were received from 419 graduates in thirty-six states and thirteen countries. Slightly less than half of the respondents, the survey discovered, were actively engaged in nursing. One-third were working in hospitals, one-quarter in public health, one-quarter in private duty, and the rest in miscellaneous fields (e.g., social service, school nursing, industrial nursing, doctors' offices).

The survey confirmed that the School's graduates were filling the most challenging and prestigious positions, in hospitals and public health agencies, and they were avoiding the least, in private duty. Private duty was fast becoming the workplace of last resort, a low-paying haven for undertrained nurses. According to the Grading Committee, half of all nurses nationwide were scrambling for this shrinking piece of the nursing pie.

A related finding was that most of the alumnae in hospital or public health nursing had taken some postgraduate courses while most of those in private duty had not. The investigators were not sure whether people who pursued private duty were by nature less academically inclined or they simply hadn't the time, resources, and energy for further study. The Grading Committee was grappling with the same question.

As expected, two-thirds of the inactive alumnae had left nursing because of marriage. Matrimony and nursing were essentially incompatible — only 13 percent of the active nurses were married. (When 1919 alumna Alice Bliss Smith was recently asked if she had practiced after exchanging wedding vows, she replied, "I don't think it ever occurred to me.") The remainder of the inactive nurses had retired because of family responsibilities, illness, and other reasons.

Two-thirds of the alumnae had chosen nursing out of genuine "interest in the profession." Others had turned to nursing as a means to earn a living (12 percent) or as an act of patriotism (10 percent). Revealingly, just 4 percent had been "called" to service, and only a handful had entered the field out of boredom with society life.

Data on the graduates' academic backgrounds were particularly impressive. Half of the alumnae had one or more years of college, compared to only 15 percent of nurses nationwide. Even the School's oldest alumnae (from the classes of 1894-99) far surpassed the national average: one-third had some college experience. And the later graduates (1920-28) were especially well-educated: two-thirds had attended college. (Many, if not most, practicing nurses in New York State at the time did not even have a high school diploma; it was not a state-mandated entrance requirement until 1932.)

Disturbingly, only one-fifth of the alumnae felt qualified to practice in all branches in nursing. Many graduates wanted to pursue a career in public health or administration, but believed they were unprepared to do so. Others wished that the School had given them more experience in surgery, contagious disease, mental health, pediatrics, or teaching. This was startling news — but not only for Presbyterian. That one of the leading diploma programs could not prepare nurses to practice effectively in all the specialties underscored the need for baccalaureate as well as master's level nursing education. The alumnae agreed: 85 percent said that if they were to start their schooling now, they would select a university-based program. But revealingly, a similar percentage stated that they would recommend their alma mater to a sister who wanted to become a nurse. To them, it seems, Presbyterian was no ordinary diploma program. They wished their sisters the opportunity of studying under an Anna Maxwell or a Helen Young.

Anyone who had followed the recent progress of the School of Nursing knew that it bore little resemblance to the average diploma program. In less than a decade classroom instruction more than doubled, to about 1,000 hours, touching upon virtually every aspect of nursing. The typical student spent another 6,500 hours in the wards of the world's most modern health facilities. And untold thousands of hours were devoted to homework.

The 1930 curriculum, under the block system, was as follows (classroom hours are listed in parentheses):

Preliminary Term

Anatomy and physiology (90)
Bacteriology (30)
Chemistry (45)
Personal hygiene (15)
Public sanitation (10)
Nutrition and cookery (54)
Elementary materia medica (30)
Ethics of nursing (20)
Elementary nursing:
    Principles and practice of nursing:
        Demonstrations by instructors (33)
        Practice in classroom (87)
        Practice on wards (55)
    Hospital housekeeping (10)
    Elementary bandaging (15)
    Principles of elementary massage (16)
Physical education (30)

Freshman Term

Ethics of nursing (6)
Elements of pathology (15)
Elements of psychology (15)

Medical nursing (30)
Surgical nursing (30)
Practical nursing (20)
Materia medica (30)
Dietotherapy (15)
Social services conferences (10)
Physical education (20)

Junior Term

Ethics of nursing (6)
Surgical specialties:
  Gynecological nursing (10)
  Urological nursing (4)
  Operating room technique including
    anesthesia (10)
  Orthopedic nursing (5)
Nursing in communicable diseases (15)
Nursing in diseases of the ear, nose and throat (5)
Nursing in diseases of the eye (4)
Mental nursing (15)
History of nursing (15)
Practical nursing (6)

Senior Term

Survey of the nursing fields and related
professional problems (20)

Clinical experiences:
  Obstetrical nursing (plus 30 hours classroom
    study)
  Pediatric nursing (plus 40 hours classroom study)
  Operating room
  Outpatient department
  Medicine
  Surgery
  Gynecology and urology
  Eye and ear, nose and throat
Clinical electives:
  Public health (three months)
  Nervous and mental nursing (three months)
  Communicable diseases (three months)

The most substantial curriculum change during the 1920s occurred in the preliminary course, "Principles and Practice of Nursing," which expanded from 30 to 175 hours. In demonstration rooms and on the wards, students learned how to admit patients, make open and closed beds, treat pressure sores, restrain patients, prepare flaxseed poultices and mustard paste, perform gastric lavages and colonic irrigations, and dozens of other tasks. "In all of these classes, emphasis is placed on the patient and the attitude of the student toward the patient," noted the School bulletin. More complex procedures were introduced in the freshman, junior, and senior blocks.

Most of the other courses were doubled in length, and new courses were added in several disciplines, including social services, psychology, public sanitation, ophthalmology, urology, and orthopedics. Nutrition courses still covered "cookery" for the benefit of future private duty nurses but also delved into physiological aspects of digestion and metabolism and "dietotherapy" (the preparation of special diets for people with diabetes, anemia, and other disorders). In addition, the faculty added lectures and demonstrations for social service students as well as fourth-year students at P&S.

Mindful of the trend toward specialization, Young strengthened continuing education opportunities for staff nurses. "This is the age of specialization," she told the 1931 graduates of Moses Taylor Hospital in Scranton, Pa. "You may not approve of it, but specialization is here to stay. Science has so advanced the practice of medicine that ... there is even now so much to learn about each specialty, that life is too short to consider learning all of them ... Choose the department that you are specially suited to, learn all there is to know about it, make the sky the limit."

Young encouraged her own staff nurses to pursue advanced study with such incentives as financial assistance, flexible scheduling, and leaves of absence, and to attend state and national conventions. Each year dozens of instructors and staff nurses enrolled in advanced-study programs. Special lectures for private duty nurses were also offered. In 1928 Presbyterian and four other area hospitals joined Teachers College in an experimental training program for head nurses. The eight-month course required thirty-six hours a week of practical work at one of the cooperating institutions plus another eight hours a week of study in such subjects as educational psychology, comparative nursing methods, mental hygiene, public health, and hospital economics. The program also required advanced study in a particular clinical area. Graduates were encouraged to continue their studies toward a baccalaureate in teaching or administration at Teachers College, where advanced standing was offered to those who passed written and practical examinations. And in 1930 and 1931 thirty head nurses at Presbyterian attended a course in public health nursing arranged with the City Health Department.

For many students, Young's advocacy of advanced study did not mean much until after they had entered the workplace. In 1938 Theodora Sharrocks '29 wrote, "When I received my Presbyterian Hospital diploma I had the feeling I had finished the course — was educated in other words ... But as the months have rolled into years, I have come to realize that a P.H. diploma is ... only a passport — not a symbol of completion." Sharrocks, who was then studying public health at Teachers College, recommended further academic study as an antidote to the inevitable nursing "rut," specifically courses in nursing education. "It is more and more true that a nurse be a teacher — of the individual patient; of the younger nurse; of the public in small or large groups."

Young also taught graduate nurses through the written word. Recognizing the need for a compact, on-the-job reference book, she recruited Georgia Morrison '13 and Margaret Eliot to help her compile the *Quick Reference Book for Nurses*, published by J.B. Lippincott of Philadelphia in 1933. The *Quarterly* called it a glorified nurses' "prayer book" with information suitable to practitioners in any part of the country, particularly those working outside of the hospital. According to the *American Journal of Nursing*, sections on general information, dietotherapy, materia medica, nursing technique, medical and surgical nursing, obstetrical nursing were of special value. "It is not intended, of course, that the *Quick Reference Book* shall take the place of the nurse's library, but for ready reference easily at hand many nurses will find it a 'good companion,'" added the *AJN* reviewer.

The book, which originally sold for two dollars, was very popular. Five thousand copies were ordered by the U.S. Army for use by medical corpsmen and nurses during World War II. "Stacked flat (one on the other), the total number of bound books of this title used by nurses would be as high as three Empire State buildings and for good measure half of the Washington Monument in addition!" the publisher boasted in 1952 after six editions — and that did not include the seventh and eighth versions, the latter printed a decade later. The pocket-sized book, it was estimated, was used by over 100,000 nurses. Almost $35,000 in royalties were collected over the years, all of which went toward the School's scholarship fund.

The 1930 curriculum was clinically as well as academically rich and varied. The faculty, however, had a tenuous grasp of the value of the different ward experiences. Each student spent thousands of hours in the wards and clinics at Presbyterian Hospital and the School's clinical affiliates over the course of the program, but what proportion of that was truly educational? Were some experiences more beneficial than others? To find out, the ubiquitous researcher Eleanor Lee enlisted eighty students in sixteen separate sites to keep daily logs of their clinical activities during the 1930-31 academic year.

To no one's surprise, the study revealed that a "preponderance" of the clinical experiences was strictly for the Hospital's benefit — 42 percent to be exact. In other words, 58 percent of time on duty was educationally valuable, only a small proportion of which involved formal instruction and supervision (8 percent) or classroom study (5 percent). The proportions varied from service to service, according to Lee's report, "A Year's Survey of Ward Teaching," published in 1932 in the *American Journal of Nursing*. Students derived the least from gynecology, obstetrics, ophthalmology, urology, and the fracture service, and the most from medicine, surgery, visiting nursing, the operating room, the outpatient department, pediatrics, otolaryngology, the diet kitchen, and metabolism.

Predictably, President Sage interpreted the study as an *affirmation* of the existing system. "An interim report," he observed, "indicates and emphasizes the academic value of much ward work heretofore overlooked."

What was a day of ward duty like? According to a log completed by "P.M.D." (Pearl M. Diament '32) in the fracture ward, it was long and tedious and sometimes valuable:

Time		Activity
7:00 am	7:15	Reported on duty — heard night report
7:00	7:55	Diets, distributed trays, feeding 2 patients
7:55	8:15	Instruction in making bed with arm in traction
8:15	9:25	Morning care of 3 patients, bed baths, etc.
9:25	9:40	Cleaned bed-side tables
9:40	10:05	Cleaning and making closed bed
10:05	10:10	Assisting and taking patient from stretcher; made patient comfortable
10:10	10:15	Gave adrenalin
10:15	10:25	Watch back brace applied
10:25	10:30	Bandaged patient's leg
10:30	10:40	Got patient up in wheelchair
10:40	11:00	Catheterized very ill patient
11:00	3:00 pm	Off-duty
3:00	3:10	Read order book and charts

3:10	3:50	Staff rounds with Dr. M. explaining cases
3:50	4:10	Learned how to measure for crutches, fit them, and teach patient to walk
4:10	4:25	T.P.R.s [temperature, pulse, respiration]
4:25	5:15	Diets, distributing trays, feeding helpless patients
5:15	6:00	Evening routine
6:30	6:40	Assisted special nurse in care of helpless patient
6:40	6:55	Cleaned utility room
6:55	7:00	Check this record with Miss Smith

Lee's study pointed to the need for a systematic program of ward teaching, wider use of the case method of instruction for individuals and small groups, regular fifteen-to-thirty-minute conferences on selected topics, and staff education in methods of clinical teaching — measures that the School adopted, at least experimentally.

Typically, the study raised more questions than it answered. What did the student need to learn on each service? How much formal instruction would that require? How much could students pick up on their own? An encouraging finding was that students showed significant initiative in seizing learning opportunities. Still, the investigators were moved to ask: "How can a questioning attitude, an interest in learning, be cultivated in students?"

The ward survey also alerted instructors to the need for a standardized and accurate means of grading the students' performance in the wards — that is, a clinical report card. "This has always been a serious handicap in the elimination of undesirable students," or in identifying those with particular strengths or weaknesses, explained Elizabeth Wilcox '27. "Certainly we need to know more about the nurses whom we are about to graduate than that they are intelligent and in good health. On the other hand, the difficulties involved in determining what we consider the essential qualifications for the good nurse have seemed so great, that many schools of nursing have hesitated to attempt it."

Consequently, in 1932 Young assembled a committee of instructors and clinical supervisors to devise and evaluate a standardized report card. The result, an adaptation of existing report cards, proved incomplete, indefinite, and overly complex. Subsequent refinements yielded two models, one for beginning and another for advanced students. The freshman-year model consisted of seven grading categories (with suggested rating words in each category): personality, attitude, personal appearance, knowledge of patients' condition and nursing principles, practical nursing skills, responsibility, care of equipment, and written work. The more detailed junior and senior-year model consisted of ten categories grouped into three sections: personality, nursing care, and administrative ability. The first section, accounting for 25 percent of the evaluation, covered various personal traits, social contacts (with patients, visitors, physicians, fellow students, hospital employees), appearance, and attitude. The nursing care section (50 percent) covered practical nursing skills, and clinical ability (knowledge of patients' condition and powers of observation). The final section, administrative ability (25 percent), dealt with responsibility, ability to plan work, adaptability, and record-keeping.

After two years of experimentation, the committee was still not fully satisfied with the report cards. Nonetheless, they did prove useful to Young in her individual student conferences and in the placement of new graduates.

Each of the studies of these years was important; together they were revolutionary. By 1932 the School of Nursing was essentially a university program in a diploma program's clothing. It would take five years, however, to sort out the financial and political details so that the School's students could officially wear Columbia blue.

13

Long May It Stand

We had a beautiful dining room, we had a swimming
pool, we had brand new equipment and a gatch on
every bed. And we had patients. It was wonderful. Miss
Young still reminded us to be ladies, to wear hat, coat
and gloves, and maybe we impressed Washington
Heights.

Margaret Wells '29 (1978)

IN THE 1920s PRESBYTERIAN HOSPITAL awoke to the disturbing reality that its
physical plant was worn and antiquated. Not a single patient-care building had been added since 1889. What was once hailed as the showcase of
hospital architecture was now a working museum piece. It was time to
rebuild or expand, particularly with the long-gestating alliance of Presbyterian Hospital and the Columbia University College of Physicians &
Surgeons near term.

Considerations of space and economics dictated the construction of a
wholly new facility in the upper reaches of Manhattan, far from midtown's pricier precincts as well as its congestion and clamor. Once again,
people ridiculed Presbyterian for selecting so remote a location, which they
jokingly referred to as "South Albany." Nevertheless, the site, a twenty-acre
parcel in Washington Heights bounded by 165th and 168th Streets and
Broadway and Riverside Drive, was well chosen, with ample room for
expansion. The powers that be were thinking big, dreaming of building
medicine's Taj Mahal. This was to be the nation's first modern medical
center, bringing together almost a dozen of America's oldest and most
respected general and specialty hospitals, outpatient clinics, and health
professional schools. The future "Columbia-Presbyterian Medical Center" (at the School's 1930 commencement, Rev. Samuel S. Drury astutely
asked why it was not named "Health Center") would include the College

of Physicians & Surgeons (established as part of King's College—Columbia's forerunner—in 1767), Presbyterian Hospital (1868), Sloane Hospital for Women (1886), Vanderbilt Clinic for outpatients (1886), Babies Hospital (1889), the School of Nursing (1892), the New York State Psychiatric Institute (1902), the New York Neurological Institute (1909), and the School of Dental and Oral Surgery (1916). Plans also called for a facility for private patients (the Harkness Pavilion), a convalescent home, and an Institute of Ophthalmology (later renamed the Edward S. Harkness Eye Institute). The sponsors declared, "It is to be an alliance, not a consolidation—in cooperation, not in competition…It will give the patient what he had in the days of the old family practitioner—a single source on which he can depend for his health."

The site of the future Medical Center, a rocky, windswept patch of land, was already rich in history. It was first inhabited by American Indians, who were forced out by the Dutch in the 1600s. Large estates dominated the terrain for a century or so, when the area's rural peace was temporarily shattered by the Revolutionary War. On what is now 181st Street, near Manhattan's highest natural point, the Union Army built Fort Washington (hence the name Washington Heights). The estates were broken up in the early 1800s, as wave after wave of immigrants arrived from Europe. In the early 1900s, 168th Street was home to the ballpark of the New York Highlanders, the aptly named forerunner to the Yankees (a historical tidbit that must have thrilled Helen Young, a dedicated Yankee fan). Across the street was the mammoth tabernacle of world-famous evangelist Billy Sunday. "Here again never ending crowds will come, this time seeking health," proclaimed a Hospital press release announcing the new Medical Center. "For all time this land is to be devoted to the trinity of medicine: teaching, research and care of the sick."

With the slogan, "Fight disease the modern way—build New York a medical center," the Hospital launched its first-ever public appeal for donations. "In this age," the fund raisers claimed, "a hospital, to become and remain an institution of the first rank, must offer its house and consulting staffs close and immediate contact with medical and surgical progress, and should combine the sickroom of the patient, the laboratory of the scientist and the class-room of the medical student and the student nurse." The estimated cost of this projected 800-plus bed colossus was $10 million.

As plans for the Medical Center coalesced, the Alumnae Association voluntarily assumed responsibility for nursing's portion of the fund-raising campaign. One million dollars was needed to construct a new nurses' residence in Washington Heights, which would later be christened Anna C. Maxwell Hall. Fortunately, half of that sum would come from the sale of the existing residence, Florence Nightingale Hall. Still, the alumnae had quite a challenge. So in December of 1924 they adroitly dispatched a cable to their champion fund raiser, who was vacationing in Europe, asking her to become honorary chairperson of the campaign. Anna Maxwell accepted, of course. Three weeks later, after an ocean crossing plagued by high winds and heavy seas, she arrived in New York, "never looking better." "We have Miss Maxwell all to ourselves again," the alumnae magazine gleefully proclaimed.

The campaign opened that February in high style with a dinner in the grand ballroom of the Biltmore Hotel. Many prominent nurses were in attendance, yet it was the students who stole the show. "They dropped the bombshell of the evening," reported Helen Young. "The student chairman, Jeanette Archer ['26] announced that the students had staged a quiet campaign, that every student had made a pledge and that their total was $25,850." That amounted to an astounding $160 per student, more than double the total tuition fee. According to Archer, the students were eager to be part of "this history-making time of the School." (Thousands more were raised in the following months.) Maxwell beamed: "This is the proudest moment of my life, to welcome this great group of Alumnae filled with enthusiasm and love for their Alma Mater."

Within months the alumnae, organized into twenty-five teams by Gertrude Drake Ballantine '08, gathered pledges worth hundreds of thousands of dollars. The largest gifts to the campaign came from two of the School's longtime supporters, Mrs. Stephen V. Harkness, who donated $250,000, and Mrs. Edward S. Harkness, $25,000. The 900 living graduates of the School contributed another $200,000. Substantial donations also came from Moreau Delano and G. Herman Kinnicutt on behalf of the Board of Managers and from Frederick Sturges, Jr. (son of the School's longtime supporter). "Needless to say we raised Our Million," Young boasted.

The nurses also raised tens of thousands of dollars to endow a number of hospital rooms for use by graduates of any and all schools of nursing.

Helen Young welcomed the impending move to Washington Heights, knowing that unlimited educational opportunities were in the offing. But she also knew there would be unfavorable consequences. There would be pressure on the School to grow in order to meet the needs of a significantly larger clinical facility. Too large and too sudden an increase in enrollments, however, threatened to dilute the quality of incoming students as well as the quality of their education. Anticipating this dilemma, in 1925 Young and Maxwell suggested to Presbyterian President Dean Sage that the School's size should be based on "concrete parameters," namely, the practical experience available in the Hospital, the number of qualified applicants, and the number of students it was feasible to instruct. A preliminary class of sixty and a total enrollment of 300 were recommended. Young and Maxwell also had a few things to say about the nurses' future quarters.

By and large Sage listened to their comments, but not everyone was receptive to nursing's point of view. According to physician Franklin Hanger,

> One of the most trying ordeals in the career of Helen Young was the break up of the orderly little community on East 71st Street and the establishing of a "Nursing Empire" on Washington Heights. Some of the master planners in this great transition complained openly that she was uncooperative, reactionary and mirthless. Naturally, she was deeply upset by the ruthless manner in which some of the fine traditions of Nightingale Hall were being scuttled by experts who were unable to make a distinction between a Supervisor and a Probationer. Many stern women would have retreated before the collusion of architects and visionaries. But she believed so strongly in maintaining a home-like atmosphere for her students, that she stood fast for points that she believed affected the dignity of the nursing profession. Eventually important compromises were reached which were to maintain the camaraderie among the residents of Maxwell Hall.

The exact location of the nurses' residence was chosen by none other than Anna Maxwell. Well before the planners or administrators surveyed the parcel of land in Washington Heights, Maxwell journeyed uptown to lay claim to the School's new home. "To give nurses what they deserve," she selected a spot high atop a bluff overlooking the Hudson River and the New Jersey Palisades, assuring students and faculty of a glorious view, fresh air, and sunshine. Nothing would change her mind—after all, the students and nurses would be there longer than any of the patients, and the doctors would be living elsewhere in their posh homes.

It was a view that did not go unappreciated. In the School's premier yearbook the class of 1936 joked, "Presbyterian Hospital was mostly selected for its reputation although a few liked the view." When Maxwell Hall alumnae reminisced, they invariably spoke glowingly of the majestic river views. "It was heaven to have a beautiful and complete room of my own overlooking the Hudson River!" exclaimed Dorothy Reid Rondthaler '29. "Pictures remain vivid in my mind's eye of the huge ice islands floating on the dazzling blue water that first Spring in Maxwell Hall."

Fittingly, there was a measure of science behind the Hall's design. Before the Medical Center's chief architect, the celebrated James Gamble Rogers, sat before his drafting table, an extensive study of women's residences in various cities was undertaken. With additional input from Young and Maxwell, he drafted plans for a fourteen-story, U-shaped structure, with a central courtyard opening toward the river. The main entrance, fronted by a circular drive, faced Fort Washington Avenue and the bulk of the Medical Center.

Rogers' design accommodated 360 students in small single rooms, each equipped with a bed, dresser, desk, chair, closet, and running water. Lav-

throughout the upper floors. There was even a rooftop area for sunbathing and sleeping (nicknamed "Tar Beach"). The Hall also included apartments for fifteen faculty members. Common areas on the lower floors included a 300-seat auditorium, a 100-seat classroom, a main dining room with large French doors opening onto small balconies, faculty offices, a reading room and reference library, a swimming pool, and a nine-bed infirmary for students "slightly ill." Ground was broken in September 1925.

Not everything proceeded as planned. First of all there were considerable objections to the residence's name. Any moniker other than "Florence Nightingale Hall" was interpreted by some as a slight to the memory of John S. Kennedy, the former Hospital president who donated funds for and named the nurses' original residence. But it was another nursing pioneer, Anna Maxwell, who would be honored this time — reportedly discouraging potential donors. Most Hospital regulars, however, were proud to honor School's founder and longtime director; Kennedy probably would have been among them.

Meanwhile, cost overruns plagued the Medical Center, whose price tag would ultimately soar to $25 million, two-and-a-half times the original estimate. Maxwell Hall was over budget, too, almost $400,000 in the red. "Dean Sage, trying every possible method to keep costs down for all construction, was particularly insistent on restricting the nurses' residence," wrote Albert Lamb. Lop off one floor, leave the top two floors unfinished, use wardrobes in place of closets, and forgo the pool and roof-top shelter, Sage demanded. Only the first economy measure came to pass, however, thanks to the ingenuity of the builder, Otto Eidlitz, the intervention of Delano and Kinnicutt (who unearthed money for the pool), and the persuasion of Helen Young. Young, an avid recreationalist, was particularly happy about saving the pool. Unusually large for its time, the pool became a prime off-hours diversion. Young even hired an instructor "so as to put the use of the pool on an educational basis and develop a high standard of swimming attainment." In Young's world, everything—even fun—had to have a structure and a goal. (She was probably influenced by the late-eighteenth century Vassar College model of education, which put enormous emphasis on physical culture in response to physician claims that young women—the country's future mothers—were predisposed to mental and physical illness and thus not fit for the stresses of higher education.)

By any standards the final version of the Hall was a treasure. Spacious, stately, and richly paneled, it was an immeasurable improvement over the previous quarters. As one alumna noted, "In the 'good old days' when the P.H. Training School inhabited the upper floors of the Hospital Buildings and nurses were pigeonholed in small cubicles, the conception of a residence like Maxwell Hall would have been merely another air-castle."

"Maxwell Hall was more like an elegantly appointed club than an institutional residence," said Helen Stoddart Mackay '28, no doubt referring to the waiters and white table cloths in the dining room and the maid and linen service in the dormitory areas.

Visitors were similarly impressed. The *New York Times* called Maxwell Hall "the last word in student housing. Architecturally it is beautiful. In its living quarters there is not only everything needed for health and comfort but every factor of the environment makes for the proper frame of mind in one whose profession will be to take not only skill but hope and cheerfulness and good taste into a sick room ... The training of nurses is one of the newer phases of education, but it has got far beyond that period in which the novitiate was looked upon as part maid servant and part student. This new home at the Medical Centre for nurses of the future is a recognition of her status."

Anna C. Maxwell Hall, rushed to completion to accommodate a new batch of probies who could not be housed downtown, was the first of the Medical Center's eleven units to open, on February 19, 1928. According to the *Quarterly,* "They arrived in a situation that seemed very remote from a real hospital; 400 workers about, furniture and equipment arriving at all hours, a large bonfire in the front yard to burn packing cases. These young women had the run of the place for twenty one days when seniors and patients arrived. Then it was necessary to assume a little more dignified manner." Actually, Helen Young, Eleanor Lee, and Margaret Eliot had moved in before the probies, but they apparently were too distracted with other matters to rein in the new students.

Admissions to the Hospital had been curtailed since the first of the year, greatly simplifying the March 26 transition from the "old P.H." to the "new P.H." With much excitement and fanfare, fifty or so patients were transferred in a fleet of six Scully-Walton ambulances and a limousine, manned by a small army of physicians and nurses, all under the command of Helen Young. Twenty head nurses flipped coins to determine who would have the honor of accompanying the first patient on the five-mile drive through Central Park and up Riverside Drive up to 168th Street. "My idea of riding an ambulance," the winner reported, "had always been to stand on the outside step and hold by one arm to a swinging strap, whipped by the breeze, streaming away from my sturdy shoulders must of course be a brilliant red lined cape. Imagine my disappointment when I was told to crawl inside and sit down!" Fifty minutes later, way ahead of schedule, the first ambulance arrived to an exuberant reception, spearheaded by Helen Young and fifteen students in their blue-and-whites. "Stretchers and wheel chairs all equipped with nurses, pillows and blankets were in eager readiness," the head nurse recalled. "Cameramen were everywhere." Several round trips later, the head nurse remarked,

> Once again the well trained hospital efficiency and cooperation left me voiceless — and again I was robbed of the joy of just and scathing criticism... [N]ot a chart had wandered from its owner, not a patient even temporarily misplaced. Of the emergency stimulants and equipment so conscientiously on hand during the day none were used except one small and unromantic emesis basin. Anti-climax enough!...
> At 3 o'clock the last of the fifty patients had left, and the old hospital at dusk, unlighted, presented a lonely spectacle. We had closed an interesting historical chapter, but we had opened a volume holding unlimited possibilities for a wonderful future.

Special measures were taken to ensure that a particular patient would be the first person ever admitted to the Harkness Pavilion, the Hospital's wing for private patients. "She arrived there about noon — with the same smile present, and the old indomitable spirit," reported the *Quarterly*. The patient was, fittingly and sadly, Anna Maxwell, who deserved as much credit as anyone for making the Medical Center possible. The ex-superintendent, now seventy-seven, had been hospitalized with cardiac problems at the old facility since October. Though quite ill, she managed to attend the Hall's dedication ceremony later in the year. "Her great influence has always been exerted upon the side of scientific progress and cooperation between the professions of medicine and nursing," remarked John Miller Turpin Finney, M.D., a friend of Maxwell's for forty years, at nursing's first commencement exercises at the Medical Center (actually held in the large armory on the corner of Fort Washington and 168th Street). "As an evidence of the widespread desire to honor her for her lifework devoted to the relief of the suffering humanity, yonder beautiful hall which bears her name has been erected. Long may it stand." Finney returned his honorarium to the School to create a library fund in Maxwell's name.

Faculty and students alike were thrilled that two of the School's longtime employees, Alexander MacKenzie and Mamie Clegg, made the move uptown, too. Both had been featured, with evident affection, in the students' Maxwell Hall fund-raising brochure. MacKenzie had been a porter and elevator man in Florence Nightingale Hall since 1908. "His genial manner, his spirit and buoyancy, endeared him to all ... " the brochure read. "He wore a white jacket, helped with luggage, kept busy with errands, and took sick nurses in a wheelchair to the hospital through the tunnel or across 71st street."

Alexander was more than a beaming face and helpful hand. To the students, he was an occasional partner in crime. "There were strict rules" at Florence Nightingale Hall, recalls Alice Bliss Smith '19. "We weren't supposed to have any conversation with the doctors—they were 'above' us. One day some of the doctors asked some of the nurses if we'd like to go out to the movies. So I tucked up my uniform, stuck it in my belt, and put on my raincoat—that's what we all did. We told [Alexander] about it and, after hours, he let us in and never mentioned it ... If we told Alexander—and no one else—what we were going to do, everything was fine. I think when we broke rules we had to wait until [Mamie] was off duty." MacKenzie retired in 1937 and died shortly thereafter.

Mamie Clegg was hired by Maxwell as a ward helper in 1895. When Florence Nightingale Hall opened nine years later, she was assigned to the front desk, a vantage point she used to keep "track of all the visitors, including the beaux, in such a personal way that you not only got your calls but she often had all the 'inside information' and the boxes of candy," noted the *Quarterly*. "She helped the beginner to avoid some of the pitfalls of the ignorant. She took care of the reception room and whisked her duster so energetically that it was said that she brushed the offending probationer not only off the chair but right upstairs."

"She loaned us nickels, many, too/And gave us hints on what to do .../She met us in a cheery mood/And ridiculed our lust for food," wrote a student from the class of 1917 in a poetic tribute. When the Medical Center opened, Clegg assumed the same role in the new graduate nurses' quarters. She retired in 1945, capping off a half-century of service to Columbia-Presbyterian nurses.

Although probies had the run of Maxwell Hall for the first few weeks, it was not long before life at the School of Nursing returned to its old, convent-like ways (Alexander notwithstanding). The School attempted to control virtually every aspect of campus life, including the time one awoke and the time one retired. "The health of the student is closely supervised," the School's bulletin warned. "A careful record is kept of hours of sleep and recreation." Furthermore, all bank checks had to be endorsed by the resident director. Stairs had to be used for trips of less than three flights. No one could visit the Hospital when off-duty without permission. Comings and goings were closely monitored, especially after the 10:30 p.m. curfew. "On our way down to the tunnel to the hospital, Miss Young inspected us, especially to check for hairnets. No hairnet—back you went," recalled Edith Wilson Stansell '30. Although the School was nonsectarian, it was not irreligious, and students of all faiths (or no faith) on day duty were required to report for pre-shift prayers at 6:45 a.m.

Nonetheless, the students were generally happy. On days off they could still sample the city's endless cultural offerings, a subway ride away. And there were many in-house diversions: drama and glee clubs; a "Forum" club for discussions of social and religious issues; student government; a lending library; a hobby show on alumnae day; swimming, tennis, clog dancing, and "corrective gymnastics"; outings to the Palisades, the Tod property in Greenwich, and the Cook estate in Port Chester, N.Y. (which had been donated to the Hospital for a convalescent home); afternoon tea served by the probies (who else?); and various other formal and informal gatherings. Or they could peruse the School's new collection of Florence Nightingale letters, donated by Hugh Auchincloss, M.D., a Presbyterian surgeon and father of Maria Auchincloss '32. The collection was supplemented with related materials gathered by Anna Maxwell, who from her sickbed had corresponded with Nightingale's niece about acquiring portraits and photos of the famed English nurse. (In subsequent years the elder Auchincloss and others added hundreds of additional items to the collection.)

And then there was the occasional visit of a dignitary or celebrity, such as the Crown Princess of Sweden, who was invited to tea while her husband was a patient at Harkness, and Eleanor Roosevelt, who spoke to a meeting of the Alumnae Association. None of the nurses would forget the day in July 1928 when Amelia Earhart, the first woman to fly solo across the Atlantic, dropped by to take in the spectacular view from high atop the

Hospital, some twenty stories up. "Naturally, as many of us as could, proudly escorted her to the entrance and the waiting limousine," one alumna wrote. "We were then surprised to see the lovely 'Lady Lindy' step from the door of the motor car and into the side car of a waiting motorcycle belonging to one of her police escorts and gaily ride away." *

While these events were memorable, what truly mattered to students was what lay across the street in the endless maze of buildings that comprised the new Columbia-Presbyterian Medical Center. Few, if any, other student nurses in the world had access to such a diverse collection of specialty wards, outpatient clinics, state-of-the-art equipment, and expert clinicians. The student nurses also had the use of the medical school's laboratories and amphitheaters for classes in anatomy and physiology, bacteriology, chemistry, and pathology, as well as its formidable library. In the Hospital proper, the School had its own practice rooms equipped with the latest hospital furniture and a special mini-amphitheater for the teaching of nursing arts, featuring "Mrs. Chase," the latest in patient dummies.

Few, it seemed, regretted the move to Washington Heights. But those who ventured downtown to the "old P.H." were shocked and saddened to see that it had been torn down to make way for expensive apartments and exclusive shops. Florence Nightingale Hall had become another piece of New York City's architectural and social history viewable only in photos and in memory. It would not be the last time the School of Nursing would lose a home to the wrecking ball.

The School adjusted smoothly to life at the new Medical Center, despite its enormous size. Several new faculty members were hired, including Dorothy Rogers '25, who took charge of the residence hall, and Manola Phillips, a baccalaureate and master's degree graduate of Teachers College, who was appointed recreation director. The School's budget was separated from the Hospital's, giving Young an added measure of independence. The move, no doubt, precipitated the increase in overall tuition from $70 to $100.

In the fall of 1928 the School accepted another batch of probies, eighty strong, the most ever, bringing total enrollment to 211. Although Young had expressed a desire to keep each new class at sixty, she had little choice but to expand, knowing that more hands were needed at the vast new Medical Center. The move from the old to the new "P.H." meant that her nursing service had to adapt almost overnight to a three-fold increase in ward beds, a five-fold increase in private beds, and a two-fold increase in clinic

---

* Presbyterian had its own aviation pioneer in Laura Ingalls '18, a New Yorker who in 1934 became the first American woman to fly solo over the lofty Andes mountains, from Santiago to Buenos Aires.

patients.* Young immediately added several dozen graduate nurses to the staff and tripled the use of special duty nurses. Still desperate for quality nurses, the superintendent wrote to inactive alumnae asking them to come back to Presbyterian, permanently or temporarily. Most wanted to, but declined the offer, citing family responsibilities. Somehow, Young managed to bring the Medical Center up to speed in eight months instead of the projected three years.

It is no coincidence that in photographs of the Medical Center's official opening Helen Young is center stage, standing in the front doorway between President Sage and William Barclay Parsons, chairman of the Joint Administrative Board (the body that oversaw Columbia-Presbyterian's creation). Young wielded enormous power as director of the nursing school and the nursing service, both of which were undergoing unprecedented expansion. Adding to her influence, she soon assumed command of nursing at Sloane Hospital and its three-month-long nursing program in obstetrics (established in 1888). Sloane, naturally, became the School's principal site for clinical experience in maternity nursing. Numerous students from other schools were also welcomed into the wards. (The only clinical component not under Young's control was Babies Hospital, which was in the capable hands of Winifred Kaltenbach '20.)

Outside of the Medical Center, Young was also gaining influence, presiding over the New York City League of Nursing Education (1930-34) and the New York State League of Nursing Education (1936-40), advising nursing educators from home and abroad, and playing a major role in the formulation of health policy, such as the New York State nurse practice act of 1938.

Young used this power, but with restraint. It was no surprise to her admirers that "some of her sternest critics became her staunchest admirers," noted physician Franklin Hanger. "It was very stabilizing to all of us to have Miss Young as Director of Nursing. There prevailed throughout the Medical Center the comfortable feeling that nothing drastic was about to happen."

A drastic thing did happen, however. As soon as everyone settled into the new quarters, the Great Depression darkened the horizon. Columbia-Presbyterian fared relatively well, though various economy measures had

---

*However, the first days in the clinic were "long and dull," remembers Magaret F. Pritchard '29, the first student assigned to night duty there. "I recall looking out the window early one morning and seeing a milk delivery wagon overturn. I thought now we will get a patient, but we did not. It took time for people in the area to learn that there was a patient service available."

to be instituted. In early 1933 the nurses, presented with a choice of staff reductions or salary cuts, agreed to a pay decrease of 7.5 percent. (An earlier round of salary cuts had affected only new hires.) One head nurse, expressing the sentiments of many, said, "we will accept another salary cut and not a change in our nursing standards now or ever." The staff did accept another (10 percent) cut, which, as promised, was fully restored (including back pay) when economic conditions improved.

The School of Nursing also held its ground, though enrollments declined about 10 percent after the swift expansion of the late twenties. The decline was due to an abnormally high rate of withdrawals and a drop in applications, a consequence of the high rate of unemployment among nurses. The alumnae, particularly those in private duty, suffered too, though not as much as other nurses. The Hospital's private duty registry was still receiving thousands of requests for nurses each year, far more than it could fill with home-grown nurses. The pay was miserable, however. Nursing's future was in organized care, in public health agencies, and in hospitals small and large.

14

A Distinct and Wholesome Protest

No individual, no student, no nurse seeking aid
through her wisdom and her knowledge left empty-
handed.

Annie Goodrich (on Anna Maxwell, 1942)

RETIREMENT SEEMED TO FREE the hidden gypsy in Anna Maxwell. From 1921 until her final illness, which started in mid-1928, the former superintendent roamed to and fro, visiting friends and relatives and former students, sight-seeing, attending professional meetings, raising funds for the School of Nursing, and delivering speeches. For the first time in her life, Maxwell, who never married (but reportedly had many offers), was unencumbered by family or professional obligations.

Her travels commenced immediately after her resignation in May 1921, when she gave an address to the nursing graduates of Moses Taylor Hospital in Scranton, Pa. That summer Maxwell vacationed in Paris, taking side trips to the countryside and the Nightingale school in Bordeaux. The following February found her in Bermuda for more rest and relaxation. Maxwell fell in love with island life and extended her stay through April. In October she took an active role in the fiftieth-anniversary pageant of Massachusetts General Hospital Training School for Nurses in Boston.

She traveled next, in March 1924, to St. Louis to discuss the emerging trend of collegiate nursing with officials at St. Luke's Hospital and the local chamber of commerce. This was followed by another European vacation, with visits to London, Versailles, Vichy (where—surprisingly, for a woman of science—she bathed in and imbibed the famous waters), and Switzerland's Rhone glacier. Upon receiving a plea from the Alumnae Association to lead the fundraising campaign for Maxwell Hall, she shortened her trip and arrived home in mid-December.

Maxwell journeyed overseas for the last time from July 1925 through November 1926. The trip began with an International Congress of Nurses meeting in Helsingfors, Finland, where she was awarded honorary membership in the Association of Nurses of Finland, and continued in Sweden, Germany, Holland, England, France, and Italy. Maxwell stayed longer than planned: various medical problems (including a heart condition) landed her in a nursing home in Rome and then in the American Hospital at Neuilly.

Back home, in improved health, she gave a radio address in mid-February 1927 about the coming Columbia-Presbyterian Medical Center. She remained relatively well throughout the following summer, when she delivered commencement addresses in the upstate–New York cities of Rochester and Plattsburgh. They would be her last. In Plattsburgh she was hospitalized with bronchial pneumonia and eventually transferred to Presbyterian Hospital. In the middle of a later hospital stay, Maxwell was transferred from "old P.H." to "new P.H.," a sad occasion with a humorous twist. As Albert Lamb recalled, "She had participated in deciding on the type of bed for the new hospital and naturally insisted on having them high enough to facilitate the work of the nurses and doctors. When we took her to her room that afternoon we did not see one of the beds she had picked out. Instead there was a very low bed which she could get out of and into without discomfort. During all of her remaining months she was a very good patient. Her old desire for organization manifested itself in her insistence on having everything in the room arranged in geometrical patterns — right angles, isoceles triangles, parallels, etc."

Illness did not silence Maxwell, who, like Florence Nightingale, was an active invalid. Wheelchair-bound, she made short visits to the nurses' residence and the wards, usually with some advice to offer. "Her criticisms and suggestions have lost none of their old time flavor, and are always constructive and helpful," noted the *Quarterly*. "In later years," reported the *American Journal of Nursing*, "when she had leisure for much travel, it was her custom to send to the editor from here, there or yonder — and in the last weary months from her bed — little notes to call attention to the significant though nonspectacular occurrence which seemed to her important. No important professional activity escaped her notice."

Maxwell reportedly devoted most of her final days toward raising an endowment fund for the School of Nursing. "Her most cherished wish … was that the school would have its own endowment," said Helen Young. "This was her earnest wish long before Johns Hopkins Alumnae started their own. Maxwell was assured by the Board of Managers that the School would always be taken care of but [she] thought it wise to have independent funds and accurately predicted that the School's need would outstrip the Hospital's means... With this thought in mind she aided and abetted the opening of the Alumnae Shop in the Hospital hoping in this way to interest the Alumnae and through them the friends of the School in the Endowment... Each morning I went in she had some new plan that would assist with one or other of these interests." One of those plans was the Alumnae Association Radio Fund, which started with a single radio donated by Maxwell. By renting radios to patients, the association raised thousands of dollars over the years, until the advent of television. Maxwell also devoted a great deal of time to the planning of the new nursing residence in Washington Heights. According to Young, "She saw completed in every detail the monument to her life and work—Anna C. Maxwell Hall."

In the fall of 1928, Maxwell's strength began to fail. Confined to her room, she was limited to receiving visitors and assembling jig-saw puzzles, a passion of her final months. "Well, why should I complain," she said to Young near the end. "I have had a long life and a merry one, and I have managed to do some of the things I wanted to do, too."

Anna Maxwell died the evening of January 2, 1929, at the age of seventy-seven. She left an estate of $48,775 to her two sisters. Services were held at Maxwell Hall and Union Theological Seminary. Maxwell was buried the following Monday at Arlington National Cemetery with full military honors. The late superintendent would probably have hated all the fuss: the carriage led by beautiful black horses, the military band, the honor guard. But to those assembled on that cold but bright and clear day—Maxwell's countless friends and admirers, the country's leading civilian and military nurses—it was a fitting farewell.

Tributes appeared in a variety of publications. In the *American Journal of Nursing*, James Miller Alexander, M.D., commented, "Her influence upon all of us at Presbyterian Hospital—physicians, nurses, and laymen alike—was very remarkable. She combined an unusual executive ability with a keen vision of the possibilities of nursing service, and a personality of rare charm ... Her contribution to the general cause of nursing education is a matter of public record, but it is the recollection of those days in intimate association with her which I shall always treasure in my memory as having been a very unusual privilege."

In the same issue, Adelaide Nutting remarked that Maxwell was of the old school, which regarded nursing as a calling and required one's complete attention and isolation from normal human interests and social relationships. However, she added,

Miss Maxwell's ordering of her own life was a distinct and wholesome protest against any such view of nursing, against any such traditions of useless self-sacrifice, of immolation on any altar whatsoever. She greatly enjoyed the pageant of life, had a keen appreciation of beauty, culture, music, art. She loved travel, and had a positive "flair" for the adventurous side of life. She had marked social gifts and was seldom too tired to use them. Though living an arduous life as the busy head of a great professional school, she found time to draw to herself a large circle of friends quite outside of professional relationships, and established for herself an honored place among them. In so doing she enlarged public respect for the work she represented. Nursing became through her a more desirable and attractive occupation to young women of good education and upbringing, and the sick benefited by a finer care, a higher degree of intelligence and devotion.

And an editorialist for the New York Times observed, "In the span of [Maxwell's] lifetime nursing came to be recognized as a profession. More than any one other human being this change was due to Florence Nightingale, but the profession had been carried to new heights of skill and devotion in America by such nurses as Miss Maxwell, who … came to be known as the Florence Nightingale of America and who died the Dean of American Nurses."

Decades later, at the 1956 commencement, Wilder Penfield, M.D, a prominent neurologist who began his career at Presbyterian Hospital, recalled a chance encounter with the retired superintendent:

Miss Maxwell I met one summer evening in the Adirondacks. Mrs. Penfield and I were drifting in a canoe on the still waters of Long Lake watching the mirrored mountains turn to deepening shades of gray and blue when we saw a row boat approaching. As it came nearer we saw that it was rowed, very swiftly, by a woman. Her hair shone white against the water, as she glided toward us with a smile. It was your own Miss Maxwell, rowing her own boat at 71 — graceful, charming, with an indestructible zest for life.

There was your nursing ideal, a woman who had given her thought and labor to the cause of nursing but whom no institution could institutionalize.

15

The Imparting of Wisdom, The Teaching of Technique

> Where can a nurse prepare as Director of Schools of Nursing, Instructor, Demonstrator, Administrator, acquire knowledge of civic and social and educational conditions to enable her to develop Rural Nursing, Community Activities and the multitudinous field of work into which she is invited? There seems to be but one answer. Admission to our universities... [N]ursing has an equal claim to the benefits of University Education as have the Law, Medicine, Pharmacy, Social Work, and other educational branches... The care of the sick, conservation of our human resources, and the protection of community health are the burdens laid upon [the nurse] by society. She must therefore secure adequate preparation to meet these professional responsibilities.
>
> *Anna Maxwell (1924)*

ALTHOUGH ANNA MAXWELL delivered the above words to the St. Louis Chamber of Commerce, in all likelihood they were aimed 1,000 miles eastward at the governors of Columbia University and Presbyterian Hospital. Consumed by the task of planning the Columbia-Presbyterian Medical Center, they had all but abandoned the School of Nursing's quest for university status.

Just a few years earlier, the School's entry into the rarefied air of academic nursing had an air of inevitability; only details and formalities stood in the way. In 1921, on the heels of the successful alliance of its medical school with Presbyterian Hospital, Columbia officials declared, "The School of Nursing is to be established as an integral part of the University on a similar basis to other professional schools." Evidently serious about this proposal, the two institutions assembled the Organization Committee of the School of Nursing, at whose core was a stellar cast of nurses, physicians, and administrators, including Adelaide Nutting and Annie Goodrich of Teachers College; William Darrach, dean of P&S; William Sloane, president of Presbyterian; Walter W. Palmer, director of medicine at Presbyterian; and Allen O. Whipple, director of surgery at Presbyterian. In a series of meetings at Sloane's Park Avenue home, the committee explored every detail of the proposed university program.

Favoring a conservative transition to academe, a subcommittee on Courses of Instruction and Teaching Staff, led by Nutting, recommended a two-track program, retaining the diploma course (in a slightly upgraded and truncated form) and adding a four-year baccalaureate course divided evenly between liberal arts and nursing. (A five-year course with extra time for specialization—similar to the joint Teachers College-School of Nursing plan then in effect—was briefly contemplated, but ultimately considered too lengthy; graduate courses in a variety of disciplines, however, were recommended.) Advanced standing would be offered to students with college experience. To maintain the School's strong clinical focus, the subcommittee suggested, "Constant effort should be made to so connect the theory with the practical training in various services, that the student may be able to apply her instruction directly to the particular problem of disease with which it deals, and thus derive the fuller benefit from her study and training."

The Organization Committee also decided that student nurses should be guided academically by Columbia and clinically by Presbyterian, patterned after the system currently in use with medical students at P&S. But there was a catch: According to Sloane's Hospital Relations subcommittee (which included Goodrich and Palmer), "the pupils of the School of Nursing would have a definite responsibility in the carrying on of the nursing work, whereas in the case of the students of medicine their direct responsibility is slight." (It is strange that Goodrich was a party to this clause; soon thereafter she accepted the challenge of establishing Yale's autonomous school of nursing.) Both the University and the Hospital tentatively accepted the committee's overall plan.

Later that year Sloane died, and with him perished any immediate prospects for academic nursing. Another fifteen years passed before the School officially entered the academic world. Why so long? According to the Hospital and the University, there were more pressing matters, namely, the planning and construction of the new Medical Center and then the Great Depression. While that is true, it is hard to understand why the people who designed and built the world's greatest health center, surmounting massive cost overruns, and survived the country's worst financial epoch did not have the administrative and financial wherewithal to orchestrate a swifter transition, especially with a school that was a university program in almost every sense but its name. The most logical explanation is that the Hospital was not yet ready to loose its exploitative hold on student nurses, and the University had neither the desire nor the fortitude to pry them away. Eventually, when faced with the choice of leading or being led into the next era of health care, the two parties relented, allowing nursing its claim to the benefits of university education.

The "villain" in this chapter of the School's history was President Sloane's successor, Dean Sage. Sage was an inexperienced hospital administrator with an inflexible perception of nursing education. Schools of nursing, in his mind, largely existed for the convenience of hospitals—a nineteenth-century attitude that was slowly but surely crumbling under the weight of progress.

Disturbed by the lack of Hospital representation on the new governing board of the proposed University School, Sage wrote to Darrach in 1924 that the tentative Organization Committee plan "would not operate to the best advantage of either the Hospital or of the Presbyterian Training School or of the Medical Centre. I think that the entire question…should be deferred for future consideration."

With reservations, Darrach concurred. "When affairs are less pressing," he said, "I should like to spend some time with you on the matter. I feel confident that we can evolve some plan whereby the traditions and high standing of the Presbyterian School of Nursing can be carried on and perhaps up in the future. They must not decline. As I explained to your predecessor, my own personal feelings are almost those of an alumnus, since I learned much from Miss Maxwell and her associates… We must realize, however, the impending changes in Nursing education and must be ready to either join the leaders or follow them closely and not be left behind smugly treasuring an honored past."

For years and years, Sage hemmed and hawed on the topic of academic nursing. In 1926, for instance, he stated that the "operation of a School of Nursing is an educational enterprise of high import," though he did little to promote the School's affiliation with Columbia. Three years later, with the rising Medical Center way over budget, he made it abundantly clear that nursing service took priority over nursing education. "Our School has practically no separate endowment," he said. "It is supported out of the hospital funds provided for the care of the sick. Obviously, the Board of Managers as trustees cannot devote those funds to an educational program except in so far as that program contributes directly or indirectly to the qualification of the pupil nurse as a hospital operative."

Sage, however, was only delaying the inevitable, which even he recognized by the 1930s. Determined not to lose all claims to the student nurses, he shifted tactics, speaking out against the creation of a fully independent school like Yale's. Such a scenario made no sense, he reasoned, since the Hospital would still require a school of its own. How else would it staff the wards? One alternative, of course, was to hire more graduate nurses, an emerging trend. That would be *less* expensive, he acknowledged to *Quarterly* readers. "But what then of the Presbyterian School?" he added. "It would simply go out of existence—a sacrifice of years of devoted labor." The School, in fact, was not facing extinction, only transformation.

Hopes for university affiliation were dashed once again by a change in command. When Darrach resigned his post at P&S in 1930, his successor, Willard Cole Rappleye, M.D., requested more time to study the situation. Meanwhile, Sage fought on, telling the 1931 graduates: "In all of [the Hospital's] multifarious and ever expanding duties the School of Nursing has an essential and active part. Hardly a problem arises from the repair of a leak in the ward piping to the operation of the laundry...that does not require for its solution the cooperation of the nursing staff. Student nurses are in daily contact with the administrative problems involved in the operation of a large enterprise...The School is indeed an integral and motivating part of a great machine of community service and as such it must develop as does the Medical Center and attain to that destiny which is dictated by the needs of the community at large."

The next May brought forth these words: "I think it cannot be gainsaid that the School, as an educational institution, properly belongs under university auspices...Medicine and nursing are equally concerned with caring for the sick. It is the purpose of each to develop that course of education which will best serve the pupil with that end in view." Why, then, did student nurses have to work their way through school and not student doctors? And then he added, "Lest you think that we may be too precipitously plunged into this new adventure..." — by that time, the idea for a university school had been brewing for a full decade.

And in 1934 he stated, "The function of the School of Nursing is not primarily to provide administrative aid in the operation of the Hospital but to properly train a professional class, utilizing the clinical opportunities of the Hospital for this purpose." But typically, he added, "The principle of promoting the welfare of the Hospital and its sick inmates through the utilization of the services of student nurses must be preserved, at least as far as Hospital funds are used for the support of the School, for otherwise there would result a diversion of funds contributed for care of the sick."

Finally, Sage noted in 1935, "Never did the Presbyterian Hospital accept the old concept of a school of nursing as a mere administrative adjunct to the hospital." Well, perhaps. But neither did it accept the new paradigm of a school of nursing as an independent academic institution.

Summing up this long episode, Albert Lamb wrote, "President Sage thus reversed his field and put the main burden of caring for the sick upon the student nurses ... [They] can properly be of great help in sharing the burden of caring for the sick. But to require the student nurses to perform work far beyond that needed for their education comes close to exploitation." Even Lamb, sympathetic to the School's plight, could not admit that it *was* exploitation.

The elephantine pace of progress toward collegiate status must have pained the School's elders. With each passing year, another top-drawer diploma program would merge with another prestigious institution of higher learning — Yale, Western Reserve, Vanderbilt, the Universities of California, Washington, and Wisconsin, to name a few. The Presbyterian Hospital School of Nursing, accustomed to setting the pace, was falling behind. (To put things into perspective, the vast majority of the nation's 1,400-plus diploma programs had few, if any, prospects of attaining university status.)

Despite Sage's attitude, the plan for academic nursing did move forward. Perhaps the most pivotal year in this long journey was 1932, when a committee composed of representatives of the School, the Hospital, and the University recommended the creation of a Department of Nursing within the Faculty of Medicine of Columbia, a relatively unexplored form of alliance of medical and nursing education.

Two other options had been considered. One was to make the School a part of Teachers College. Presumably, this was rejected because the college was a rather independent part of Columbia University, it was geographically and academically isolated from the Medical Center, and its nursing focus was educational, not clinical. The second—and least probable—alternative was to create an independent nursing school; nursing had always fallen under the control of medicine and that was not likely to change now. This attitude was best expressed by George E. Vincent, Ph.D., LL.D., former president of the Rockefeller Foundation, at the 1936 commencement. "You are an auxiliary to the medical profession," he said. "It is your loyalty to the great common cause which includes at times protecting the medical profession in your calling."

The University's official defense of a nursing "department" went as follows: "There is universal recognition of the dependence of nursing and of nursing education upon the medical sciences and clinical medicine. It would seem logical that the content and methods of training for nursing should be guided in large part...by the medical faculty, leaders of which are familiar with the fundamental sciences...and with the medical, public health, hospital, and community needs." A subsequent University memorandum added, "By placing the program within the Faculty of Medicine, the other departments of that faculty will take a more active interest in and responsibility for supporting and forwarding the highest type of preparation for nursing; and, conversely, give to the medical staff, medical students and students of public health administration a better and more sympathetic appreciation of the problems involved in this professional field."

Although the University was not ready to give nursing its full independence, it at least acknowledged that apprenticeship training was no longer tenable. "By emphasizing the educational features of the course, by providing study periods, and by relieving the students from unnecessary duties and the use of their time in activities which contribute little or nothing to their education and experience, a contribution of fundamental importance to the entire health program could be made," the memorandum added.

It wasn't only paternalism that figured in the decision against an independent program. Nursing still lacked the scientific rigor of other disciplines, which Columbia President Nicholas Murray Butler pointed out to the 1933 graduates: "Today, you women are joining a profession which is well on the way to becoming learned. It has some distance yet to go in academic organization, but the ideal is there, the conviction is there, and all there remains is to find ways and means to put these into practical effect and to add one more to the systematic callings of men, the professions which require and rest upon the scientific body of fundamental knowledge."

The School also had to get its admissions process in order. Students — probies as well as seniors — were dropping out in record numbers, generally due to ill health or poor academic or clinical performance and occasionally due to marriage, which was not allowed. During the 1931-32 academic year, 64 of 298 pupils (21 percent) departed — well below the statewide rate, though still unacceptable. Ten years earlier, only 9 percent had left. As Helen Young had feared, the Medical Center–inspired rush to expand had upset the School's balance.

Presbyterian's budgetmakers, already beleaguered by the Depression, were not pleased. The loss of a student meant the loss of a (part-time) ward nurse for almost three years; her spot could not be filled midstream. At President Sage's request, a new admissions subcommittee was asked in 1933 to reduce student turnover and develop "eligibility and adaptability" tests for applicants. Acting on a tip from Allen Whipple, the subcommittee invited Johnson O'Connor of the Human Engineering Laboratories at Stevens Institute of Technology, Hoboken, N.J., who had devised aptitude tests for engineers, business executives, and other professionals, to try his craft on nurses. Over the next three years, he analyzed sixty alumnae in various fields and an untold number of students in order to fashion tests for would-be nurses.

Meanwhile, the subcommittee (composed of Mrs. Edward T. H. Talmage, a member of the Board of Managers and head of the Nursing Committee since 1930, a Mrs. Staunton Williams, and alumna Marguerite Wales) recommended that the School establish a registrar's office with a full-time secretary. The post went to Margaret Conrad '20, who had recently returned to the School as an assistant director.

Positive results began to appear by the fall of 1934, even before the admissions reforms were fully instituted. There were no dropouts in the first month of the new academic year, a period in which at least a few pupils usually fell ill, flunked out, or found the experience distasteful. "The students who actually enter have made a very definite decision and seem better adjusted," noted Conrad.

By 1936 each applicant was required to submit a brief biographical essay, two letters of reference, a letter from her school principal regarding her class standing and fitness for nursing, and evidence of various vaccinations and inoculations. She also was asked to spend a day at the School, which included a thorough physical examination (formerly required after acceptance), a personal interview, luncheon in Maxwell Hall, and a battery of aptitude tests measuring vocabulary skills, mental acuity, personality, clerical accuracy, and mechanical ability. Each application was reviewed by a five-member admissions committee. Withdrawals declined precipitously, averaging under 9 percent for the next four academic years.

Young turned to the alumnae, the School's unofficial recruiters, for assistance with another admissions dilemma. As the Depression dragged on, more and more nurses around the country found themselves unemployed. Prospective nurses started to panic, loath to enter a field with such dim prospects. As one applicant to the School wrote: "Still another reason for the delay was that I have been thinking a great deal about choosing nursing as a profession. I have been discouraged and greatly disturbed all during the past week and have spent several sleepless nights in thinking the matter over. Last Saturday I spent the evening in the company of our family physician and he is very much against my taking up the profession. Among the objections advanced was that at the end of three years of training I should find myself among the vast multitude of unemployed nurses and would have a very difficult time. At the age of twenty-five I should be perhaps in a rather tragic situation." This was quite different from the unbridled enthusiasm of applicants from the previous decade, typified by Delphine Wilde '26, who had written, "When I had to go into the hospital in June for an operation, friends said that my experience would cure me of my 'nursing mania'—but it only 'aggravated' it."

In a 1935 issue of the *Quarterly*, Young informed alumnae recruiters that unemployment was a problem only among nurses who were "unemployable ... on account of personality, lack of education, lack of suitable cultural background or home advantages ... Even in New York City where the employment situation is greatest there is a serious need for better qualified candidates for all types of positions." Negative publicity, she added, "is influencing the intelligent group in this country with the result that many are advising their friends and acquaintances not to consider nursing." Bolstering her argument, she noted that almost every member of the class of 1933 who sought a job in nursing had found one.

In a second letter to the alumnae, Young described the successful applicant. She was in the upper 10 percent of her high school class with a B-plus average or better and in good overall health (not prone to colds in winter, growing pains, headaches, or other minor ailments—or to complaining about them). Preferably, she had some college education. The School was looking for "well adjusted, well informed young women with a splendid cultural background acquired either from environment or books ... But we have not a successful nurse yet ... One important characteristic ... is her ability to work with a group for the good of the patient ... This is not the profession for the lone worker but rather for the person who can be part of the whole," wrote Young, alluding to the trend toward interdisciplinary care. The ideal candidate was patient, humane, selfless, outgoing, and inwardly and outwardly confident.

Around this time, the New York State Department of Education recommended a two-year moratorium on nursing school admissions in order to alleviate unemployment. The idea was quickly quashed by nursing educators, presumably with help from hospital administrators. The department ultimately decided that it was better to raise entrance requirements and recommended aptitude tests akin to Presbyterian's.

In 1934 the proposal for a Department of Nursing was accepted by the managers of Presbyterian Hospital and the trustees of Columbia University, clearing the way for detailed planning. By mid-decade, a final blueprint was adopted, but money troubles delayed the plan for two more years. (Were it not for Sage's 1935 heart attack, the plan might have been delayed even longer.)

Finally, in 1937, sixteen years after the idea was first broached, P&S Dean Rappleye announced, "Beginning July 1st, the Presbyterian Hospital School of Nursing will become the Department of Nursing of Columbia University with that autonomy, educational independence, and unity which every major department of the university enjoys. Under the new arrangement, the basic course in nursing will become an integral part of a larger educational plan design not only as a sound preparation for the usual practice of bedside nursing but also as a foundation for advanced training in the fields of public health, school, industrial, and hospital nursing school administration and other phases of nursing practice and education."

Despite the new "Department" moniker, the School continued to be known as the Presbyterian Hospital School of Nursing. Indeed, official publications usually listed both names, reminding readers of the program's illustrous origins and its current university status. (Much later, in 1961, the Alumnae Association changed its name to the Columbia University–Presbyterian Hospital Alumnae Association; the School pin was updated in 1976, with the Columbia crown replacing the ornate "PH" monogram.)

When Columbia's newest department was announced to the public in 1935, reports appeared in all the metropolitan papers and not a few national journals. The *New York Times* noted, the new program "indicates great progress toward replacing the apprenticeship system with true education. Until recently ... students have been enrolled to do the work of the hospital. Training and education have been inevitably subordinated to hospital chores. During the boom years, when hospitals increased rapidly in number, exploitation of student nurses also increased ... Medical students receive much of their training in hospital wards. But every detail of their work has a place in their education and none of it is done to save money for the hospital. Nursing remains the only profession in which the apprenticeship system still prevails."

The *Times* added that although Presbyterian was not the first nursing school to move into academia, "it has long functioned as a real school, with a definite three-year course of practice and theoretical instruction ... The Presbyterian Hospital School of Nursing remains unchanged in its new

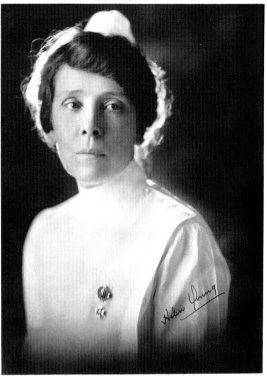

Helen Young '12

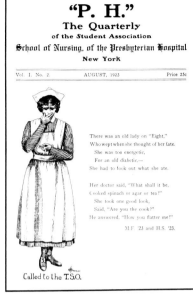

"P. H."
The Quarterly
of the Student Association
School of Nursing, of the Presbyterian Hospital
New York

Vol. I. No. 2.   AUGUST, 1923   Price 25c

There was an old lady on "Eight,"
Who wept when she thought of her fate.
    She was too energetic,
    For an old diabetic,—
She had to look out what she ate.

Her doctor said, "What shall it be,
Cooked spinach or agar or tea?"
    She took one good look,
    Said, "Are you the cook?"
He answered, "How you flatter me!"

M.F. '23 and H.S. '23.

Called to the T.S.O.

Student publication, 1923

Left: *(Left to right) Dean Sage, Helen Young, and William Barclay Parsons at the opening of Columbia-Presbyterian Medical Center, 1928*

Right: *Mamie Clegg*

Below, right: *Alexander MacKenzie*

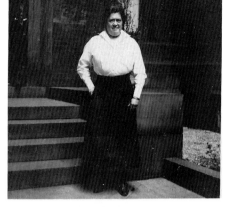

Bottom: *Breaking ground for Maxwell Hall, 1925*

Below: *Maxwell Hall under construction, 1927*

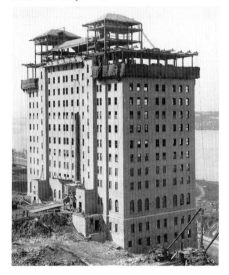

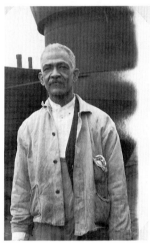

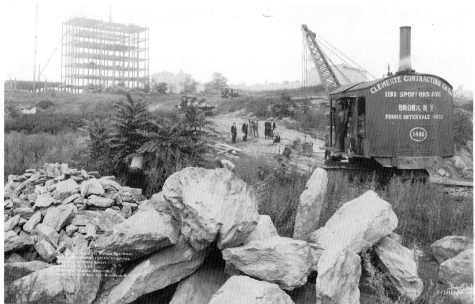

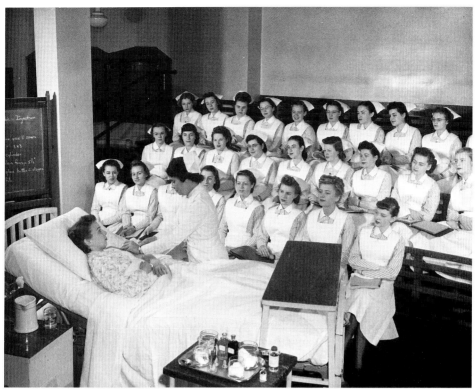

Helen Pettit '36 demonstrating nursing technique to class of 1948

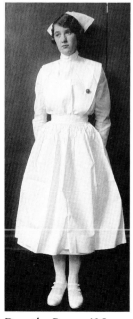

Dorothy Rogers '25, 1943

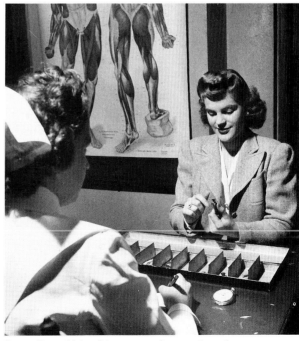

Susan Petty '44 taking aptitude tests for admission to School of Nursing, 1942

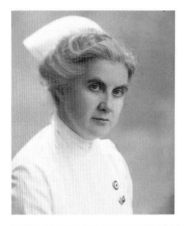

Left: *Margaret Conrad '20*

Below: *Conrad under the arch of diplomas at commencement, a tradition originating with Anna Maxwell's farewell commencement in 1921*

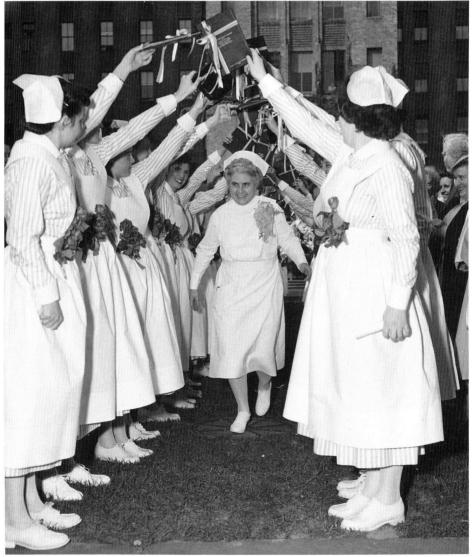

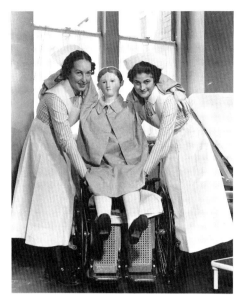

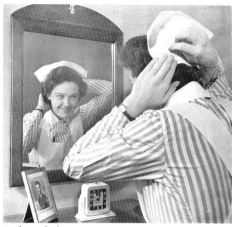

Left and above:
Student nurses, 1940s

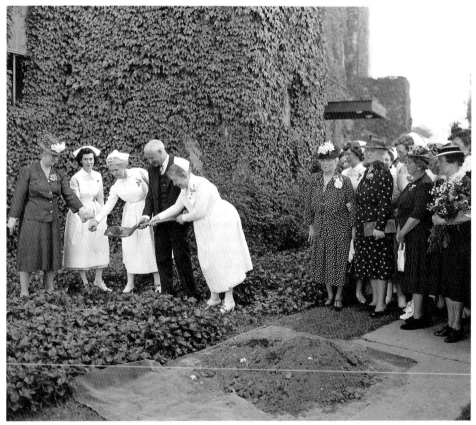

Burying the fiftieth-anniversary time capsule outside Maxwell Hall, 1942; Group at left includes (right to left) Helen Young '12, P&S Dean Willard C. Rappleye, Margaret Conrad '20; Group at right includes (front row, left to right) Harriet MacArthur '95, Sara Strain '01, Severina Wilson '01, Emily Clatworthy '98

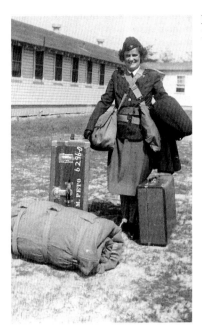

Left: *Lt. Col. Marjorie Peto '26, 1942*

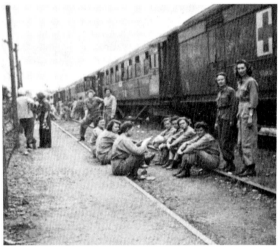

Right: *Nurses of Second General Hospital at the end of World War II, 1945*

Below: *Test run of Second General Hospital in Columbia-Presbyterian Medical Center's back yard, 1942*

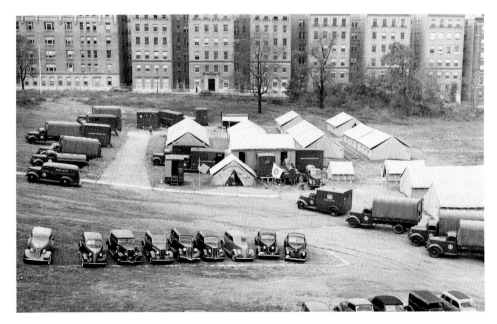

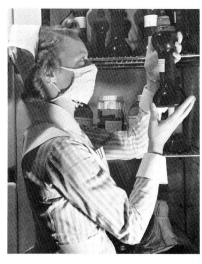

Left: *Nurse in Columbia-Presbyterian's pioneering blood bank, circa 1942*

Below: *Second General Hospital evacuating patients in Lison, France, circa 1944; Geraldine Keefer Schwarz '39, behind stretcher, facing camera*

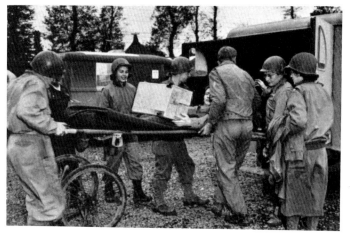

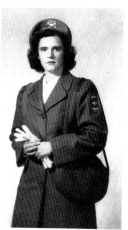

Above: *Joan Tompkins Wheeler '46, Cadet Nurse, circa 1945*

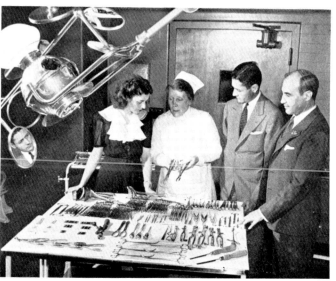

Left: *Helen Young presenting surgical instruments to Duchess of Leinster of Great Britain for use in World War II, 1940*

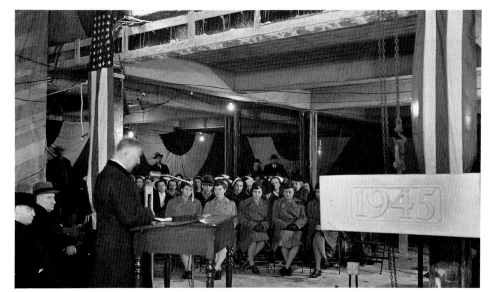

Above: *Laying of cornerstone for Maxwell Hall's new wings, 1945, attended by (left to right) New York City Mayor Fiorello LaGuardia, P&S Dean Willard C. Rappleye, and Presbyterian President Charles Cooper and (seated, front row), Margaret Wells '29, Aileen Hogan '40, J.M. Ada Mutch '36, Laura Smith '32*

Right: *Completed Hall, 1950s*

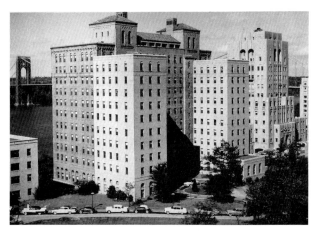

Right: *Dwight D. Eisenhower, Columbia University president, congratulating 1949 graduates Ethel Rematore Weisman, Norma Shisler MacKenzie, Mary Whitesell Mogavero, Nora Ruane Mulvihill, Barbara Smith Redmond, Dorothy Delamaster, Helen Hulburg, Phyllis Partridge, and Olive M. Benn*

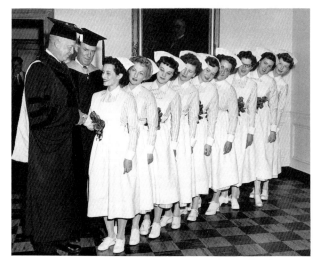

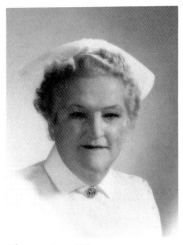

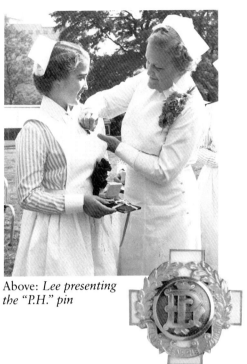

Above: *Lee presenting the "P.H." pin*

Eleanor Lee '20

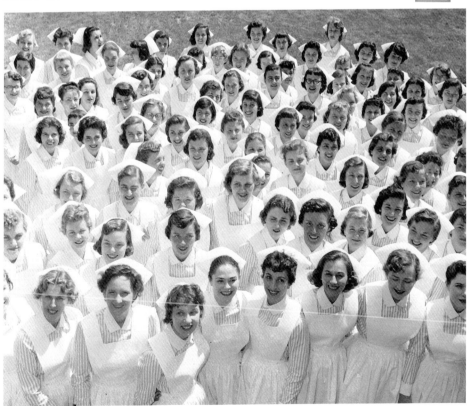

Class of 1958

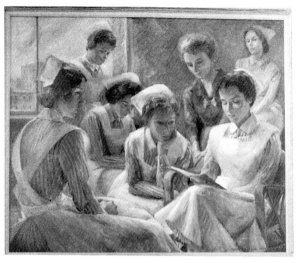

Top: *"Senior Seminar,"* 1959 oil painting by Gene Ritchie Monahan, depicting 1960 graduates (left to right) Patricia Gleason Daugharty, Pamela Scott Heydon, Margaret (Peggy) McEvoy, Jean Monahan Glazier, Lois Mueller Rimmer, Paula Grossman Mosher, Yvonne Corpuz Conrad

Middle: *Faculty member Beatrice Dorbacker '50 demonstrating proper way to feed patients, 1955*

Bottom: *Class of 1954 on rear steps of Neurological Institute*

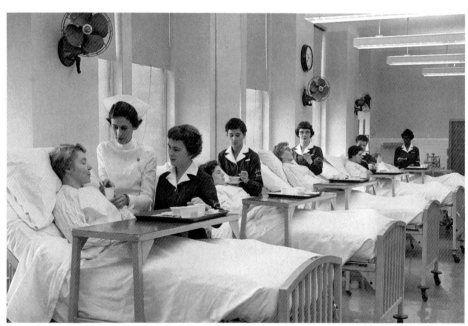

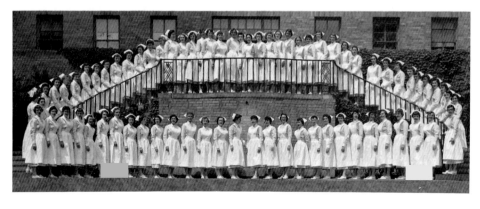

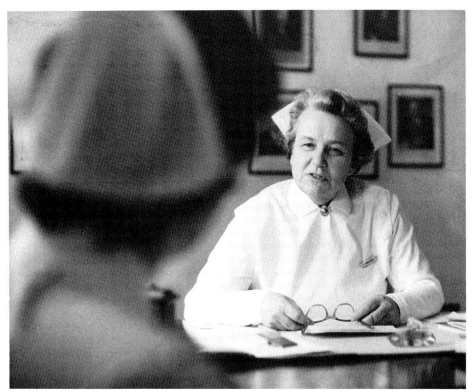

Elizabeth S. Gill '37

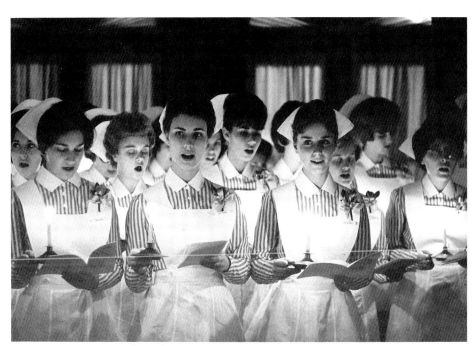

Dedication ceremony, class of 1963

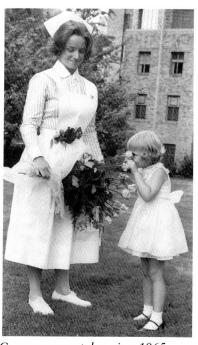

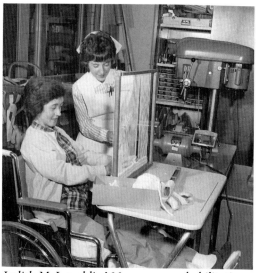

Judith McLaughlin '66 on neuro-rehabilitation unit, 1965

Commencement day, circa 1965

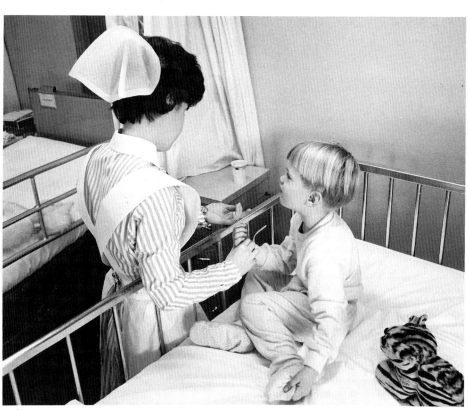

Pediatrics, circa 1965

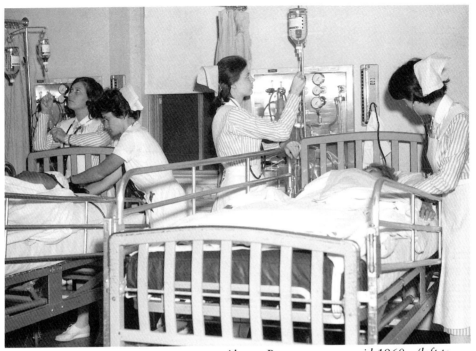

Above: *Recovery room, mid-1960s; (left to right) Layne R. Garside '68, faculty member Holly Howard Stover '61, Joy Davis Gould '68, and Carolyn Hames '68*

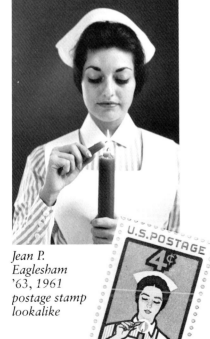

Jean P. Eaglesham '63, 1961 postage stamp lookalike

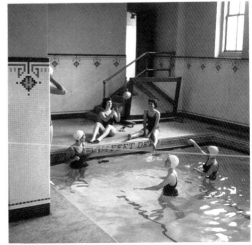

Maxwell Hall pool, circa 1965

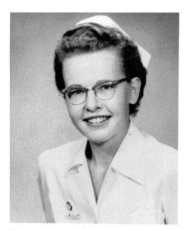

Mary I. Crawford

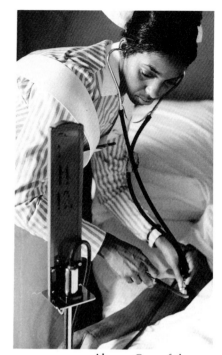

Above: *One of the first minorities to enroll at the School of Nursing, mid-1960s*

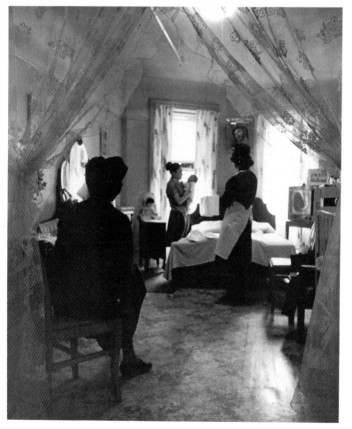

Left: *Public health nursing, 1960s*

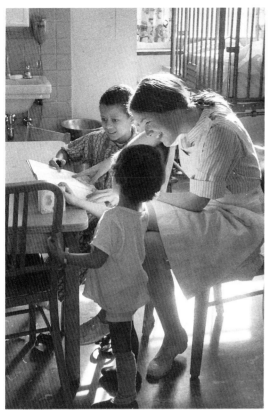

Pediatrics, 1970s

Helen F. Pettit '36

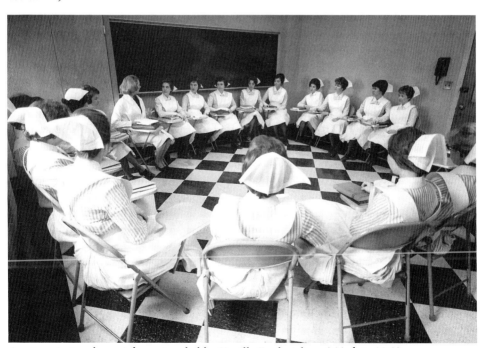

Seminar in psychosocial nursing, led by Keville Frederickson '64, late 1960s

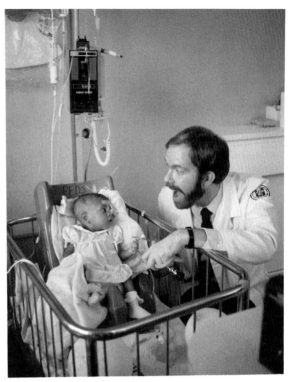

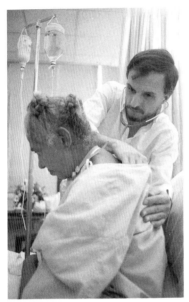

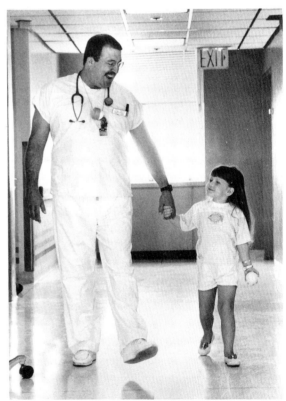

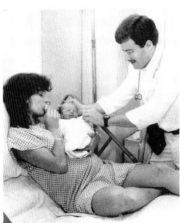

Men in nursing: (Clockwise, from top left) Frank Hunter '84, David Ekstrom '75, Jack Gentile '91, and Bill Bradley '91

affiliation. The same courses … will be given by the same doctors and nurses. The field work will continue to be done in the hospital wards, laboratories and diet kitchens as heretofore. But the entire emphasis on nurse training is changed as the school becomes a department of a university medical school and ceases to be a department of a hospital."

Indeed, the new Department was very much like the old School. "We are not planning any radical changes at the present time," Young wrote to the alumnae. The curriculum, which had been undergoing constant revision for well over a decade, was up to date. Admission policies had recently been upgraded, which meant that the same high-quality students would be enrolled, except that now they would be placed in three different tracks, depending on their academic preparation: (1) As before, students with baccalaureate degrees were awarded nine months credit and thus could complete the nursing program in two years and three months (assuming they had taken courses in natural sciences, psychology, and sociology or economics). Upon graduation, they received a baccalaureate degree from the University and a diploma from the Hospital; (2) Those with at least two years of college were enrolled in the traditional three-year program and would receive both the degree and the diploma; and (3) Those with a high school education were enrolled in the traditional three-year diploma program; they could acquire their B.S. with two more years of study in the Department of Nursing Education at Teachers College. Individuals in all tracks were registered as Columbia students. The first two groups were awarded sixty credits toward the 120-credit baccalaureate degree.

New students now entered only in the fall, instead of twice a year. After the preliminary term (comparable to the old probationary term), baccalaureate and diploma candidates were taught in separate sections, with the former receiving more theoretical material, laboratory exercises, seminars, case-study conferences, and clinical experiences. The groups were reunited in clinical specialty courses and other senior-level courses.

By the late thirties the number of hours that most students spent in the wards had dropped to 4,500, from a high of over 6,500 earlier in decade. Classroom hours remained the same, about 1,000. The typical weekday included four hours of classes and three hours of ward duty. Three more hours each week were spent in conferences and special demonstrations. Although students still had to work several hours every weekend, their overall burden was much lighter, which reportedly reduced fatigue and improved concentration.

Among the curriculum highlights of this period were new affiliations with the Neurological Institute and the New York State Psychiatric Institute and a revised affiliation with Henry Street, which was seeking to reduce its teaching commitment. In the new arrangement, students were sent to the Settlement House for two intensive weeks of training, which was prefaced by substantial academic preparation and six weeks of experience at Vanderbilt Clinic. The change was ideal for short-course students (those with previous degrees), whose cramped schedules heretofore prevented any public health experience. "Henry Street," one such student commented, "has made me realize that patients must have a mental recovery as well as a physical one before they can be restored to society. In returning to the hospital, I have tried to set each patient apart and realize his situation and difficulties. It has almost made me believe that some illnesses have their basis in difficult backgrounds."

The faculty were unaffected by the new affiliation with Columbia, too. Virtually the entire staff was retained—much to Sage's dismay. In a letter to Rappleye, he grumbled, "I know from past experiences that there is a strong urge on Miss Young's part to take care of old timers and that that urge often prejudices her judgment as to their qualifications." Five teachers were appointed as assistant professors of nursing—Mary Elizabeth Allanach '21, Ardis E. Duggan '25 A. Winifred Kaltenbach '20, Eleanor Lee '20, Florence L. Vanderbilt '27—and twenty-one others were appointed as instructors. Salaries ranged from $600 to $2,400 a year. Joint appointments were given to Hospital personnel with educational responsibilities, which included supervisors of all the clinical services and many head nurses.

The Department's top appointment, professor of nursing and executive officer, with a salary of $3,500, went to Margaret Conrad, a seasoned clinician, teacher, and administrator who was intimately familiar with the ways of Presbyterian Hospital.

Financially, there were significant changes. The final agreement stipulated that the Hospital's contribution to the School would be limited to its current outlay. Any additional educational expenses would be assumed by Columbia. The Hospital would retain control of the School's $1 million endowment, the income from which could be used to defray its educational expenses. All tuition fees, which would be raised to $300 for baccalaureate candidates and to $150 for diploma candidates, would go to the University.

The estimated annual expenses for the new Department were $110,600, including $90,000 for salaries, $14,000 for office and infirmary supplies, $5,000 for compensation to medical instructors, and $1,600 for the school physician. Income would amount to $65,000—about $52,000 stemming from the Hospital and $13,000 from tuition fees. That left a shortfall of $45,000, which would come out of Columbia's coffers.

Margaret Elizabeth Conrad was born in 1894 in Blue Earth, Minn., and educated in public schools in Massachussetts and New Hamsphire. Upon graduation from Mount Holyoke College (Mass.) in 1917, she taught history and Latin at South Hadley Falls (Mass.) High School for one academic year. Answering the nation's call to duty, she enrolled in the Vassar Summer Training Camp and, with twenty other young women, went on to the Presbyterian Hospital School of Nursing, graduating in 1920.

Her nursing career began at Massachusetts General Hospital, but in six months she was back at Presbyterian as instrument nurse in the operating room and subsequently as night director in the wards. Her oscillations between the two states would continue for another thirteen years.

Conrad's rise to nursing's upper echelon was swift. By 1924 she was superintendent of Holyoke Hospital, a post she held until the decade's close. Predictably, she returned to her nursing alma mater, this time to study anesthesia under Anne Penland from 1929 to 1930. Next on the itinerary was New England Hospital for Women and Children in Boston, where she became principal of the nursing school. By 1933 she was back in New York, as one of Helen Young's assistant directors. The title of registrar soon was added to her credentials.

Apparently, Conrad was popular with the students. In 1938 the student editors of *Student Prints* commented, "Titles of honor add not to her worth who is herself an honor to her titles." To many she was the quintessential nurse, particularly to those who witnessed her response to an accident at Maxwell Hall during a social gathering. "Miss Conrad took over the situation," recalls Helen Pettit '36. "They saw her ability to function clinically quickly and to feel for the person who was hurt. They were impressed; I don't think that class ever forgot."

Although Conrad was a caring clinician and capable teacher, she could be an insensitive manager, sometimes brusque and nondiplomatic. "I don't think she was comfortable in some of her other roles," says Pettit. "But she had many loyal supporters."

Conrad also served as vice president of the New England Hospital Association, chairwoman of the Massachusetts State Commission of the Red Cross Nursing Service, New York State representative on the National League of Nursing Education's Committee for Revision of the Nurse Practice Act, director of the New York State League of Nursing, director of the New York Branch of the American Association of University Women, and chairwoman of the Post War Planning Council of the New York City Nursing Council. A perennial student, she took numerous graduate courses in education at Boston University and Teachers College.

Notably absent from the new faculty roster was the name of Helen Young. In 1937, when the Department of Nursing was officially opened, Young relinquished her educational responsibilities to Conrad but retained control over the Hospital's nursing service. At age sixty-one, Young was still sharp-minded and productive—otherwise she would not have been given charge of nursing at the Neurological Institute the following year—but it was time to turn the School over to the next generation.

Following the division of nursing service and education, relations between the Hospital and University remained cordial and cooperative. As long-time colleagues, Young and Conrad made the transition with no difficulty and co-taught the School's two courses in nursing ethics. "The one thing which seems to be most difficult to explain [to a visitor] is the harmony between the University and the Hospital officials and staff," said Conrad. "It appears that frictions exist in most [other] places." (Later, administrators of both institutions came to the conclusion that nursing's two elements ought not to be divided, and with Young's retirement the roles of director of nursing service and nursing education were reconsolidated under one person, Conrad. And to bring Conrad into closer contact with professional services at the Hospital, the Board of Managers gave Conrad a seat on the Medical Board.)

Properly, Young's contributions to academic nursing did not go unnoticed. "The program as evolved here would never have been possible without the leadership of Miss Young, whose unselfish devotion to the large interests of the profession has brought the plan to fruition," Dean Rappleye noted.

"The whole transition was accomplished with no interruption to nursing in the Hospital, largely because of the cooperation between Miss Young and Miss Conrad... Nothing so attests to Miss Young's stature as a splendid woman, nurse, and educator as her gracious cooperation in surrendering her leadership of the School," added Albert Lamb.

And President Sage remarked, "Many have labored valiantly for the success achieved... There is one, however, who stands out above all the others and that is our director, Miss Helen Young. During the years of Medical Center expansion each burden imposed upon shoulders already overladen has brought from her the simple reply, 'We can do it.' High spirit, loyalty and devotion has she lavished upon her task. To her and to her predecessor, Miss Anna C. Maxwell, the school owes not only what it is but what it will become."

"She guided us through the period of expansion ... without sacrificing [the Department's] simplicity, its directness of contact or its friendliness...

We consider her truly a second founder of our School," offered Conrad. Similarly, Marjorie Peto '26, a faculty member under Young, said: "As the hospital and school grew she continued to recall names and take a personal interest in each nurse."

Young was presented the Columbia University Medal for Excellence in 1937 "in glad recognition of a quarter-century of unselfish and untiring professional service of the highest character." Later, in 1953, she was awarded the Columbia-Presbyterian Medical Center Distinguished Service Medal.

Young retired in 1942, capping off thirty-three years of service to Presbyterian Hospital. The Board of Managers voted to give her a yearly retirement income of $3,200 plus a one-time $5,000 payment of appreciation.

In retirement, Young continued to work on nursing's behalf, serving as treasurer of the Alumnae Association, as a nurse recruiter with the National Committee of the Red Cross Nursing Service during the Second World War, and as the School's constant friend and adviser. Visitors to her apartment at the Medical Center were subject to her perpetual teachings on subjects great and small. She would dispense advice on how to run a nursing school or how to ripen a pear. Frugal as ever, she abhorred the thought of spending money to have her portrait painted. She loved to take leisurely drives out to the country, with her longtime friend and colleague, Anne Penland. Clear of mind and sound of body until her last days, Young died in Harkness Pavilion in 1966 at the age of ninety-two.

"The School of Nursing has come of age," Sage declared after the affiliation with the University was formalized. "It is about to graduate from the academic guardianship of the hospital and take its rightful place in the world of University Professional Schools." The School was well situated, but it had not yet taken its rightful place. Nowhere elsewhere in the University were students expected to work like apprentices. The extent of noneducational ward duty had been reduced, but not eliminated. Presbyterian still depended on student nurses to help run its wards, and it intended to keep it that way as long as possible. The final agreement gave the Hospital representation on the new School of Nursing Committee and stipulated that Columbia could not appreciably lower enrollment or ward hours without Presbyterian's consent — or the University would have to bear the substantial cost of hiring additional graduate nurses or other personnel.

Columbia wanted to end the whole dilemma of exploitative ward duty, but it couldn't afford to do so immediately. A 1936 administrative memorandum stated, "If funds can be secured to support a staff of instructors supplementary to those already provided by the hospitals in the present plan of nursing training and to allow the employment of graduate nurses to relieve students in the wards and clinics of the hospital, it is our belief that the educational program outlined will make a contribution of the first magnitude to nursing education." In the spring of 1938 the two parties agreed to a fee of $140 per month per graduate nurse needed for relief. That semester, $4,480 in fees were paid to Presbyterian. At the same time, the Hospital adopted an eight-hour-a-day limit for staff nurses, necessitating the hiring of forty-four additional graduate nurses. Piece by piece, year by year, the School was severing its apprenticeship roots.

The tone for the new Department of Nursing was set by Virginia Gildersleeve, dean of Barnard College, in a 1936 speech to the Professional Women's Club of New York City. Referring to Columbia's new venture in nursing, she observed,

> Everyone's education should consist of two parts: liberal and vocational; or the imparting of wisdom, and the teaching of techniques. This means the general development of your intelligence and your spirit on the one side; on the other, the placing in your hands of tools, professional or vocational tools, that enable you to express your intelligence and spirit in service to your fellowmen. In this sense the art of nursing is a tool, so is the art of journalism, so is the art of politics, and so the lovely art of music. Without some such tool or medium of expression your intelligence and your spirit may be wasted, and not translated into action or into beauty.

The first university class included twenty-eight baccalaureate candidates (including twenty with previous degrees) and fifty-three diploma candidates (ten of whom had a year or more of college). Following a year-old tradition, each new student was greeted in Maxwell Hall by her "Big Sister"—a senior who would take her under her wing, doing "all that one would wish to do for a real little sister," explained Aileen Hogan '40. "This quite often was the beginning of a very real friendship. There is the fun of introducing the little sister to the magic of New York…, the cheering note at the desk, the extra letter in the mailbox, the sandwich and the coffee the night before anatomy quiz." Less than three years later, in June 1940, thirteen of those little sisters were awarded the School's first baccalaureates in nursing.

All was well within the School of Nursing as it entered the new decade. Located in the midst of a great medical center, with ready access to the best minds and resources in American health care, the School was secure and confident, eager to explore uncharted territories of academic nursing. Great changes were afoot—though for reasons that no one had imagined.

16

Destinations Unknown

> War, grand and glorious on the Generals' maps, is full of mud, bugs and other desperations for the individual soldier, and we were soldiers along with ten million other Americans in uniform, who did the best we could about it.
>
> *Lt. Col. Marjorie Peto '26 (1947)*

A FEW WEEKS AFTER Japan's surprise attack on Pearl Harbor, Charlotte Kerr '39 wrote to her fellow alumnae in the *Quarterly:* "The New Year has dawned on a sad world, but the 'P.H.' family in Honolulu is well and busy. We are glad to be here now because there has been much to do—and there will be much more to do in the future. As you could easily guess there were not enough nurses here to carry the huge load thrust upon us on December 7th. But we all pitched in and did our best." Kerr's remarks seem eerily casual, as if she were describing a bad traffic accident and not an unprecedented attack on American soil that had taken thousands of lives and triggered the country's entry into a world war. But at Columbia-Presbyterian, Kerr had been taught to handle pressure and calamity with professional calm. And in Eleanor Lee's class in nursing history, she had learned that nurses were expected to rise to the nation's defense, that a generation earlier Presbyterian nurses had served in the First World War, and a generation before that in the Spanish-American War. After another cycle of war and peace, it was her time to serve.

America may have been unprepared for Pearl Harbor, but it was not unprepared for war. In the wake of Hitler's stunning 1939-40 European blitzkrieg, the country began to mobilize—nursing included. The profession's major organizations quickly united to form the National Nursing Council for War Service, recognizing that the existing loosely organized system of recruiting and training nurses was not up to the demands of wartime. Furthermore, enrollments were on the decline. With Hitler dreaming of a thousand-year Reich and Hirohito of a pan-Asian empire, tens of thousands of additional nurses would be needed to see an end to this doubled-edged nightmare.

Patriotism went only so far in drawing women into the field. Most of them wanted nothing to do with the armed forces or with the healing arts — a dilemma that only worsened as the war intensified, when women could easily find employment at better wages in businesses and industries stripped of their able-bodied men. All the while, the military persisted in giving nurses "relative rank" with substandard pay and benefits (an injustice rectified very late in the war).

Nonetheless, nurses did not let the country down (although most Americans thought they did, unaware of the depth and breadth of the field's wartime contribution, a contribution unmatched by any other profession). Twenty-nine percent (65,000) of all active R.N.s volunteered for military service. Thousands more joined civil defense units. Tens of thousands of young women enrolled in the U.S. Cadet Nurse Corps. Hundreds of college women enrolled in the Red Cross Nurses' Training Camp at Bryn Mawr College. Thousands of inactive nurses came out of retirement. Nursing schools trained tens of thousands of volunteer nurses' aides. And countless student nurses assumed extra duties in wards and clinics around the country.

The School of Nursing was involved in virtually every facet of nursing's remarkable wartime campaign. Its most public contribution was to the Second General Hospital of the U.S. Army, Columbia-Presbyterian Medical Center's overseas military hospital unit. For more than three years, stretching from the day of infamy to the days of victory, the unit served in England, Ireland, and France, in modern hospitals and muddy fields, sometimes perilously close to the front and always within range of Germany's bombs and rockets.

On the homefront, the School recruited and educated a record number of student nurses; participated in the Bryn Mawr and Cadet Nurse Corps programs; offered courses for nurses' aides, retired nurses and graduate nurses; joined civil defense emergency units, and participated in war-related clinical research. The faculty contributed countless hours to national and local nursing organizations while students raised money for war relief and worked extralong shifts.

As 1940 unfolded, preparations for war were on everyone's mind at Columbia-Presbyterian Medical Center. At commencement in May, James

Wadsworth, a U.S. Senator from New York, lectured, "Sometimes we have been led to believe we can run the world. That is not so. We are not the master of world events. We must strive, however, to be the masters of our own destiny. To do so, we must be strong. And to be strong we must be willing to work and sacrifice... I cannot escape the conviction that here at least is a group prepared to serve." The senator was right. There was no shortage of volunteers when, at the request of the U.S. Army surgeon general, the Medical Center reestablished its military hospital unit (dormant since the close of the Great War, when it was called Base Hospital No. 2). Seventy-two alumnae who were on the Columbia-Presbyterian staff or the School faculty, or both, eventually joined the unit. Another 200 graduates served in other units spread all over the globe. During the war, it could be said, the sun never set on the School of Nursing.

In June the Medical Center, with substantial help from the Department of Nursing, staged a carnival on the lawn of Maxwell Hall, raising over $7,000 for the Red Cross War Relief Fund. In the years to follow, students raised thousands more for various causes, including the rebuilding of L'Ecole Florence Nightingale in Bordeaux, which the School had helped establish after World War I. They also collected books for the troops and old clothing for the Red Cross. They diligently saved paper, old boxes, metal, string, toothpaste tubes—anything that could be recycled—and, without complaint, accepted added burdens in the wards. "With women of today assuming an even more important status in daily life, the residents of Maxwell Hall have increased their activities in proportion," Martha Pearson '42 remarked at the time.

Also in 1940, two faculty members were given leaves of absence to serve overseas: Delphine Wilde '26, who became head nurse of the American-Scandinavian Field Hospital, and Sheila Dwyer, who joined the staff of the American Hospital in Britain. "Each of us has been issued a gas mask and a tin hat," Dwyer wrote to her friends at the Medical Center. "You may tell Miss Penland that I know just how she felt about her tin hat when she first went to the front in the last war. Personally, I think the only suitable garment is a complete suit of armor... I have discovered that the expression, 'The Presbyterian Hospital in the City of New York,' is international. So many people have asked, 'Are any of you from Presbyterian,' that I expect to be knocked over the head by jealous co-workers any day now."

All the while, the Second General took shape under the direction of surgeon William Barclay Parsons (who was soon called to the Pacific theater and replaced by Rudolph Schullinger, M.D.) and nurse Marjorie Peto '26, instructor of nursing and supervisor of the men's surgical service. Together, they assembled a healing battalion of approximately fifty physicians and one hundred nurses and a handful of ancillary personnel.

Another commencement arrived before the Second General set sail. War, of course, was the topic of discussion at the 1941 exercises, and no one was better prepared to address the implications and consequences of international conflict than guest speaker Walter Lippmann, the foremost journalist of his day and advisor to presidents. The venerable newsman stated,

> Yours is one of the very few professions in all the world of doubt and struggle which transcend the conflict and evoke respect and gratitude from all men everywhere. Thus you will have that most enviable of all possessions—the conviction that during your hours of activity you are able to do very well something which indisputably needs to be done. Most of your fellow citizens, indeed, most of mankind, lack this conviction, and that I venture to say is the ultimate cause of the tragedy through which mankind is living; that progressively among civilized men there has fallen apart the conviction that there is work of infinite value to be done and that it is the vocation of man on this earth, to see, to understand, and to do that work. For without such a conviction there can never be the confidence to go on where the work is hard and painful, nor steadfastness in danger, nor consolation in sorrow, nor, in the end, victory.

Lippmann's words were moving, doubly so in light of recent news. On May 19, 1941, the war was no longer an abstraction. On the front page of the *New York Sun* that day, an across-the-page headline in 108-point type screamed: "Sunken Steamship's 170 Americans May Be Prisoners on Nazi Raider." The ship in question was the *Zamzam*, an Egyptian steamer whose passenger manifest included two new alumnae, Katherine J. Saliari '40 and Marietta Papasaphiropoulo '40, who were returning to their native Greece. Both were briefly imprisoned by the Germans. Saliari lost her passport and money in the mishap, but was more troubled by other losses. "The most important and valuable thing I lost was my diploma and nurses' pin," she wrote.

Weeks after the *Zamzam* was sunk, three other 1940 graduates, members of a Harvard–Red Cross epidemiology team, were aboard ships that were torpedoed somewhere between Greenland and Iceland. Five nurses died. Fortunately, alumnae Martha Reis, Susan Ralph, and Marion Weismer were rescued by an English tanker. But three more School pins descended to the ocean floor. The various sunken pins and diplomas were replaced at the war's close. "I was so thrilled to be able to wear my pin again after so many years," Saliari exclaimed.

Ending months of anticipation, the Second General Hospital was called to duty in late January 1942, with orders to report to Ft. Meade, Ga., for basic training. The School was a hive of activity; within two weeks, one hundred nurses had to be examined and fingerprinted and measured and sworn in. The Hospital generously gave the nurses full pay for February plus a two-week bonus (the physicians received a four-week bonus) and promised that their jobs would be there when they returned. Ready and eager to serve, First Lieutenant Peto and her troop of second lieutenants hopped on a south-bound train.

All that rushing, it turned out, was for nought. Four months of fitful training were to follow. Priceless lessons in how to survive a mustard gas attack or evacuate casualties from the front were mixed with lazy after-noons of roller skating and off-base excursions. Despite the occasional hike and drill (led by a foul-mouthed officer right out of central casting), the Army's newest recruits were neither toughened nor disciplined by the experience. "We were to learn though, the hard way," recalled Peto in her moving and humorous wartime memoirs, *Women Were Not Expected* (1947). As the "training" dragged on, with no definite end in sight, the nurses worried that they would miss out on all the action. "After thirty-eight months overseas, it was amusing to remind them of their fears along this line," Peto later noted.

Finally, "on June 30, 1942, the 2nd General Hospital nurses staggered up the gangplank of the *Duchess of Bedford*, dressed in navy blue woolen uniforms; each carried a pistol belt, canteen full of water, first-aid kit, gas mask, musette bag, overcoat, steel helmet, and a suitcase that weighed at least 25 pounds," the chief nurse recorded. "The temperature that day, 98 degrees." With 4,000 other military personnel, the unit sailed to "desti-nation unknown," variously rumored to be Alaska, Ireland, Australia, or England. Liverpool, it turned out, was the port of call (coincidentally, where Base Hospital No. 2 disembarked). They were among America's first medical units to arrive.

Housing for the nurses was cold, dirty, and dismal. "Women were not expected and no provisions for their accommodation had been made," explained Peto. But there were larger worries. "One night German bomb-ers flew over the bivouac area and dropped their bombs on nearby Birmingham; the din was deafening and great flames shot into the sky."

Within weeks, half of the Second General was dispatched to a hospital in Northern Ireland. The work was relatively light; most of the patients had jaundice and were more in need of diversion than expert care. The nurse in command was Peto's assistant J. M. Ada Mutch '36 (a full-time instructor back at Columbia). Mutch was later appointed chief nurse of the 120th Station Hospital in Bristol, England. With the rank of major, she served as a regional supervisor in Northern Ireland, Le Mans, Rennes, and, finally, Vittel, where she commanded 800 nurses. Six months later, Mutch's splinter group rejoined the Second General in Oxford, where it had assumed control of Churchill Hospital from the staff of the American Hospital in Britain.

Life in wartime Oxford was relatively normal. The weather was cold and rainy, the housing inadequately heated, the food bland and boring, the hours long, and the patients mostly routine (save for a number of frostbitten flyers). Under the grim English skies, which held the constant threat of rain and air raids, the nurses worked hard and played even harder. After one particularly long day of nursing and night of dancing, one nurse wrote home, "Soon we are going to wish we had stayed in the States so we could feel sorry for the poor ANC [Army Nurse Corps] overseas!" According to Peto, "Other nurses threatened to go to bed for good when the war was over, just as Florence Nightingale had done." The full measure of war's horrors had yet to test Columbia-Presbyterian's finest.

In the meantime, the Army struggled to mold a bunch of civilian nurses into a platoon of soldiers. Oxford's 500-bed Churchill Hospital, under the Second General, had become a medical marvel but a military embarrassment—at least commanding officer Colonel Paul M. Crawford thought so. A career military man, Crawford thought it vital that nurses know the proper way to salute, wear a military uniform, drill in formation, and address an officer. However, as Peto noted, "the nurses were inclined to think the war was not to be won nor men's lives saved with correct sentences" or with other seemingly trivial matters. They did value order and discipline, but not when it interfered with their primary role. "The nurses should know how to drill," the lieutenant acknowledged, "but to be made to drill two hours a week in a functioning hospital seems unnecessary. When the drill has to be conducted in … the main plaza, often one prays for rain. Perhaps that is why it rained so much when the Second General was in England."

Later, Peto and thirteen other nurses from the unit were sent to a "battle school for nurses" at the American School Center in Shrivenham. Valuable lessons were learned, though according to the chief nurse, much time and energy were wasted on the familiar or the unfathomable. "Up at 5 A.M.," she wrote, "to scrub my floor with scouring powder, polish my shoes, then dress for Inspection … I have a demerit for having my helmet strap inside instead of outside and I got three demerits the other day for something my shoes did. The rooms were microscoped; everything must be in its proper place and folded as directed. Then drill for an hour; an exam on gases and how to inspect a mess. I've just learned, too, how to wash dishes. At one time I thought I was a nurse."

Peto's humor and healthy skepticism of all things military were among the many traits that endeared her to her charges. Even as she rose through the ranks, all the way to lieutenant colonel, it was her other title, chief nurse of the Second General, that mattered most. At the Medical Center, this 1926 graduate of the short-lived Presbyterian Hospital–Teachers College joint-degree program had been a supervisor and an instructor—in other words, a leader, a teacher, a mentor. At Churchill Hospital, "Petie," as she was affectionately known, assumed the same roles. She was a comforting link to home.

When not soldiering or nursing, the nurses tried in vain to teach basic nursing skills to enlisted men on the hospital's staff. Fittingly, the soldiers wanted to be nurses as much as the nurses wanted to be soldiers. The situation might have been humorous had it not detracted from the nurses' time at the bedside.

Slowly, the months passed, with no end to the ordeal in sight. Spirits were lifted with the delivery of gifts from the School and visits from dignitaries and celebrities, including Eleanor Roosevelt, General Eisenhower, Lady Astor, John Masefield (Britain's poet laureate), Al Jolson, and Bob Hope (a cousin of Lt. Elizabeth Habif '41). There was also time for dances, bicycle rides in the countryside, punting on the Cherwell river, and relaxing in the nurses' own club, "The Vestals Retreat." Another highlight, at least for Peto and four compatriots, was afternoon tea at Buckingham Palace with the King and Queen of England, Princesses Elizabeth and Margaret, Prime Minister and Mrs. Churchill, Lord and Lady Mountbatten, and other notables. "The King was good-looking and easy to speak with, not stiff or formidable," Peto recollected.

Two years after its arrival in Oxford, in June of 1944, the Second General was ordered to another "destination unknown." The unit camped briefly in Circencester and then Tidworth, with little to do but conduct drills and pass the time. Eventually, seventeen of the nurses were dispatched to form the nucleus of a new hospital in England. The rest went to France, landing on Utah Beach in Normandy weeks after D-Day, the launch of the momentous Allied invasion of France. "The trip over had been quiet," Peto recalled, "the channel had barely a ripple and the combat suits and full field regalia which everyone was wearing seem somewhat incongruous in the pleasant atmosphere. Normandy however was a different matter, one could see instantaneously that life was grim, tense and businesslike and that the war was not very far away. This fact was emphasized the first morning. Bivouacked in a field near Carentan the nurses could see and hear the terrific bombing of St. Lo, they could see the bombs drop and feel the earth respond."

While the Second General constructed its new home, a sixty-acre, 1,000-bed field hospital in Lison Gare, the nurses were temporarily scattered about the countryside in evacuation hospitals. Louisa Kent '36 remembers being pressed into duty the moment she returned to the new facility: "I was assigned to a ward with sixty post-operatives, seriously wounded... There were five ward men ... and three nurses; we ran all night ... We gave penicillin, sulfa, plasma, blood, oxygen, etc., on and on, over and over ... This went on for seven nights."

Oxford, their former haunt, was beginning to look like paradise. Now, they were crowded in tents in an enormous apple orchard muddied by incessant rains and plagued by bees and mosquitoes and fleas. Trenches served as latrines and helmets as sinks. The food was dehydrated. "Walks in the country were not safe because the countryside was full of land mines," Peto wrote. "Restlessness and monotony developed ... [A]s it got cold everyone went around saying the other fellow had 'orchard neurosis.'"

In time, half of the hospital came to be filled with German POWs. "They received excellent nursing care," Peto insisted. "Although few nurses knew how to speak the language they managed to convey their thoughts to these ardent Nazis."

By November the hospital was turned over to the 189th General Hospital. Peto and sixty of her nurses were immediately called to newly liberated Paris to assist with the massive and rapid evacuation of patients to Britain. Others went to Revigny for the Battle of the Bulge, and still others to Nancy to organize a 1,500-bed hospital, which would become the Second General's next home. Most of the unit's nurses were reunited there at the beginning of 1945.

"Living took on some degree of normalcy," wrote Peto about the time in Nancy, but the nursing did not. As the Allies pushed into Germany, cas-

concentration camps in Poland and Germany. "From a professional standpoint the nurses were doing the most satisfactory work of their enlistment; the wounded were in need of expert handling and tender nursing care and the nurses of the 2nd General were happiest when the demands on their skill was the greatest; morale was way up. This was what they had enlisted for."

Peace came to Europe on May 8, 1945. "The $64 question at 2nd General after V-E Day: When are we going home?" Peto wrote. But departure was still months away. As the patient load slackened, the chief nurse was assigned briefly to teach English to French nurses' aides and then, for some obscure reason, to study French history at the Sorbonne in July.

Several alumnae had very different perspectives on the war. Elizabeth Colmers Standen '40, whose family fled from Nazi Germany to America in the mid-thirties, wrangled her way into the Army because she "had a debt to pay to this country" (as a public health nurse, she was supposed to remain stateside). She served in Rheims and then in Paris, leading a venereal disease control team. Near the end of the war, she visited Etretat, home to Presbyterian's World War I military hospital. "One day I walked down to the village," she said, "and in the store I saw the picture of our nurses marching along the streets of Etretat—the same picture we have in Maxwell Hall. Among the women who helped clean our quarters was one who remembered our nurses well... Now we are using an old civilian Hospital erected after the last war and, I am told, largely equipped by Presbyterian —so, you see, P.H. is all over the world."

Halfway around the globe, Dorothy Davis '40, a civilian nurse attached to the U.S. Army when the Japanese attacked Pearl Harbor, was imprisoned (along with her father, mother, and sister) by the Japanese in Manila for twenty-one months. She was later awarded the Bronze Star. Second Lieutenant Beatrice Chambers '35 spent forty-two months in four different prisons in the Philippines, including the notorious Bilibid camp. Chambers bided her time caring for fellow internees as well as the Japanese guards in a makeshift prison hospital. "Occasionally a native woman in labor would be allowed to come to our hospital for help... [They] left only at the point of a bayonet," she recalled. "Most of our trouble was due to deficiency diseases and boils. Teeth went bad very quickly and ... [were] extracted without a sedative." In early 1945, her prison camp was liberated by General Douglas MacArthur, who personally awarded Chambers the Bronze Star and several other medals and ribbons.

Finally, in early October 1945, the nurses of the Second General, many with four battle stars on their sleeves, and 8,000 troops started the long journey home aboard the *General Meigs*, which was bound for New York but diverted to Virginia by a longshoremen's strike. During a short stopover at Camp Patrick Henry, "it was a Resumption of the Incomprehensible," Peto wrote in response to a lecture on how to behave in America, with emphasis on comportment with the opposite sex. "After having traveled on land

and sea with men, bivouacked with them, nursed and cared for them when they were wounded, watched them die, and after having worked with them for three and a half years, the advice sounded ludicrous, anti-climactic."

In Manhattan, the nurses of the Second General were feted at an open house at Maxwell Hall in October and at a testimonial dinner at the Waldorf-Astoria in March. Their leader, Lieutenant Colonel Peto, was awarded the Bronze Star for meritorious service, for her "outstanding skill and sound judgment" while overseeing the care of 22,000 sick and injured soldiers.

The nurses were saluted once again in 1949 by commencement speaker Dwight D. Eisenhower, then president of Columbia University. "I am coming here as a soldier of the past war to try to tell you just a little of what the nurse meant to American victory," he said. "I had to bear the responsibility for the lives, the comfort, the health, the convenience, everything that affected three million men, three million Americans, in an atmosphere and an area of tragedy and of drama. Naturally, anyone bearing such responsibility on his shoulders had to have tremendous and well-organized assistance. Among those I had, none was more necessary, none more brilliantly performed its work than the nursing corps."

Eisenhower might have mentioned the brilliant work performed at home, too. Washington Heights was never attacked, and no one had to live in muddy pastures or care for Nazi prisoners, but the wartime contributions of domestic nurses were no less vital to the Allied victory—a central point of the 1943 commencement address given by William A. Neilson, president emeritus of Smith College. "There are not going to be enough of you, and I don't need to talk of the more picturesque and heroic sides of your opportunities that have ... become conspicuous to the public eye during the war," he said. "That needs no emphasis; rather I would emphasize the importance of the work that remains for those of you who do not go to the South Pacific islands or to Africa; those of you who are here to look after us old men and women who cannot be allowed simply to disappear in neglect; those of you who are needed to look after the wives of the men who are abroad and their babies."

Indeed, at home there were many old men and wives and babies and very few nurses to care for them. At Columbia-Presbyterian, the country's largest voluntary hospital, with a patient census between 1,100 and 1,200, one-third of the nursing staff was away on military service during the war. Additionally, turnover of remaining employees was alarmingly high. Since new hires were nearly impossible to find, there was but one solution to the staffing shortage: ease the nurses' burden. Under Margaret Conrad (who after 1942 was in charge of nursing education and service at the Medical Center), nursing administrators reduced standard nursing procedures to a minimum and assigned auxiliary workers—Red Cross Volunteer Nurses' Aides—to take over every possible nonprofessional duty. Under the direction of Margaret Eliot '21, assistant director of the nursing service, hundreds of these aides delivered over 100,000 hours of labor in total.

Hospital President Dean Sage criticized the Department of Nursing for not making fuller use of auxiliary workers. "As a matter of record," Albert Lamb rebutted, "the School of Nursing had introduced auxiliary workers in 1921 and had continued to urge extension of this program without sympathetic support from the administration until the Hospital was caught by the war."

Another method of easing nursing's burden was early ambulation of the surgical patient, as early as a day or two postoperatively, a seemingly dangerous idea that had proved successful in overseas military hospitals. "We opened our eyes in shocked horror at the program ... " noted the student editors of the 1946 School yearbook, "but quickly adjusted our nursing techniques and watched our patients progress with pride."

Conrad also arranged refresher courses for inactive nurses, which lured many retirees, homemakers, and career-changers back to the wards of Presbyterian and other institutions. "It was in December 1941 that I had a yearning to do some nursing in addition to my primary job of housewife," said Marion Wood Otis '31, echoing the sentiments of many alumnae.

Civil defense needs added yet another burden to the nurses of Columbia-Presbyterian. Looming over everyone's head was the prospect of enemy attack. Even before Pearl Harbor, New York City assembled a number of disaster response teams, including one at the Medical Center, which was comprised of twelve doctors and twelve nurses plus an anesthetist and two orderlies. The organizing committee included Margaret Eliot, Margaret McCurdie '22, and Nellie Estey '20. Weeks before the Japanese attack, the unit participated in a city-wide drill, rushing down to Union Square and then to Pier 87 on Manhattan's West Side.

A larger emergency team, called an Extemporized Military Hospital Unit, was assembled at the Medical Center in 1943 under the auspices of the U.S. Public Health Service and the Office of Civilian Defense. The nurses of this unit, thirty-six in total, were led by G. Harriet Mantel Deleuran '33, instructor in nursing, and Helen L. Fimbel '37, head nurse in the Vanderbilt Clinic emergency ward. The Medical Center had its own air raid precautions and drills. At Maxwell Hall residents were instructed to keep on hand a heavy coat, shoes and socks, a flashlight, and a blanket. In the event of an emergency, they were to extinguish all lights and cigarettes, close all shades, and assemble in designated interior corridors. Forty students were to report for duty in the Hospital.

On the clinical front, several nurses, led by Helen Stoddart Mackay '28 and her assistant, Jean P. Harris '40, were involved in the emerging specialty of blood banking. Just before the war, Columbia-Presbyterian physician John Scudder started experimenting with the preservation of blood, with great success and with enormous implications for military as well as civilian medicine. Heretofore, most transfusions went directly from donor to recipient, and blood storage was an uncertain art. According to Lamb, Mackay's "insistence on absolute cleanliness contributed greatly to [the bank's] success."

One of the blood bank's first assignments was to collect blood for the English during the 1940 Battle of Britain. The following year, at the request of the surgeons general of the Army and Navy, the bank launched a pilot blood collection program, sending mobile units, largely nurse-staffed, throughout the metropolitan area. The nurses were supervised by Margery Temple '38 and, later, by Vivian Olson Bradshaw '40, who ultimately commanded four mobile units and one hundred nurses. Bradshaw eventually transferred to the West coast to conduct blood drives for the Pacific theater. She also wrote a manual on nursing techniques that was adopted by Red Cross blood-collection centers nationwide. Another bloodmobile nurse, Ruth Derr '31, journeyed to China (where she was born and raised) to supervise a new blood bank in Kunming for Chinese soldiers being trained by the U.S. Army. She was the first and perhaps only American woman in World War II to hold a commission in the Chinese army.

In 1944, in another war-related research project, Conrad dispatched four nurses and several seniors to Bellevue to organize and maintain a malaria research unit. After Japan seized Java, producer of 90 percent of the world's quinine, the search for an alternative anti-malaria agent became a high priority. Veronica Kish Goddard '41 was the unit's head nurse.

While nursing administrators struggled to staff their wards and agencies, nursing educators struggled to expand and fill their classrooms. Early on, the military abdicated any responsibility for nurse recruitment and training. Fortunately, Congress did not. Pushed by the Nursing Council and Congresswoman Frances Payne Bolton, federal legislators allocated $1.8 million for nursing education in 1941. Schools of nursing were pressured to increase enrollments, shorten their courses, and lower their admissions and educational standards—anything to get more students in the nursing pipeline.

Margaret Conrad was hesitant to apply for funds. In a letter to P&S Dean Willard Rappleye, she stated, "The appropriation is not large, and we are not among the most needy institutions in the country." Not only that, she added, "I do not believe we should plan to enlarge our student enrollment without careful study of the consequences... Our clinical facilities would not be adequate for the necessary experience for an additional class without discontinuing some of our present affiliations in services vital to the program of other schools." (By this time over a dozen schools of nursing in the Metropolitan area and upstate New York had come to rely on the Medical Center as a clinical resource. On a typical day over a hundred affiliating students could be found on the pediatrics, obstetrics, and neurology wards, gaining practical experience under the tutelage of the School's clinical faculty.) "I cannot approve the admission of students beyond our capacity for class room, laboratory, practice, supervisory and housing facilities," Conrad stated.

She had even deeper concerns. "The acceptance of federal funds," she explained, "would open the door to some degree of government supervision of our educational program—a situation which [Columbia University] President [Nicholas M.] Butler has prophesized with gloom and regret."

Surprisingly, "Dean Sage stood solidly with the School of Nursing in resisting pressure to meet the demand for more nurses by reducing the content of the course of instruction at the School," Lamb reported. "He also agreed with School officials that although more practical nurses [new and controversial additions to the nursing field] were needed, the School could not offer such training." Sage's 1942 annual report added: "It is inadvisable to add uncorrelated courses to the now overburdened shoulders of teaching staffs of schools of nursing, particularly those of university grade. Nor can the two curricula be integrated without disservice to both."

Conrad, however, was not unyielding. The School did perform its patriotic duty, but on her terms. Enrollments were increased (by 25 percent), the curriculum was shortened (but not compromised), and federal programs were conjoined.

One of the School's earliest efforts to boost enrollments was the Bryn Mawr College Summer School of Nursing, a reprise of the World War I–era Vassar program. In 1941, with support from the American Red Cross and the U.S. Public Health Service, Columbia and a handful of other top nursing schools joined with Bryn Mawr College and Women's Medical College of Philadelphia to create an intensive pre-clinical course in nursing for college women. As before, the idea was to offer educated young women a speedier route into the nursing field. After a three-month summer course, the women enrolled in shortened nursing programs at the participating schools.

Again, the program was a success, drawing more than 500 inquiries immediately after its May 23 announcement. A mere thirty-four days later, the program opened with thirty students, five of whom went on to Columbia. Roughly 135 more Bryn Mawr alumnae enrolled at the School in the years to follow. The summer school was led for most of its five-year run by Margaret Conrad, who was succeeded by Elizabeth Wilcox '27, instructor in nursing.

Though Bryn Mawr was a worthy effort—college women were needed more than ever in the profession—thousands, not hundreds, of new nursing recruits were required. Consequently, Congress, again with Bolton in the lead, passed legislation creating the U.S. Cadet Nurse Corps in 1943. For the first time the federal government got serious about nursing, offering full scholarships to current and future nursing students. In return graduate Cadets promised to serve in essential military or civilian nursing positions until the end of the conflict. Nearly 180,000 women took the government up on its offer (though nearly a third dropped out, many after the hostilities ceased). Over $160 million were funneled through the Public Health Service to the Cadets Corps from 1943 to 1948.

Cooperating nursing schools had only to shorten their programs from the usual thirty-six months to between twenty-four and thirty months; they did not have to alter admissions policies or curriculum content. Conrad had no qualm with those conditions, and ultimately graduated 116 cadets (many of whom were alumnae of the Bryn Mawr program). Another junior block was added in the summer to accommodate the extra students, who were indistinguishable from their peers until they ventured outside in their official gray uniforms, festooned with scarlet epaulets and felt berets. Very few of Columbia's cadets withdrew, even when the war ended. A handful found that they weren't up to the task, and one discovered that medicine was a better vehicle for her talents.

In 1944 Conrad received a telegram from Thomas Parran, surgeon general of the Public Health Service, congratulating Columbia's cadets. "I am deeply gratified at your inspiring response to your country's call for service," he wired. "By performing nursing duties in hospitals where you are studying you are helping to relieve critical shortages at home. You are preparing yourselves for vital service as graduate nurses and good citizens in the post war world to come. The nation salutes you for your two-fold contribution to its health and welfare. You have enlisted in a proud and challenging profession. May you always serve with wise hands and stead-fast hearts."

Unfortunately, none of the cadets was ready in time for the Germans' last major European offensive, in late 1944. "Give us nurses — 10,000 over-night," the Army cried, as casualties reached all-time highs. An enraged Walter Lippmann charged the Army with gross neglect of its wounded. "The last thing our people will put up with is that sick and wounded American soldiers should suffer because the Army cannot find enough women to nurse them," the newsman lectured. "Yet, I am reporting only the stark truth, which is well known to the Army and to the leaders of the medical profes-sion, when I say that in military hospitals at home and abroad our men are not receiving the nursing care they must have, and that with casualties increasing in number and seriousness, this will mean for many of the men that their recovery is delayed, and even jeopardized." Tens of thousands of nurses, he claimed, were being wasted in nonessential positions.

Weeks later, President Roosevelt shook the nation with an unprece-dented call for a draft of nurses, arguing that "volunteering has not pro-duced the number of nurses required." The public, unaware of nursing's unmatched contribution to the war, favored this action. To set the record straight, Conrad wrote in the Quarterly, "The first publicity campaigns ... gave the impression that American nurses had failed miserably, as a profession, in meeting the needs of the war ... The true picture is [that] ... nearly 50% of the eligible nurses have already volunteered. Their record in service has been one of inspiring courage and devotion in all circum-stances. The unexpected need for the additional ... nurses should not dis-tort the true facts."

Roosevelt's proposal, however, never became law, as the Allies rebounded on Europe's Eastern and Western fronts and sufficient numbers of nurses sought military commissions.

The alumnae, particularly members of the class of 1920, also deserve mention for their varied domestic contributions to the war effort. Ger-trude Banfield, for example, was director of recruitment for the American Red Cross, which oversaw all military nurse enlistments. Under her com-mand, 110,000 nurses were certified for service. She was assisted by class-mate Priscilla Barrows. Another 1920 graduate, Marguerite Wales, was educational director of the Red Cross, responsible for nationwide expan-sion of its home nursing classes, which enrolled hundreds of thousands of women. Dorothy Deming '20, a noted public health nurse and author, revised the Red Cross Home Nursing Manual. During a seventeen-month leave of absence, Eleanor Lee '20 worked for the New York City Council for War Service as chairwoman of a special student recruitment committee and for the New York Red Cross as director of local recruitment. Margaret Conrad, it should be noted, was also a member of this accomplished class.

In retirement, Helen Young became treasurer of the Council for War Service, organized in 1942 to recruit nurses for domestic and international service. Through the Council, the public was urged to forgo all unessential nursing, retired nurses were encouraged to return to work, and employers were urged to make wider use of practical nurses.

Dorothy Watkins Conrad '22 helped the Public Health Service and Congresswoman Bolton establish the Cadet Nurse Corps. And Ina Simpson '95 somehow found the energy to volunteer for the British War Relief Society, for which she was awarded the King's Medal.

Thankfully, this would be the last time that the School of Nursing and its graduates would be called to destinations unknown.

17

An Army of Officers?

You could not have entered your professional practice at
any more momentous moment and challenging period
in the history of this nation and of the world.

Annie Goodrich
(Commencement exercises, 1946)

DESPITE THE BURDENS OF THE WAR, life at the School of Nursing maintained
a degree of normalcy in the 1940s. During this frenzied decade time was
found to observe the School's fiftieth anniversary, produce two well-received
books, expand Maxwell Hall, and enrich the curriculum.

The School's golden anniversary, which coincided with the start of the
war, could not have come at a more inopportune time—at least for those
anticipating a joyous celebration of everything the School and its 2,000
graduates had done in the half-century since 1892. On the other hand, there
was no more appropriate moment to honor an institution that for the third
time in three generations was putting the nation's goals before its own. So,
during the busy spring of 1942 the School set aside a week for anniversary
observances, beginning with a memorial service for Anna Maxwell at her
grave in Arlington National Cemetery, attended by some two dozen students, relatives, and friends of the School's founder—including her sister,
Mary Lapham, and her niece, Diantha Laurientias—plus a contingent of
nurses from the Second General Hospital (then stationed in Georgia).
Unfortunately, tire and gasoline rationing forced the School to cancel a
scheduled picnic in nearby Westchester County, but a special alumnae
dinner at the Waldorf-Astoria went on as planned. Some 600 guests were
treated to a student dramatization of the School's history, "Without Regard
to Race, Creed or Color," whose title was borrowed from Presbyterian
Hospital's original motto. Celebrants were also invited to a special panel

discussion on "Nursing Participation in National Defense" at Maxwell Hall.

Later in the week Annie Goodrich paid tribute to Maxwell, her old friend, at the annual meeting of the Alumnae Association. All present adjourned to the ivy bed in front of Maxwell Hall's south wing to bury a time capsule of School memorabilia. One of those buried items was the newly published *History of the School of Nursing of the Presbyterian Hospital, New York, 1892-1942*, by Eleanor Lee. Among many favorable reviewers was Adelaide Nutting of Teachers College, who called the book "a highly valuable chronicle of events." The librarian of the Army Medical Library, Harold W. Jones, said it was "a splendid historical contribution." Julia Stimson, president of American Nurses' Association, added: "I...find it not only a valuable historical document but an extremely interesting story." And Ada L. Comstock, president of Radcliffe College, opined, "I am especially interested in the book now, when war has emphasized the importance of nursing as a career for college women." All 1,500 copies of the two dollar book, which was commissioned by the Alumnae Association, were sold, with all profits going to a student scholarship fund.

Even better reviews greeted *Essentials of Nursing* by Helen Young and Associates at Columbia-Presbyterian Medical Center. The publisher, G.P. Putnam's Sons, was eager to prepare a successor to Maxwell's widely used textbook on practical nursing, which it had first published in 1907. *Essentials of Nursing*, edited by Lee, consisted of sixty-two alumnae-written chapters on virtually every aspect of nursing, with line drawings by Helen B. Pristop.

"These days of first aid consciousness and preparation make [the book] appropriate to any householder or anyone who hopes to be of help in possible emergencies," noted the Book-of-the-Month Club. Instructors around the country also offered praise. Myrtle Peterson, a nursing instructor at Kansas City General Hospital, wrote, "It is difficult to enumerate all the good points of this book. Every time I pick it up I find another reason of wishing to adopt it for my next class." A teacher at McKeesport Hospital, McKeesport, Pa., Sarah H. Smith, added, "I have long been wishing for a text which was simple enough for the new student and yet scientific and advanced enough for use for the entire three years of training and I think *Essentials of Nursing* will meet these needs." And the *American Journal of Public Health* commented, "There is significance in the fact that the central theme of *Essentials of Nursing* is the patient. All through the book emphasis is placed on contact with the patient, and the reaction of the patient to treatment is given importance."

Young's text was an instant hit. By the end of the year eleven schools of nursing, including Bellevue, were using the three dollar book. The U.S. Army purchased 1,700 copies. Another 12,000 copies, in a special German-language edition, were sent to the American Zone of Occupation, where local nursing schools adopted the book as their primary text. It was also translated into Korean and microfilmed for use in China. A second edition appeared in 1948 and a third in 1953. All royalties went to the Helen Young Scholarship of the Alumnae Association.

A little more than a decade after it opened, Maxwell Hall could no longer accommodate the School of Nursing. No one had anticipated that another world war would force the School to expand so fast or that the Medical Center would attract so many nursing students from affiliated schools. In 1942 the maids' quarters on the second floor were converted into student rooms, but that only delayed the Hall's inevitable expansion. Three years later the original architect, James Gamble Rogers, was sent back to his drawing board with a request to add space for over one hundred students, twenty faculty members, conference rooms, offices, a private dining room, an expanded infirmary, and a library. Rogers' solution was to add two wings to the front of the Hall—which actually were part of the original design but fell victim to cost overruns—lending the building an "H" shape as seen from above. Proceeds from sale of the Tod property in Greenwich, Conn., which had been bequeathed to the Hospital, were used to finance the addition. Construction commenced in late 1945, when New York City Mayor Fiorello LaGuardia was invited to lay the cornerstone of the new wings. The revamped Hall, completed the following August, had room for 475 students.

Even with all of the war's distractions, the School's emphasis on academic excellence did not waver. According to the New York State Board of Nurse Examiners, during the years 1935-44, the School compiled the highest passing rate on the state licensing exam, surpassing 107 nursing programs. Of 730 Columbia students examined in that period, only nine failed, for a passing rate of 99 percent. Statewide, only 88 percent of examinees passed (fewer if Columbia's students were excluded from the total). The board also praised the School's unusually low withdrawal rate, under 8 percent (one-quarter the national average), which it believed was indicative of careful student selection as well as student satisfaction.

A different measure of the School's academic progress was the growth in enrollment. From 1939 to 1945, one of the most competitive recruitment periods in nursing history, the School boosted overall enrollment by one-third, from 279 to 369, *and* nearly doubled the percentage of degree candidates, from 34 percent to 63 percent.

The board credited several curriculum features for the School's exemplary performance, including a requirement that students compile monthly case studies during clinical rotations. The studies, the board said, were "well done, some showing scholarly thought and procedure."

Another laudatory feature was the School's Out-Patient Nursing Service, created just after war to replace a two-week field experience with the Visiting Nurse Service of New York (formerly, Henry Street), which the longtime affiliate could no longer afford to maintain. The program's chief objective was to demonstrate the importance of continuity of care and the role of the public health nurse; patients were selected for their instructional value (which is not to say the program had little clinical value—over 1,000 patient visits were made in the first academic year). After two weeks of duty in Vanderbilt Clinic, students, dressed in special gray uniforms with black bow ties and arm bands and gray felt hats, ventured into the homes of clinic patients, delivering follow-up care and teaching patients how to manage on their own. The field experience was guided by Margerete Martin Reiser '39, a former Henry Street nurse; the overall program was supervised by Constance Hamon '29 and Delphine Wilde '26.

The outpatient services of Vanderbilt Clinic had become indispensable to the swelling immigrant population of Washington Heights and Inwood — a fact not lost on novelist John Steinbeck, chronicler of the dispossessed, whose family routinely relied on Columbia-Presbyterian doctors and nurses. In a special report on the clinic, he noted, "The Medical Center is the middle of a web that weaves throughout the whole city; that penetrates thousands of homes; that, beyond treatment, gives the lift here and the encouragement there, instruction and advice. Teaching has become one of its greatest functions."

The Board of Nurse Examiners also praised the School's two-week-long skills classes, one focusing on the administration of medications, the other on the application of surgical dressings. Students were individually supervised and had to master the skills before assignment to night duty or special services. Also noteworthy were exams in anatomy and physiology and materia medica, repeated at six-month intervals to keep constant tabs on the students' expanding base of knowledge. Finally, the board lauded the School's administrative organization, which encouraged broad faculty participation in curriculum issues.

Several senior electives were instituted in this turbulent decade, further strengthening the curriculum. An early addition was a two-month clinical experience at the Neuro-Psychiatric Institute of the Hartford Retreat in Connecticut. In 1942 the short-course for college graduates was lengthened from twenty-seven to twenty-eight months to bring it in line with national standards and free time in the crowded schedule for hands-on study of psychiatric nursing. The following year the School offered an elective in ward organization and management, taught by supervisors and head nurses. In 1946 the faculty inaugurated a three-month elective in orthopedic teaching at New York Orthopaedic Hospital, the newest member of the Medical Center family of specialty hospitals and institutes. And in 1949 the School started electives in cancer nursing at Memorial Hospital in Manhattan and in rural nursing with P&S's newest teaching affiliate, Mary Imogene Bassett Hospital in Cooperstown, N.Y. (whose nursing service had been shaped by Katherine Danner '06 and Lillian Douglas '17). Under the new affiliation, faculty member Elizabeth Wilcox was appointed Bassett's director of nursing and promoted to assistant professor of nursing.

While the Board of Nurse Examiners found much to applaud, it also found much to criticize. It faulted, for example, the students' crushing forty-eight-hour-a-week schedule and short vacation allowance ("necessitated" by the shortage of staff nurses at the Medical Center). Margaret Conrad — whose title had been upgraded to associate dean (nursing) in the Faculty of Medicine, putting her on the same level as other program directors at the University — was told informally that the School "worked [its] students harder and gave them less time off duty than any other school in New York State." It was not a compliment. Conrad herself lamented the long hours (though they did benefit her as director of the nursing service). In a memo to P&S Dean Rappleye, she wrote, "The amount of serious, independent intellectual effort which can be achieved beyond this schedule is obviously minimum." She also complained of the Hospital's continuing habit of shifting students on the wards without regard to their educational needs. The students' weekly workload was subsequently reduced to forty-four hours—but only after Rappleye made certain, as he assured Presbyterian President Charles Cooper, that it would not disturb Hospital operations.

The board also criticized the small size of the teaching and supervisory staffs, the inadequate integration of basic science material, particularly chemistry, into the rest of the curriculum, and the poor correlation of clinical and classroom instruction in dietetics, which were sometimes separated by months.

Yet another problem was faculty insularity. According to the National League of Nursing Education (NLNE), the ideal faculty included members of various ages, specialties, and educational backgrounds. The School's faculty met the first two criteria but not the third — almost all of the instructors were home grown. In rebuttal Conrad argued that many had extensive professional experience elsewhere, and that the clinical staff— the supervisors and head nurses—was quite diversified.

Finally, the School was cited for not having enough classroom and laboratory instruction — 1,068 hours instead of the NLNE-recommended 1,200 to 1,315 hours — which Conrad feared would cost the School its accreditation. Cooper, for one, wasn't worried. "It seems to me," he told Rappleye, "that the important fact is the excellent record made by your graduates ... [which] clearly indicate[s] that the School is turning out a superior product." Nursing's new accrediting body, the National League for Nursing (NLN)—comprising the NLNE, the National Organization of Public Health Nurses, and the Association of Collegiate Schools of Nursing—agreed. In 1950 the NLN recognized the School as a bonafide collegiate program in nursing.

Conrad must have believed all along that the program was sound. Otherwise, she would not have diverted resources to an ambitious one-year clinical master's degree program, the first of its kind, which debuted in mid-forties. "There is a need for advanced instruction in a number of clinical fields above and beyond the ordinary professional course and the usual experience as a nurse, paralleling in many respects the program of graduate medical education," she wrote. The faculty originally envisioned a master's program offering opportunities to specialize in any one of ten different branches. Each student would be required to complete two semester-long courses in the specialty of one's choice, two courses in educational psychology, one course in sociology and related subjects, a thesis, and 750 hours of clinical experience. The plan called for affiliation with Teachers College or a comparable institution. Experienced nurses with no formal academic training would be allowed to enroll, but not as degree candidates.

Deprived of economic sustenance, the program died in infancy. Records indicate that there were but two graduates: Elizabeth O'Connell '47, who specialized in pediatrics, and Martha Moore Bradley '48, who concentrated in neurology. Several courses were offered through Teachers College, including "Foundations of Education."

Though Conrad did not agree wholeheartedly with the Board of Nurse Examiners' assessment, she subscribed to its general intent, which was to strengthen nursing education. Others were inclined to weaken it—anything to get more "bodies" at the bedside. To everyone's surprise the nurs-

ing shortage intensified in peacetime. Many military nurses retired instead
of returning to civilian practice. Some chose to marry and raise a family or
to pursue different (and more lucrative) careers, a trend exacerbated by the
G.I. bill. Others found they had no taste for general duty nursing, which was
more rigid and controlled than military nursing. Many civilian nurses also
retired, opting for the domestic life. At Presbyterian Hospital staff turnover was a devastating 75 percent in 1947.

While more and more nurses left the field, fewer and fewer entered it.
Demographic trends were not in nursing's favor. Not only had the pool of
young women reached its lowest level in the century, so had the average age
at which women married.

Ironically, many felt that there never was a better time in which to practice nursing. At the 1946 commencement, Annie Goodrich called the post-
war period the most "momentous" and "challenging" moment for nurses
in history. School of Nursing recruiters told would-be nurses, "In an era
when a strong emphasis on destruction is inevitable, nursing offers constructive activity with health as a positive goal. As Walter Lippmann noted,
'Health is the greatest single asset of an individual or a nation.' " Although
Columbia nursing enrollments remained high after the war, young women
in general were not swayed by these arguments. Marriage, not nusing (or
any other profession for that matter), seemed to be on their minds.

Complicating matters, the dwindling supply of nurses was met with an
increasing demand for specialized, labor-intensive health care as well for
more public and community health services. "The type as well as the amount
of care has changed radically in the past few years," remarked Conrad. "The
presence on our services of several abdominal perineal resections, lobec-
tomies, corneal transplants, and other complicated cases where formerly
one was an unusual occurrence, and the frequency of such treatments as
penicillin and streptomycin, make the demands on the nursing staff more
complex and urgent." An added factor in the nursing shortage was the
shrinking work-week, which at Columbia-Presbyterian dwindled from
fifty-four hours in 1928 to forty-four hours in 1950.

Thus, just when Conrad and her peers began to realize the promise of
academic nursing, physicians and administrators renewed their calls for
more expedient (i.e., simpler and quicker) nurse training. As a St. Louis
hospital administrator declared, "One definitely doesn't need a Ph.D.
degree to carry a bedpan." It was not the first time, nor would it be the last,
that such sentiment was expressed. Such complaints were echoed at
Columbia-Presbyterian. "In a sense nursing schools today are turning out
an army composed entirely of officers," commented a special Medical

Center committee convened in 1947 to devise clinical and educational solutions to the nursing shortage. The committee recommended that the School should explore a "drastic revision of nursing education which would provide nurses qualified to care for patients after one year's training, with longer training reserved for those nurses desiring administrative, teaching or other advanced positions." They also suggested that the School equalize the number of students on clinical rotations *so as not to disrupt the nursing service.*

Conrad, the committee's nursing representative, fumed. In a dissenting report she wrote, "The recommendations ... seem to me to be based on a misconception of the current studies of nursing curricula, and of the entire process of professional nursing education. I cannot, therefore, endorse them in any way. While the preparation of auxiliary workers in nursing is unquestionably essential, it should not be confused with professional nursing education ... [and] does not belong under University auspices." Everyone agreed that health care needed more "soldiers," but Conrad believed it needed quality troops, not just green privates, and it needed more officers—team leaders, as they came to be called in the emerging model of hospital nursing, who commanded a unit of registered nurses, practical nurses, nurses' aides, nursing students, attendants, orderlies, and volunteers.

As to the second proposal, Conrad reminded the committee that the Hospital and the University had agreed a decade ago that clinical assignments would be based on academic needs, leaving students "free to pursue the course of study best suited to their professional development. Should we now reverse the matter and manipulate an obviously successful curriculum in order to produce a simple design or table of some sort, or to please the graduate nurses?"

The committee might have anticipated Conrad's vigorous defense of the curriculum. Two years earlier she had quickly condemned a University of California Hospital survey on the nursing shortage circulating among the Hospital's top administrators. The survey seemed to advocate greater reliance on auxiliary workers in lieu of professional nurses. Conrad had no quarrel with such workers insofar as their limitations were clearly understood, especially in acute care. "It is evident that [the survey author] has no conception of the contribution to modern medical care made by the professional nurses in this country," she wrote to Rappleye. "If they are given the status of servants, this situation will deteriorate quickly." Conrad pointed out that Red Cross Volunteer Nurses' Aides, whose wartime service was highly valued, were generally women of substantial intelligence and cultural background, and were not typical auxiliary workers in any sense.

No further mention of the committee appears in the School's records. Apparently, the matter was dropped, perhaps in response a new nation-wide study of nursing education, *Nursing for the Future,* which predicta-bly concluded that nursing education was in a miserable state and nursing schools should be allied with colleges and universities, not hospitals. According to Esther Lucille Brown of the Russell Sage Foundation, the study's author, "only a mere handful of schools have kept up with the advance in medicine." By her calculations only 146 (13 percent) of the nation's 1,200 nursing programs were "good or excellent."

By the late forties Presbyterian Hospital authorities ought to have known that they could push Margaret Conrad only so far. What were they think-ing when they locked horns with her over policy regarding (of all things!) the nursing uniform? The uniform was, on one level, a protective smock, to be kept scrupulously clean so as not to infect patients (a holdover from the days before antibiotics, when cleanliness was of paramount impor-tance). But the uniform, especially Presbyterian's blue-and-white-striped classic, was also a symbol of the wearer's selfless devotion to the care of humanity. So when the directors of the Neurological Institute proposed in 1948 that uniformed staff nurses be allowed to venture outside without benefit of a cape or cloak, so long as they remained in the vicinity of the Medical Center, Conrad was furious. The rule was evidently intended to facilitate movement to and from the Institute, whose connecting tunnel followed a circuitous route through Maxwell Hall.

Interestingly enough, the roles had been reversed in 1934, when the Hospital chastised Helen Young for letting nurses venture into the streets in uniform. "We request that this practice be stopped," an administrator wrote. "Beginning December first, the officer at the door will be instructed to stop all employees leaving the building in their uniforms."

Now, with the tables turned, Conrad responded: "Our regulation...is based on two things: A careful technique which prohibits wearing on duty articles of clothing which have been worn on the street; and a strong tra-dition which discourages the exhibition of the uniform in public." Fearing a slippery slope, she argued that it was impossible to allow just one group of nurses uniformed egress; all nurses, particularly those living a block or so from the Medical Center would expect the same privilege. "The Hos-pital has invested a great deal of money in our fine tunnels, and we con-sider them a safeguard in many ways."

The Hospital did not budge—and neither did Conrad. The debate spilled over into 1949. Towing the nursing line, Margaret Eliot, assistant director of nursing, argued, "1. ... There would be no way of stopping nurses from going to nearby apartments, Broadway, and stores in the neighborhood. 2. We feel the dignity which the uniform should carry with it would be lost. 3. With the high winds ... nurses would have a very poor and disheveled appearance and the uniforms would not be acceptable on duty. 4. The Harkness entrance would become very congested ... 5. Hazards to health would be unjustifiable."

The arguments fell on deaf ears. By early 1950 Hospital administrators were content to let staff nurses cross Fort Washington Avenue cloakless. (This didn't affect student nurses, still firmly under Conrad's control.) Conrad couldn't understand their reasoning, contending that it was nonsensical to let nurses to cross Fort Washington to reach the Neurological Institute, but not 165th or 168th streets to reach their apartments. A city street was a city street, windswept and dirtstrewn. But the bottom line was that she did not want any nursing stripes on the street.

In May, after learning of the Hospital's steadfast decision to permit uniformed excursions, Conrad submitted her resignation. In her mind the debate had mushroomed from a minor squabble over policy to a major debate over authority. "Since [our recommendations] bear no weight and receive no support, but are pointedly ignored ... the situation is obviously an impossible one," she wrote to Rappleye. "Certainly it is reasonable to assume that authority for such details as this should be delegated to the Nursing Department." And to Presbyterian's executive vice president, John S. Parke, she added, "The protection of our uniforms as strictly indoor bedside uniforms has been a strong tradition in the Presbyterian Hospital since the founding of the School. It is impossible for me to agree to its abolition."

Conrad was not alone in this matter. In the wake of her resignation, letters of protest were filed by senior nursing administrators, the executive committee of the Alumnae Association, representatives of supervisors and head nurses, and the Hospital Medical Board. All parties were in general agreement that the administration had bypassed the usual lines of authority, setting a dangerous precedent. The students also protested, though they apparently did not know the full story behind the resignation. (A loyal Medical Center employee, Conrad apparently told most people that she had quit in order to care for her ailing father.) Nonetheless, the students took particular pains to quell rumors that they disliked Conrad and favored her departure. "We ... all admire and respect Miss Conrad as a person for her ability and integrity," they stated. "We consider her one of the outstanding leaders of nursing in the country today and we are proud to own her as our

Director of Nursing and our friend."

Unmoved, the Hospital accepted Conrad's resignation and issued the new uniform rule in August. Conrad's clinical duties were assumed by Margaret Eliot, who was appointed acting director of nursing at Presbyterian Hospital, and her educational duties by Eleanor Lee, who was appointed acting executive officer of the Department of Nursing, Columbia University; both appointments were effective at the beginning of 1951.

At the annual meeting of the Alumnae Association in 1951, the following tribute to the newly departed director was read: "Miss Conrad's high regard and loyalty for nursing principles and her indefatigable efforts in upholding these principles have made her a prominent figure in the nursing profession ... We honor Margaret Conrad as a nurse, a teacher and a leader of broad vision and great integrity."

Conrad, only fifty-six, was not yet done with nursing, and capped off her career as director of nursing at Alfred University in upstate New York from 1952-54. In retirement she lived in both Guilford, Conn., and Keene, N.H. She continued to work for the Alumnae Association and helped organize the Nutmeggers chapter of Connecticut alumnae. She also served on the board of trustees of Norwich (Conn.) Hospital, was active in the Mt. Holyoke Club of New Haven, and taught home nursing for the Red Cross.

Among several awards and honors bestowed on Conrad was an honorary doctorate of science from her alma mater, Mount Holyoke College, awarded in 1948. "Your career in short is the perfect demonstration of what we preach ... for broad service to your fellow men, for rich tending and understanding in pursuit of science and learning," remarked the school's president, Roswell G. Ham. In 1977 she received the Alumnae Association's first Distinguished Alumnae Award. And the following year she was presented the Alumni Medal of the Columbia University Alumni Federation for fifty-five years of distinguished service to the University.

Margaret Conrad died in 1983 in Middletown, Conn., after a brief illness. She was eighty-eight.

18

The Hub of the Health Care Wheel

> I reported for my first time on a ward with very little
> thought about the noble position I would assume. Pre-
> vious advice about the confident nurse who inspires
> confidence in the patient disappeared into the darkest
> corner of my mind and I was possessed with severe
> shakes and a lack of confidence which only a first expe-
> rience can produce.
>
> *Anonymous student (1952)*

SHORTAGES STILL PLAGUED the nursing profession at mid-century, foment-
ing anew the debate over how much education nurses truly needed. Hospital administrators and physicians, tired of continual understaffing, which
was hindering both patient care and medical progress, were willing to accept
any type of bedside practitioners, be they nurses' aides or practical nurses
or diploma nurses. Baccalaureate-prepared practitioners, they believed,
were a luxury the country could ill afford.

The Medical Society of the County of New York, for example, asserted
that university nursing programs were "wasteful" because of their high costs
and attrition rates and because "bedside nurses do not need full collegiate
education." The graduate of a baccalaureate program, the society contended, "often becomes an executive or teacher, heavy on theory and light
on practice, who knows less about fundamental nursing jobs than those she
directs or teaches ... [T]he soundest approach to executive and administrative nursing is through the ranks rather than through the college classroom... While nursing requires the intelligent application of many and varied
disciplines, it is not an intellectual pursuit."

The society acknowledged the need for intellectual leaders, but argued
that "this leadership should always be oriented toward the job to be done,
which is primarily the care of sick patients... It is distressing to observe the

distracting influences on nursing as a whole of this relatively small group, some of them not nurses, who are now more concerned with the theoretical aspects of nursing problems than with the fundamentals." The society also asked, deploying an old scare tactic, if all nurses obtained degrees, "would the sick patients receive care?"

In reality, many collegiate programs were glorified diploma programs offered in a university setting, turning out the *traditional* nurse who was heavy on practice and light on theory.

There were other problems with the society's thesis, not the least of which was that it was based on nursing care as it was practiced in the 1920s. However, nursing practice in the 1950s was infinitely more complex, and demanded greater, not lesser, skills—clinical and administrative. As Kalisch and Kalisch note, "The primary responsibility of the registered nurse had changed from direct nursing care and maintenance of the environment to administration of complex systems, supervision of workers with diverse skills, and provision of comprehensive nursing services." In the evolution of patient care nurses closely followed physicians up the technological ladder, assuming many of their once-exclusive tasks and responsibilities. This generation's nurses were much like the previous generation's physicians, and no one had argued that *they* didn't need a college education.

At a 1953 conference commemorating the Medical Center's twenty-fifth anniversary, Margaret Arnstein '28, chief of the Division of Nursing Resources, U.S. Public Health Service, explained,

> When the thermometer was first used in clinical practice the physician took all the temperatures. Likewise when the blood pressure apparatus was invented... [N]urses were taught to do them in order to give the doctors more time to do the still newer procedures constantly being developed... In 1928, no nurse ever did a venipuncture. Today in many hospitals and clinics nurses draw all bloods and often, under only general supervision, give intravenous fluids. In 1928, the nurse did not usually give intramuscular injections; today she feels sometimes that this is all she does... Those of us who are out of nursing school 25 years are as lost in the tangle of tubes running into and out of patients... as we would be in a tropical jungle. Even those out of school only five years find they must master new procedures and understand new medications which are now in common use ... Education must equip today's graduates to satisfy the requirements of current practice. But it must also instill in them the desire to continue to learn for in this way they can understand new findings as they occur and be ready to meet the demands of practice tomorrow.

The postwar boom in health care was inescapably obvious at Columbia-Presbyterian Medical Center. In the 1950s alone it opened the city's first nursery for premature infants, several specialized recovery and intensive care units, a diagnostic unit for ambulatory patients, rooming-in facilities in obstetrics, new units for communicable disease, dermatology, medical metabolism, otolaryngology, and short-term psychiatric care, and an expanded orthopedic service. These changes had enormous implications for nursing. In the late twenties, when the Medical Center had about 800 beds, the 225 or so students and faculty members of the School of Nursing were an indispensable part of the nursing service, which had only several dozen full-time staff nurses who were assisted by a few dozen aides, clerks, and orderlies. Now, with a bed count of almost 1,600, the Medical Center was staffed by almost 500 general duty nurses, 100 practical nurses, and 400 auxiliary workers. The School's 350 students were rightly relegated to an ancillary role, delivering about one-fifth of the care. They were never adequate substitutes for experienced graduate nurses; now the disparity between the two could not be ignored.

A unique perspective on nursing's evolution comes from Helen Ellis Thorne, who dropped out of the School in 1937 to marry a P&S intern. A quarter-century later she resumed her nursing studies at Grace-New Haven Hospital School of Nursing. "One often hears the sad lament: 'Where has the good old fashioned nurse gone?'" she wrote in the *Alumnae Magazine* (the renamed *Quarterly*). "Actually, she is right here at the patient's bedside, capable of doing a great deal more, trained to detect many more signs and symptoms of many more complications, capable of doing many duties that were once the doctor's responsibility. She gives many more medications and knows not only the reason for giving them but also the dosage, toxic effects and action desired. She is responsible for carrying out many more orders, giving varied treatments and knowing why and how to do them."

In this atmosphere, did the Medical Society really want fewer first-rate nurses? Physicians like F. Randolph Bailey at Presbyterian Hospital did not. "How helpful it is when a nurse calls your attention to an anxiety a patient feared to tell you about, or to a sign you have missed or to the omission of a zero in an order you have written for Digoxin," he remarked in 1956 to the incoming class.

The society was correct in saying that collegiate nursing programs experienced a higher attrition rate than lesser programs and that their graduates were less likely to pursue positions at the bedside than practical or diploma nurses. (Although this wasn't true at the School of Nursing, which experienced an attrition rate of less than 16 percent from 1937-60, roughly half the rate in diploma programs.) Thus, one could conclude that baccalaureate education in general was more costly in the simplistic terms of each bedside nurse produced. But was it wasteful and superfluous? The society itself believed that 20 percent of all nurses should be prepared at the baccalaureate level. Others favored a higher ratio, up to 30 percent baccalaureate-prepared nurses and 20 percent master's-prepared nurses. The reality was that only about 7 percent of nurses had college degrees (not all of them in nursing) and only 1 percent had master's degrees. More highly educated nurses *were* needed. The best solution, then, was to endorse several types of nursing education, not only the most expedient (and inferior) ones. Had hospital and physician associations lobbied at mid-century for —instead of against—federal support of nursing education, that might have happened. (But, then, this wasn't a debate over educational philosophy, it was a struggle for power, which the medical men were gradually losing to unions, federal agencies, health insurers, and nurses. And the medical men knew that with advanced education comes autonomy.)

Another misconception was that baccalaureate nurses were generally disinclined to bedside nursing. At a Medical Society–sponsored symposium on the nursing shortage, Agnes C. Gelinas, chairman of Skidmore College's nursing program, remarked, "I would say that every nurse that I have had contact with in collegiate education wants to go into nursing because she wants to give direct care to patients." An exaggeration perhaps, but not a egregious one. At the School of Nursing, for instance, four-fifths of the baccalaureate graduates from the Classes of 1940-60 went directly into clinical positions, usually at Presbyterian Hospital* (comprising about one-third of the general duty staff)—interestingly enough, a higher proportion than in the pre-baccalaureate years. One third of them stayed at the bedside; the rest became administrators or teachers or school nurses—but somebody had to, and who better than nurses familiar with practice and leadership fundamentals? If hospital administrators had concentrated on making the clinical setting more agreeable and rewarding—with better hours, pay (nurses had the lowest median income of all profession women in 1959), working conditions, auxiliary support,

*The yearly influx of School of Nursing graduates didn't thrill some staff nurses, according to a 1952 survey of Presbyterian nurses. The following complaints were heard: "Too much bias in favor of opinions and methods of Presbyterian Hospital graduates"; "Less condesension toward nurses without degrees needed"; "Show less favoritism to Presbyterian graduates"; and "Presbyterian Hospital graduates have superiority complex." Though the disgruntled were few in number, nursing service director Margaret Eliot made an effort to make the Hospital a friendlier place to "outsiders." And fortunately, the negative comments didn't deter nurses from applying for work at Presbyterian. In fact, the survey, published in the *American Journal of Nursing*, stimulated recruitment because so many staffers had stated that the Hospital was *the* place to practice.

opportunities for clinical advancement, social activities, continuing education programs and incentives—more baccalaureate nurses might have stayed at the bedside. By implementing these measures Presbyterian Hospital reduced staff turnover from 52 percent in 1950 to 33 percent in 1954.

An increase in auxiliary support, long overlooked by hospital administrators, was one of the quickest and most efficient means of easing the shortage. "A study conducted by the Public Health Service... showed that as much as half the time of staff nurses in some hospitals was spent on work that could be reassigned to clerks, maids, and messengers," noted Oveta Culp Hobby, secretary of the Department of Health Education and Welfare, at the 1955 commencement. "Hospitals across the country are using the research findings... to relieve professional nurses of duties others can perform, and to give patients more complete nursing care."

Finally, contrary to the Medical Society's beliefs, collegiate nursing programs were not "heavy on theory and light on practice." Nursing, still an embryonic profession, was properly groping for answers, questioning its practices and methods. If some educators were accentuating research, it was because this fundamental was so long neglected—but they were not necessarily doing so at the expense of clinical training.

At Columbia, for example, patient care remained center stage. "We have never lost sight of our main purpose: to provide comfort (physical and emotional) and cleanliness for the patient, and to carry out the program of medical care around the clock," noted faculty member Dorothy Reilly '42. Reilly spent most of the decade engrossed in research, but her subject was how educators could make optimal use of the clinical setting, "the great asset we have in preparing the professional nurse." Moreover, the fruits of her inquiries—dubbed "action research"—were implemented as they unfolded, not relegated to obscure scientific journals. If the School of Nursing was an ivory tower, it was situated right in the middle of a hospital ward.

The Medical Society made no mention of one sure way to reduce attrition among nurses: raise the legal age of marriage to thirty. (The medical men were powerful, but not *that* powerful.) In the placid, nuclear-familied fifties, a time when more than half of *all* college women dropped out to marry or to improve their chances of marrying, many nurses viewed their jobs as a convenient bridge between childhood and motherhood, not as a career. In its yearbook the class of 1952 expressed "a burning desire for a nursing career," yet it also congratulated faculty member Harriet Mantel Deleuran '33 "for running the gamut of degrees, R.N., B.S., M.A., and for finally obtaining the most desirable degree of all, MRS." Almost always, the "MRS" degree led to postgraduate work in parenting, not nursing.

At the 1951 commencement the Reverend Paul Austin Wolfe of the Brick Presbyterian Church remarked, "One of the problems of this country is how to have a sufficient number of nurses. It is not only how to educate you, but how to keep you in nursing after you are educated. I have got the answer. Don't build the tunnel to Bard Hall"—the medical student residence.

Deleuran, incidentally, was reportedly the first teacher allowed to remain on the nursing faculty after marrying. "She went over Miss [Eleanor] Lee's head to the dean of the medical school and got him on her side," recalled Lois Mueller Rimmer '60, who taught at Columbia during the sixties. "That was the old mentality. One of the things that bothered me about the leaders of the School—they were nice, dedicated women—was that they were all single. It was almost if you wanted to be a good P.H. nurse, you had to remain single your whole life. It was hard for a lot of the girls to find positive role models. We were all interested in getting married, that was our object. Many of us saw nursing as something we were going to do until we got married, and maybe work at now and then, but not for the rest of our lives."

The "dream" of having it all—marriage, children, an education, a career —was for a generation yet to come.

The challenge for nurse educators in the postwar era, then, was to prepare nurses for practice in highly complex settings yet remain true to nursing's elementary principles. As Reilly wrote, "The nurse must master a great variety of skills. She must acquire more technical knowledge ... [and] be informed about the dynamics of human behavior and about the complexities of social structure, so that her contribution, rather than depending on intuition, may be based on conscious knowledge...Moreover, she must be able to assume responsibility for the performance of ancillary personnel ... [T]he nurse is responsible for patient care in a broader context than formerly and therefore is no longer performing total care, but is, rather, the hub from which the whole wheel emanates."

By the early 1950s the faculty had a good grasp on curriculum fundamentals (if not all the details), which were presented at the Medical Center's twenty-fifth anniversary conference. Those fundamentals, according to Helen Pettit, director of education, consisted of patient care (which she called ministration), teaching, communication, and research. "The professional nurse will never be very far from the patient..." explained Pettit. "I think it is fair to say that the most essential contribution of the professional nurse as she ministers is accurate observation based on knowledge and experience, followed by considered judgment and appropriate action

—in this most important ministrative function, she can be replaced by no one."

Another role of the nurse, she continued, is to "help others help themselves stay well or get well. This involves teaching in a formal or informal way." And teaching, Reilly added, goes hand in hand with communication. "Although the nurse may teach specific skills," she said,

> such as insulin administration, colostomy irrigation, crutch walking, and various health habits, the majority of her teaching skills falls into the area of interpretation... [Of the] various members of the health team who contribute to the patient's recovery ... it is often the nurse who serves as interpreter of their aims, for she is the one that is most consistently in contact with the patient. The significance of the patient's disease to his daily living, the role of the many agencies that can contribute to his recovery, the meaning of various doctor's orders and the plans for follow-up care are all areas in which the nurse often serves as interpreter.

Finally, Arnstein told the conferees, nurses need to be researchers. Talk went only so far, she said. "We need to study how nursing affects the patient, and not continue to sit around tables discussing at great length whether so many hours at such and such a ratio of professional to nonprofessional nursing care is adequate."

"Research sounds so profound," noted Pettit, with an appropriate note of wonderment. "It is, but we are getting used to the word at least."

With two major studies already underway, the faculty of the School of Nursing was indeed getting used to the word. Perhaps the most important research project of the decade was "Nursing Student Responses to the Clinical Field," supported by a $20,000 grant from the China Medical Board of New York, one of eleven grants awarded to schools of nursing for curriculum development. It was the first grant ever awarded directly to the School. Free to examine any element of the curriculum, the faculty decided to determine how to get the most out of the School's "greatest asset"—the clinical field. A central challenge was to find a balance so that students were neither exploited nor isolated in practice settings. According to Reilly, the project's director, "Nursing history gives us a great deal of evidence that... we have failed because of exploitation of students in meeting service demands. As a result, the pendulum has swung the other way, as some educators feel that a service should be able to function whether or not the students were there. This approach is controversial and needs a great deal of thinking... If the student is in excess of the nursing service needs, will she continue to feel that what she is doing is essential and therefore a source of satisfaction to her?"

For three years, starting in 1953, the faculty observed first- and third-year students as they gained hands-on experience in medical-surgical nursing. The study was richly rewarding, Reilly reported, precipitating "fundamental changes...in the clinical field and the classroom." Many of those changes were precipitated by data collected by the students themselves in diary form. Entries such as "The ward behind those swinging doors seemed like another world and it was the hardest thing to do to walk across the threshold as if I knew what I was doing" and "I felt like a complete stranger even though I had been fully prepared for what I was to perform" led the faculty to conclude that "students should receive more preparation for role conflicts and special problems which arise in a new and demanding situation." During the study the investigators initiated a new orientation program featuring role playing and panel discussions, which reportedly gave "a better sense of security to students and improved their initial contacts with patients."

The diaries also highlighted the need for a regular forum in which students could discuss problems and methods of problem-solving. Instructor-student conferences were promptly instituted, reportedly improving students' understanding of their clinical roles, enhancing their performance, and increasing their knowledge. (A wider counseling program, geared toward helping new enrollees in general, was inaugurated in 1955, bringing small groups of freshman, juniors, and instructors together for weekly meetings.)

Reilly's inquiry led to a complete overhaul of the first-year curriculum. The revised freshman year began with two new ninety-hour survey courses. One, "Basic Science 35," which combined separate courses in anatomy, physiology, chemistry, microbiology, and nutrition, was designed "to promote understanding of the normal structure and function of the body, the environment in which man lives and the factors underlying the promotion and maintenance of health." Content was spread among six units: the body as an integrated whole; the erect and moving body; maintaining metabolism of the body; digestion; excretion and reproduction; and nervous control of coordinating mechanism of the body. The second survey course, "Nursing 35," offered concurrently, introduced basic principles of nursing "with special emphasis on physical and emotional health, the interaction of the community and the individual in relation to health, the significance of illness to the individual, his family and the community." The course also included supervised practice and clinical instruction involving mildly ill and convalescent patients, which gave students an earlier-than-usual exposure to the wards and opportunities to see correlations between theory and practice.

The two survey courses—comparable to the probationary or preclinical periods of earlier years—led directly into "Medical-Surgical Nursing 45-46," two consecutive courses similarly "integrated" with principles of basic science. Nursing care in seven categories was covered: general physical states; infections; cardiovascular and renal disorders; tumors; collagen disorders; psychosomatic disorders; and endocrine disorders. Material from formerly individual units in diet therapy, materia medica, and pathology was also included. "The approach is one of total patient care and consideration is given to the patient as a person," explained Harriet Deleuran, assistant professor of nursing. "The psychodynamics of patient care are discussed and aid the student in understanding the patient's reactive and adaptive mechanisms to illness. Consideration for the patient's socioeconomic aspects of daily living help to interpret the community in its public health role." The courses carried over into the second semester, basically completing the first year of the curriculum.

"I think last year's students thought we carried the integration a bit too far when in one day we [had] a lecture by Dr. Ferrer on surgery of the biliary tract, Dr. Cosgriff on diseases of the liver, nursing care of patients with liver disease, then [went] over to Maxwell Hall for dinner and found on the menu—liver," joked Rosalie Lombard '51, associate in nursing.

Overall, the new curriculum gave students earlier introductions to medical-surgical, obstetrical, and pediatric nursing, which Reilly's study indicated they could easily handle.

Reilly and her colleagues also examined the value of regular conferences between nursing students and other health professionals. Meetings between nursing and medical students demonstrated that "through joint discussions barriers could be broken down as each group developed a greater understanding of the other's role, and that joint discussions could lead to a more unified and comprehensive approach to patient care." Unfortunately, because of scheduling constraints, such conferences could not be adopted permanently into the curriculum. Another type of conference, between house officers and nursing students, satisfied the students' desire for more specific information about patient conditions and approaches to care. Physicians and administrators were surprised to learn of the students' great thirst for medical knowledge.

The faculty also examined the value of first-year clinical "field trips." Two sites were chosen, the recovery room (to sensitize students to the patients' immediate postoperative needs) and the emergency clinic (to broaden their concept of illness and illustrate the range of patient experiences at the Medical Center). Because of student input, the visits were amplified to include participation as well as observation. In the end the students "enjoyed as well as profited" from the experiences and faculty learned which activities were most valuable. The trips became a regular part of the curriculum.

In a final part of the study, third-year students were assigned to share in the clinical teaching of first-year students. The experiment was a success for both beginning students, who received more individualized instruction, and advanced students, who honed their leadership skills. As a consequence the faculty added a senior elective in teaching, with this experience as a prerequisite, for those contemplating a career in education.

"There are still many questions to be answered before we can make the most effective use of the clinical areas," concluded Reilly. "What does the student learn, both tangible and intangible? How long does it take for these learnings to occur? What about incidental learnings? When does learning stop and service begin?" But at least the faculty were asking questions and approaching problems rationally and scientifically.

A second study with weighty curricular consequences was a 1951-53 demonstration project in natural childbirth. The project was rooted in what might be one of the first grassroots protests against high-tech, in-hospital deliveries. Childbirth was fast becoming a "medical problem," often necessitating surgical, medical, or pharmacological intervention. But not all women welcomed the physician's intrusion. When a number of pregnant women who planned to give birth at Presbyterian's Sloane Hospital for Women requested classes in natural childbirth, it was decided to explore a return to basics.

The logical place to turn for guidance was the Maternity Center Association (MCA) of New York, a pioneer in nurse-midwifery. Margaret Hogan, an MCA nurse-midwife, was recruited to head the project and given a joint appointment with the School of Nursing. Like MCA, she was guided by two principles: childbirth is a family affair and pregnancy should be natural and normal. Accordingly, she said, "The philosophy of natural childbirth accepted [for this study] was that there is no such thing as success or failure. Each person is an individual with certain basic physical and emotional characteristics. The only evaluation of success was whether or not patients were satisfied with their experiences."

Though Hogan was given relatively free rein in the obstetrics service, she had to overcome significant barriers — administrative and attitudinal. One was a rule prohibiting husbands from the labor room. One obstetrician remarked, "They'll just be in our way and the next thing you know we'll find them in the shower with us." Many of the nurses were similarly closed-minded. "Don't you think that all [the wives] want their husbands in the labor room for is to see them suffer," commented one. Another added, "It will lower the birth rate and the couple will never have another baby."

But reason and science prevailed, permitting the project to go forward. Many staff members reacted positively to Hogan's ways, particularly the anesthesiologists. A common reaction was that the fathers contributed "a great deal of emotional support to their wives." Students, who understandably preferred to work with cooperative rather than frightened or disoriented mothers in the labor room, were very enthusiastic. Overall, Hogan contended, the study improved the professional atmosphere. "It is perhaps one of the best illustrations of the democratic method of health education when doctors, nurses, and parents work together."

As for the patients, the study revealed that mothers who received childbirth education had more spontaneous deliveries and required less medication than mothers who did not take the classes. But most important, the mothers got what they wanted: a safe birthing alternative. The classes were incorporated into the obstetrics service, and a midwife, assisted by two MCA midwives-in-training, was added to the staff to establish an antepartal clinic. Not everything went smoothly, however. According to Mary Crawford, an MCA nurse-midwife involved in the clinic, "following the first delivery the roof blew off the institution. The resident insisted the nurse-midwife use the Ritgen's Maneuver which she did not know how to do and [the] patient sustained a third-degree laceration."

Nonetheless, the potential of organized midwifery, which had long flourished in Europe, could not be denied. In 1955 the School of Nursing joined with MCA to establish the country's first graduate program in maternity nursing. The eleven-month program, which was also supported by the Columbia's School of Public Health and Administrative Medicine and Presbyterian's obstetrics and gynecology service, was, according to the School bulletin,

> based on the concept of maternity care as a continuous, integrated service, starting with the first awareness of pregnancy and continuing throughout the puerperium. The complete service (envisaged) includes not only expert obstetric care, but education of the parents for their role, preparation of the mother for the labor experience, skilled attendance and

emotional support throughout labor, and integration of maternity care with good family living.

Education in nurse-midwifery qualifies the professional nurse to function as a specialist on the obstetric team, and with medical guidance, to manage antepartal, intrapartal, and postpartal phases of normal pregnancy and labor, and to give and supervise care to the newborn.

The curriculum was split evenly between courses in maternity nursing and in public health and hospital administration. Presumably, the School was intent on training nurse-midwives who could navigate through an unfriendly, disease-focused health care system or function independently of it. Graduates of the program were awarded a master of science degree from Columbia University and a certificate of nurse-midwifery from MCA. Four students enrolled the first year, each of whom was supported by $3,000 traineeships from the U.S. Public Health Service. Nurses without baccalaureate degrees also could enroll, but only in the clinical course and as candidates for the certificate. Five such students were accepted the first year.

The program was directed by Hattie Hemschemeyer '28, assistant professor of nursing at Columbia and associate director of MCA. Crawford, who played a large role in the program's development, was appointed assistant professor of nursing. (In the early fifties, as a participant in a Teachers College demonstration project, she helped start the first hospital-based nurse-midwifery education program at Johns Hopkins.) Three other members of the faculty were certified nurse-midwives.

In the mid-sixties, Harlem and Kings County Hospitals were added as clinical affiliates in midwifery. And in 1969, with support from Charles M. Steer, M.D., acting director of obstetrics and gynecology, Presbyterian Hospital established its own midwifery service, which allowed the School to offer a full-fledged internship. It wasn't an easy sell. As Steer told the Medical Board, "The midwives actually perform a number of functions which we normally consider to be those of the physician. They perform physical examinations, pelvic examinations, and give a good deal of advice. They perform deliveries, including the making and repair of episiotomies. They administer local anesthetics and ... certain drugs." He counseled the board not to confuse the issue with "administrative and professional matters." The bottom line was that patients would receive "closer and better care."

A few other research projects deserve mention. One was a study of teaching in mental health, funded by a five-year grant (1956-61) from the National Institutes of Health. The primary result of the study, led by Anne M. McQuade and then Betty B. Jones, both assistant professors of nursing, was the integration of mental health concepts and experiences into all parts of the program. Psychiatrists and social scientists were recruited to participate in various classes and patient care conferences, and an introductory course in social work was added. All students by this time were getting three months of hands-on practice in psychiatric nursing. In a related study, Deleuran toured seven European counties to observe the teaching and practice of mental health in hospitals, clinics, and health agencies.

Mental health thus became one of three basic "threads" woven into the curriculum. The second thread was public health. (The third, communicable disease, was the subject of an earlier program-wide study.) Two factors were placing greater burdens on the community-based nurse, including the trend toward shorter hospital stays, which meant that patients were being discharged sicker than usual, and a new emphasis on preventive health, which called for more teaching and screening — the public health nurse's forte. "Today, we know that health is not only the absence of disease, but complete mental, physical and social well-being of the individual," wrote Constance Cleary, assistant professor of nursing. "We must begin to give [students], as early as possible, a broad understanding of the individual within his family and community groups."

Even though public health was one of nursing's oldest branches, educators here and elsewhere did not have a firm grasp of what public health nurses needed to know, or of how and where to teach it. To settle these issues, the Public Health Service awarded study grants to a handful of nursing schools, including Columbia. In the School's study (1957-60), led by Eleanor Lee and Anne McQuade (who was succeeded by Gloria Dammann), several experimental patterns of field study were tested with three different agencies, the Visiting Nurse Services of New York and Brooklyn and the Bureau of Public Health of the New York City Department of Health. The students' progress was monitored with detailed written tests, diaries, structured interviews, group conferences, and other means.

The results led to numerous curriculum changes, including a new unit in human behavior — an expanded version of existing courses in personal hygiene and psychology — which focused on the effects of illness and hospitalization on patients and on helping patients cope with these experiences. Another new unit addressed basic nursing communications skills, such as interviewing, listening, observing, and recording. Moreover, new courses in public health theory, public health administration, public health nursing, social work, and continuity of patient care were initiated. It was not long before the School required all students to get hands-on experience in public health; such training had become too vital to be an elective part of one's education. Before the study ended, the public health program was accredited in 1959 by the NLN Collegiate Board of Review.

Two years later the curriculum was amended so that second-year students devoted roughly half of their spring semester to courses in public health, including a two-day-a-week, twelve-week field placement in which they met with one or two patients per day. This was supplemented by a concurrent course and clinical experience in outpatient nursing or continuity of care.

As the curriculum progressed, the faculty (who now numbered about sixty — half of whom were full-time — plus several part-time physician lecturers) realized that students with little or no college background were an anachronism in what was essentially an upper-division university nursing program. Beginning with the 1953-54 academic year, no one was accepted without at least sixty liberal arts college credits (including many science prerequisites), which meant that all enrollees were candidates for the baccalaureate degree. Not only did this sever the School's last formal link to its diploma-program origins, it ensured a certain level of scientific competence in the entire student body. This, along with various curriculum accelerations, allowed the program to be shortened from thirty-six to thirty-two months later in the decade. In 1961, the program for short-course students (those with prior degrees) was condensed from twenty-eight to twenty-four months, the equivalent of two academic years and two summers.

All these curriculum improvements cost money, of course, which no doubt prompted the School to raise its fees. Tuition and other charges amounted to $1,260 a year for the 1959-60 academic year. About one-quarter of enrollees received some scholarship funds, and all were given opportunities to earn pocket money by working as babysitters, typists, and library helpers.

Still, the University was not yet satisfied with the School's academic standards. In a candid and sobering report, the President's Committee on the Educational Future of the University concluded in 1957 that "the Department of Nursing is maintaining commendable standards and is one of the leaders among such institutions ... Despite its high standards, high for most schools of nursing, the level of preparation is frankly lower than in other units of the University, though the upward trend has been noted ... [T]he further progress of this necessary adjunct to medical science, so important in its own right, ... will necessitate a constantly forward-looking educational policy ... Apparently, insofar as the present pattern falls short of the ideal, it is in the academic immaturity and lack of intense motivation of some of the students admitted." The committee recommended "constant vigilance against slipping into overemphasis on routine training in mere techniques." It also noted that the curriculum's

> intellectual level is somewhat low and far less challenging then it should be in view of the relatively high average capacity of the students currently entering the program. The plan itself appears to be somewhat haphazard and could be better designed if there were more close conferring at the instigation of the administration between the various [basic science and clinical] teachers on whom any effective integration ultimately depends...
>
> [P]rofessional esprit would be enhanced (as it is in good medical teaching) by presenting the nursing career, like other professional careers, as a profession based upon a fundamentally scientific approach with ever-changing frontiers. This picture of nursing should stimulate the more ambitious and capable student by suggesting the possibility of more specialization.

As the School of Nursing diversified and expanded, it bore less and less the stamp of its leaders. At the turn of the century, schools were inseparable from their directors and flourished or floundered because of their strengths or weaknesses. Names like Hampton and Maxwell and Nutting and Goodrich attracted students from around the country. But the growing complexity of health care gradually diminished these educational cults of personality. By mid-century a successful program rested on the shoulders of its entire faculty. It was the aggregate reputation of the teaching staff and the alumnae, among other things, that brought in new students and research support.

That is not to say a school's director became superfluous. As always, the stronger and more visionary the leader the better. The School of Nursing was fortunate to have Eleanor Lee as its leader during the 1950s. Lee was born in Boston in 1896. Her father was a veterinary surgeon, presumably the source of her interest in health care. The Lee family resided in Jamaica Plain, away from the city's busier quarters, and summered in the Cape Cod town of Falmouth. Eleanor attended the Winsor School and then Radcliffe College, graduating in 1918. Her route into nursing ran through the experimental Vassar Training Camp for Nurses and then Presbyterian Hospital.

After graduating from Presbyterian in 1920, she worked briefly at the Hospital as a head nurse in a surgical ward, then departed for Boston's Peter Bent Brigham Hospital, where she taught courses in anatomy, bacteriology, chemistry, hygiene, drugs and solutions, and materia medica. Following a short stint at Teachers College, she returned to Presbyterian as an instructor in 1924. Lee soon became one of the School's most influential curriculum reformers. In 1929, just after she was appointed director of education, she was awarded a Rockefeller Foundation fellowship for an observational study of nursing programs and services around the country. In subsequent years she had a hand in nearly all of the School's major curriculum projects, including the block system of instruction, the demonstration project in outpatient nursing education, the case method of ward instruction, the early-1930s survey of ward teaching, the formulation of standardized clinical report cards, and the public health nursing field study.

All the while Lee improved her own educational credentials, taking a number of courses in educational psychology, nursing supervision, and public speaking at Teachers College. When the School affiliated with Columbia University — another milestone she helped bring about — Lee was appointed assistant professor of nursing. At the peak of the Second World War, Lee took a leave of absence to assist the recruiting efforts of the Army and Navy Nurse Corps and the American Red Cross. Later in the decade she used a spring sabbatical to visit women's colleges and nursing schools in the South.

Lee was fondly remembered as a teacher. She taught in all phases of the program, but she was particularly known for her history of nursing course. "She made it come alive for us," remembered her successor, Elizabeth Gill '37. Lee's fascination with nursing's past spilled over into two other roles, curator and writer. For decades she oversaw the School's extensive Florence Nightingale collection. A busy scribe, Lee penned two histories of the School of Nursing (published on its fiftieth and seventy-fifth anniversaries, respectively) and four articles for the *American Journal of Nursing*. She also edited two nursing texts, Helen Young's *Essentials of Nursing* and the faculty's *Quick Reference Book for Nurses*.

Lee was appointed acting executive officer of the School after Margaret Conrad's resignation in 1950. The appointment was made permanent in 1955, when she also assumed control of the nursing service from Margaret Eliot. Three years later she earned the additional title of associate dean (nursing).

Lee was active in several professional organizations throughout her career. For ten years she served on the New York State Board of Nurse Examiners. She also contributed to the New York Counties Registered Nurses' Association as treasurer and vice president, to the New York State League of Nursing Education as a member of the board of directors, and to the Visiting Nurse Service of New York as a member of the education committee.

In 1954 she was twice honored. She was elected to the Phi Beta Kappa society at Radcliffe College "in recognition of her high attainments in liberal scholarship" and was awarded Columbia's Bicentennial Medal for spearheading the School's contribution to the University's bicentennial fund drive.

Lee, at first glance, did not strike people as a leader. As Gill recalled,

> When we were students we were inclined to think of Miss Lee as a rather quiet, reserved and perhaps shy person. As we came to know her, however, we thoroughly enjoyed her delightful sense of humor and we recognized her great friendliness and interest in us. She was interested in each one of us — who we were, and what our goals were … She had a razor-sharp mind and I have never seen anyone who so quickly took up a new idea or a new suggestion, followed it through, and if it was a good one, put it into action … She was a tower of strength, generous with her praise and quick to encourage — many a student remained in school to finish her program because of Miss Lee's encouragement and help over the hard spots. Her boundless energy and enthusiasm spilled over and often caught us up in it, causing us to undertake rather cheerfully things that we had no intention of doing.

In Dorothy Reilly's view, Eleanor Lee "was the major force in moving the School out of a 'diploma' mentality." Because of her retiring personality, however, she never received proper credit. "She was a woman of ideas. But she couldn't sell herself." Reilly explains that it was Lee who reorganized the curriculum in the mid-fifties to ensure that classroom theory and clinical experiences always ran concurrently, who put the program on a true academic schedule so that students graduated in June and had a Christmas vacation, and who abolished the rule requiring students to make up clinical hours lost to illness, a holdover from the days of apprenticeship training. Lee, at least, was aware of her limitations and delegated responsibility. "She operated more with honey than with vinegar," Helen Pettit says. "She could 'trick' you into doing anything."

Lee retired in 1961 at the age of sixty-five with the first-ever title of professor emeritus of nursing. A good portion of her retirement years, spent in Cambridge and Falmouth, Mass., were consumed by her final literary project, *Neighbors 1892-1967*, her second installment of the School's history. She also served on the board of managers of the Home for the Aged in Boston.

Eleanor Lee died suddenly on May 31, 1967, during a visit to Maxwell Hall, where she had intended to help the School prepare a historical exhibit for its seventy-fifth anniversary celebration and to sign copies of *Neighbors*, slated to be published the next day. She was survived by two sisters.

"Her sudden death was an unbelievable shock to all," wrote Pettit. "For Miss Lee a lingering illness would have been intolerable. Illness or injury that kept anything from getting done was unnecessary and above all interfered with living. She seemed to think of it as an insult. This she wasn't asked to suffer."

Slowly, perhaps imperceptibly to students of the time, campus life evolved in the 1950s. At the beginning of the decade, Columbia's nursing students were still cloistered in Maxwell Hall, still governed by strict rules of behavior and dress and ingress and egress. (Nursing students around the country were similarly restricted, except in a few collegiate programs.) Infractions were dealt with swiftly and sometimes harshly. In 1952 a second-year student was forced to resign for violating curfew and staying overnight in the apartment of a medical student. School authorities went so far as to track her down at the man's apartment, where they found her asleep on the sofa. The student blamed a sudden illness for her inability to call in as required. Unsympathetic or unbelieving, the School asked her to resign. (Apparently, the young woman did not collect her "inheritance" from the previous class, whose tongue-in-cheek "Last Will and Testament," published in the yearbook, read: "To the underclassmen we will leave our ways and means of getting in and out of Maxwell Hall — and there are many.")

The following year, the School organized a "Mothers' Club," inviting mothers who lived in the area to help "make Maxwell Hall a home away from home." But increasingly, the students did not want a surrogate home — they had all experienced the liberating and relatively liberal college life; they were adults and wanted to be treated as such.

Thus, the rules were gradually eased. (They had to be, for nursing schools were facing stiff competition from liberal arts colleges, where campus life was far less authoritarian. Regimentation in society in general was on the wane.) The Hall's visiting hours were extended. Late passes were given out whether or not one had classes or day duty the following morning. Permission to marry was granted — on an individual basis — to seniors (a privilege briefly allowed during the Second World War). "A student contemplating marriage during her program in nursing should consider seriously whether or not she is able to meet the demands of both responsibilities," warned the student handbook. "Many an evening I would walk through the lobby and see a young lady nervously waiting to see Helen [Pettit] because she was planning to marry and it was required she discuss her plans and future in nursing with Helen," remembered Constance Cleary. "I don't know of any student who was not allowed to marry — but it sure made her think through why she was doing it."

With the new freedoms came new responsibilities, as a section on "Decorum" in the handbook reminded the undergraduates:

> The word nurse means a great deal to many people and as a result certain demands are made of her. It is hoped that quite soon you will become aware of what the residence community as well as the community as a whole expects of you. In most instances this cannot be clearly defined but will be obvious if you look for it. It is challenging, as it suggests the trust that is placed in you ... The community as a whole and members of other professional disciplines associated with us in the Medical Center look to us to maintain with them the high standard of the health profession. Too, many of our patients come from the immediate vicinity which makes it most important that we always represent ourselves as we truly wish them to think of us. They entrust themselves to us often.

Typically, as the rules grew more lax, the students grew bolder. Books disappeared from the library in record numbers. Late pass violations proliferated. Fire alarms were plugged with towels and extinguishers emptied all over the floor. Men were sneaked into the Hall. "Even when I was in School, girls had boys in their rooms," remembers Lois Mueller Rimmer '60. "There was one guy who used to pretend that he was a janitor, push a broom down the hall, and then disappear into this girl's room. All the girls knew it."

Margaret (Peggy) McEvoy '60 admits to sneaking in late at night on more than one occasion, harboring a pet cat in her room, and hiding a friend's motorscooter in a locker room — all in violation of Hall rules. "Peggy and I would ride around on the motorscooter wearing our dark glasses and black [school uniform] stockings and our mothers' fur coats," remembers Jean Monahan Glazier '60, her partner in crime. "We were real rebels." The School was evolving, yet it wasn't quite ready for the likes of McEvoy. "At the end of school," she remembers, "everybody had an interview in which they tried to get you to stay on, to work at Presbyterian Hospital. When they came to mine, all they could say was, 'Gee, maybe we could find some place for you in the outpatient clinic.' "

McEvoy and Glazier were part of a small clique that hung out in the Greenwich Village studio-home of Glazier's mother, Gene Ritchie Monahan, a well-known portrait painter. Down in the Village, amongst the beats and the poets, they saw that there was life beyond 168th Street. No wonder they rebelled in the cloistered atmosphere of Maxwell Hall. (Monahan, incidentally, painted a compelling portrait of Jean and six of her friends, "Senior Seminar," which she donated to the Medical Center for a fundraising event. The oil painting was purchased by the children of Mrs. Henry P. Davison to honor their mother's longtime service as a Presbyterian trustee and chairperson of the School of Nursing committee. To everyone's delight, the work was given to the School, where it still hangs.)

McEvoy and Glazier and their friends weren't the administration's only headache during this era. In 1958 a group of students circulated a petition on nuclear weapons (presumably against), throwing Lee for a loss. Past students had been politically active, but always under the faculty's aegis, and never on non-nursing matters. This was a first, and the School had no relevant policy. Lee turned to P&S Dean Willard Rappleye, who advised against sanctioning their actions. But he added, "Of course, we have no control of what the students do on their own." It was a prescient remark. College administrators around the country would soon realize what little control they did have.

The clash of old and new came to a head in June 1960, when the School attempted to bar a pregnant *married student* from participating in the graduation ceremonies. "The class got really angry and said that if she couldn't march, the rest of us couldn't," recalled Rimmer. "So they backed off and let her march." (Another member of that class reportedly got pregnant and went to Puerto Rico for an abortion. Presumably, the School never learned of this.)

Finally, a century after Florence Nightingale gave birth to modern nursing education, students nurses had gained a measure of freedom.

Also in 1960 nonagenarian Harriet Beatrice Gibson '94, the sole survivor of the first graduating class, died at her home in New York City. Her death was reported in the *Quarterly,* but its symbolism went unnoticed. Gibson was not among the School's leading lights — her one position of note was as first directress of the Alumnae Association's residential clubhouse, founded in 1897. But her passing signaled the end of one era and the start of another. As Bob Dylan would sing in a few years, "the times are a-changin'." The question now was whether the School would recognize those changes and evolve accordingly.

19

You Say You Want a Revolution?

It has not been easy to "change" because we feel our
program has produced excellent nurses for many years.
Editors, The Alumnae Magazine *(1966)*

PEOPLE FONDLY REMEMBER the 1950s as a time of domestic peace and prosperity, when everyone seemed to be busy pursuing the American dream. Society was subdued and orderly and static, and people knew their place —a comforting thought to some, though not to others. On the dark side of this well-mannered paradise, women "belonged" in the home, blacks in the back of the bus, and nurses at the bedside at the physician's beck and call.

But something happened as the next "decade"—roughly starting with Vietnam and ending with Watergate—unfolded. With bewildering speed, the United States disunited, not geographically but socially and culturally and politically. Young were pitted against old, students against administrators, hawks against doves, blacks against whites, feminists against chauvinists, hippies against straights, rich against poor, us against them. It was the decade of sex and drugs and rock and roll, of numbing violence and race riots and political murders. If the 1950s were a Norman Rockwell painting, the 1960s were a Jackson Pollock, a dizzying, psychedelic swirl.

Few institutions escaped the storm that was the sixties. Universities like Columbia reeled as students found that confrontation won them more attention than conversation. The School of Nursing, buffered from the tempest on the Morningside campus by a distance of fifty blocks, emerged from the decade relatively unscathed—but not unchanged, and perhaps a bit the worse for wear. Tradition, at once the School's strength and weakness, took a battering. The blue-and-white-striped student uniform, resplendent to some, belittling to others, was ultimately shelved. The normally docile student body stirred to life, calling on the faculty to resolve incongruities between classroom theory and clinical practice, between the ideal and the real. Students and instructors alike, emboldened by the women's movement, broadened their professional horizons, less content than ever to assume the nurse's traditional role. In the face of physician cries for better "trained" (but not better "educated" nurses), the School continued its long climb to the heights of academe and added a second clinical specialty to the graduate program. For the first time, blacks were enrolled, followed soon thereafter by men, ending the School's unintentional segregation. Finally, as social mores relaxed, so did the restrictive rules of Maxwell Hall, liberalizing the cloistered life of the student nurse.

Nonetheless, many were left unsatisfied, viewing the changes as largely cosmetic. The undergraduate program, they contended, remained too task-oriented, while the graduate program barely expanded. What the School needed was a new paradigm of nursing education that gave more emphasis to theory, research, and leadership and decision-making skills, that was based on *nursing*—not medical—science, and that yielded nurses who could practice autonomously, as peers — not handmaidens — of other health professionals.

The never-ending nursing shortage spilled over into the 1960s, still clouding the debate over the necessary breadth and depth of nursing education. More than ever, educated nurses were needed at the bedside and throughout the health care system—a view shared by the Surgeon General's Consultant Group on Nursing. In 1963, following the tradition of the Goldmark, Grading Committee, and Brown studies of nursing education, the group called for substantially more monetary support for collegiate nursing education as well as for nursing research, particularly in the areas of methodology and teaching. At least 75 percent more baccalaureate-prepared nurses and 194 percent more master's-prepared nurses would be needed by the end of the decade.

No doubt, the group was moved by the growing complexity of health care, epitomized by the emergence of the technology-driven critical care unit (CCU). The death rate among severely ill heart patients, it had been found, could be reduced dramatically through immediate detection and treatment of cardiac abnormalities. Nurses were called the most important factor in the CCU environment, more important than electronic monitors or physician specialists. In response to these and other developments, Congress passed the Nurse Training Act of 1964, allocating almost $290 million over five years.

The following year, the American Nurses' Association released a controversial position paper calling for all nursing education to be moved out of hospitals and into institutions of higher learning. They were understandably impatient with nursing's progress. Even after decades of educational reform, two out of three practitioners were entering the field with less than a baccalaureate.

Many physicians welcomed the trend toward academic nursing, including Dana W. Atchley, professor emeritus of clinical medicine at P&S. At the 1961 nursing commencement, he noted, "I now feel that while carrying out orders is essential, the orders should be understood, their meaning and purpose should be clear and many of them [nurses] should apply a technical competence derived from such understanding." He also called for a closer and more egalitarian "partnership" between doctors and nurses.

Many other members of the medical world were less understanding, including Douglas Damrosch, M.D., an assistant dean at P&S. In a letter to the editor of the *New York Times,* he wrote,

> Today's nurses are unable to assume the responsibilities expected of a graduate professional nurse and are thoroughly and completely miserable when faced with the necessity of having to put into practice the theory which they learned from books, demonstrations and seminars, without having had the opportunity to develop competence in the protected and supervised structure of the hospital school of nursing ... [T]here seems to be a blind and uncritical faith in a system which to all purposes is replacing the professional competence with a smattering of nursing skills, a smattering of liberal education and an academic degree.

He did acknowledge the weaknesses of diploma programs, but wanted them strengthened, not closed — even though studies showed that baccalaureate graduates adapted to the rigors of practice in only six months, as compared to twelve months for associate degree graduates and eighteen months for diploma graduates.

Damrosch found an ally in the Medical Society of the County of New York, whose nursing committee chairman, Vincent J. Tesoriero, complained to P&S Dean H. Houston Merritt that academic nursing was preoccupied with the emotional and sociological needs of the sick, fostering "an attitude almost of impatience toward the more basic need for attention to the physical requirements of acutely ill patients... If nursing is to gain the stature to which it aspires, it must realize that it can never do so by neglect of the *very center of its responsibility.*"

It could be argued, however, that *medicine* was neglecting its responsibility. In their rush to embrace specialized, high-technology health care, physicians inadvertently depersonalized the practitioner-patient relationship and disrupted continuity of care. Nursing, however, was unwilling to view the patient as a collection of physiological systems and, in order to fill the vacuum left by the demise of the general practitioner, proceeded to carve out new roles for the professional nurse, most prominently, the nurse practitioner.

As Francesca Castronovo, a former faculty member, explained at the 1973 commencement, "In such areas as clinics, chronic care facilities, ghetto communities and rural areas, most quality care can be directed and implemented primarily by nurses. With additional education in physical assessment and diagnosis, many of the responsibilities formerly met by the general practitioner can be assumed by the professional nurse. Finally, nurses can now move from dependent and sometimes subservient roles to ones that allow development and utilization of your intellectual and leadership abilities. That tired old cliche, 'if you are bright you should become a doctor' will finally meet its demise."

Nursing's new role was further articulated by Lucile Petry Leone, former assistant surgeon general and chief nurse officer of the U.S. Public Health Service, at the 1967 graduation: "Nursing is a channel between science and people. It is said that more advances have been made in the last three decades than in all previous centuries, and of all the scientists who ever contributed to health research, 90 percent of them are now at work. Advances will be even more rapid in the future ... Nursing is one of the essential forces which guarantees that human values and spirit are not lost in the progress which science makes ... Our job as health workers is to push the frontiers of science ahead and, at the same time, reduce the lag in application and practice of new knowledge."

The medical community, not surprisingly, interpreted the various trends in nursing as territorial invasions. "It is the physician who bears the ultimate responsibility for the safety of human beings under our laws, and properly so," Tesoriero countered, extolling the nurse as physician handmaiden. "The fundamental role of the nurse must necessarily be to help the patient receive the care which has been decided upon by the physician."

Current practice, however, demanded novel roles for the nurse. While Tesoriero and his kind complained, study after study confirmed the value of the nurse practitioner. Further support came from the 1970 National Commission for the Study of Nursing and Nursing Education, an independent body with diverse professional representation. Arguing that the physician shortage was more harmful than the nursing shortage, the commission concluded, "it makes sense to have the nurse take over as many functions from the doctor as she can capably handle," and to have nurses in general relieved of burdensome non-nursing functions (housekeeping, recordkeeping, ordering, and supply handling), said to consume up to 75 percent of the nurse's time. "The industrial, social, electronic, and biomedical revolutions are already underway within our health care system. As these changing patterns broaden health care opportunities so will they increase its problems ... It may be that nursing, in particular, holds the key to maintenance of individualistic concern for people and their health problems, and this capacity must be zealously enlarged."

In this new model of health care, the commission added, nurses would be more likely to find a satisfying lifetime career in the field, which would increase retention and stimulate recruitment, two keys to easing the nursing shortage. "While the controversy has raged over the best form of institution for preparing nurses," wrote the commission, "the high school graduates of this country have given their own response to the situation— a slight but steadily decreasing interest in going into nursing at all."

The School had faced trying times in the past, including two world wars and a depression, but never a time so disorienting, so variable. Almost simultaneously, the School was unmoored by the students', women's, and civil rights movements, each characterized at times by an "us-versus-them" attitude that made constructive debate and compromise all but impossible. To confuse matters further, nurses and physicians were jousting over control of the practice setting, and nurses were enmeshed in internecine warfare, divided into the camps of the progressives and the traditionalists.

If any Columbia students of the sixties had reason to rebel, they were the undergraduates of the School of Nursing, probably the most conservative segment of the academic community. Socially, the School was run circa-1930s style (which was true at many women's colleges, too). Afternoon tea was still in vogue. Rules prohibited men from visiting dorm rooms and students from venturing to Broadway in anything less formal than a blouse and skirt. "Miss [Florence] Vanderbilt ran the door like a very strict mother superior," recalls Bettie Springer Jackson '67. In an age when students elsewhere were dropping acid, fighting hand to hand with police, and occupying administrative offices, students at the School of Nursing were getting into hot water by breaking rules of etiquette. Jackson, for example, made the "mistake" of breaking an ankle while jogging (not the universally accepted activity it is today) and limping back to Maxwell Hall in the midst of an important afternoon tea. "I went up to student health to ask for help," she says. "I had not done the right thing. I should have known to take myself over to the emergency room. There wasn't a lot of bending and patience with aberrant behavior—as mildly aberrant as mine was."

Students had to face the added indignity of watching the women's movement—their natural ally, it would seem—pass them by. Feminist leaders simplistically denigrated nurses as victims of male oppression, ignoring their rich and long history as social pioneers. How much self-esteem could impressionable young student nurses have after hearing Wilma Scott Heide, president of the National Organization for Women (NOW) and a nurse herself, exclaim, "Nursing, in my view, and that of feminists and behavioral scientists, reflects the secondary status of women. To the extent that physicians are male and nurses female, you have the prototype of the male-female relationship of the culture at large. The doctor is presumably in charge, the nurse serves." That was essentially true, but what about nurse practitioners and clinical nurse specialists, promising and groundbreaking new role models? Worse yet, Carol Kalinoski, vice president of NOW's New York chapter, asked, "If you're really keen on medicine, why not be a doctor?" displaying a profound ignorance of what nursing was all about. She would have better served nurses and womanhood in general by asking, "Why not change the nature of health care?"

It is doubtful that Kalinoski and her like-minded NOW colleagues would have felt this way if they had seen some of the essays submitted by Columbia's nursing applicants. A typical essay read: "I was persuaded by a number of teachers and counselors that my grades were 'too good to become a nurse. Why not aim to become a doctor?' ... Starting right in with a premedical program, and attending lectures by doctors and other professionals in the medical field, I quickly became disillusioned and soon realized what I had believed all along: I did not want to be a doctor. I did not want to see patients on hourly visits simply to examine, diagnose and prescribe; rather I wanted to be involved in the day-to-day care of these patients, in seeing them heal before my eyes. I wanted to be a nurse."

(The same feminist disdain for nursing exists today, contends Ellen Davidson Baer '62, Ph.D., a faculty member at the University of Pennsylvania School of Nursing. On more occasions than she cares to remember, she has been denigrated by ostensibly liberated women for being "only" a nurse. On a recent op-ed page of the *New York Times*, she lamented that this behavior "has come to exemplify for me the terrible paradox of feminism, which glorifies women who emulate masculine behavior while virtually ignoring women who choose traditionally female roles and careers ... [N]urses are women whom people can denigrate and still get away with it…Professional nursing requires brains, education, judgment, fortitude, inventiveness, split-second decision-making, interpersonal competence and day-to-day determination. When feminists or their families are sick, they want their own nurses to have all those traits, but they don't want to assign those attributes to the group as a whole.")

Though they had every reason to, Columbia's nursing students did not revolt. Possibly, they were intimidated by the School's conservative mien, or they were inherently conservative themselves. But more likely, they did not see themselves as powerless victims of an unfeeling establishment. On the Morningside campus and around the nation, undergraduates were calling for an end to sundry social injustices: the Vietnam War, the inequality between blacks and whites, men and women, rich and poor. Frustrated and rebellious, they took to the streets, engaging in civil, and in many instances, uncivil disobedience. Nursing students shared many of the same concerns, but not their sense of impotence. They were learning that nurses — and women, no less — could affect change within the existing system, however imperfect. History told them so. For three-quarters of a century, the School and its alumnae had been involved in social issues, making a real difference in the lives of people from all walks of life.

That is not to say the students were untroubled. There was much they wanted to change. And now, aroused by the various social movements, they were more willing to take a stand. In 1963, for example, the administration barred a student from graduating because she had broken a leg and failed to complete a public health requirement. The senior class protested by refusing to report for immunizations — an action almost without precedent.

Later in the decade, students brought about a substantial relaxation in the rules governing Maxwell Hall. Men, for the first time, were allowed on the upper floors until midnight on weekdays and two a.m. on weekends. Gentlemen callers, however, had to sign in and out and be escorted up and down. Alcoholic beverages were also permitted. "Nursing students are at least Juniors in college and have already adjusted to 'men and booze,'" Mary Crawford, then the School's director, explained to the dean of P&S. Each student was allowed a limited number of 6 a.m. late passes. Short-course students (those with a previous college degree) were allowed to live off campus after the second semester (mainly because space was tight, not because the administration had become more liberal). A few years later, students had a hand in a number of curriculum changes, including a switch to pass-fail grading in all psychosociology courses.

They had worldlier concerns, too. On two occasions, nursing students voted to strike in sympathy with other protesters and to voice their displeasure with "the state of world affairs." "The faculty was in an uproar and didn't know what to do with them," remembers Sarah Cook, an instructor during the second occasion (and today associate dean for academic and clinical affairs). There were all kinds of meetings, involving students and faculty from all parts of the Health Sciences campus. "They were pointless," recalls Helen Pettit, then professor of nursing. "We didn't know how to answer them, and they didn't know what to ask. They wanted to demonstrate, but didn't know what to do. They didn't have the leadership like they had on the downtown campus." Nursing students and faculty on several occasions met to discuss the ethics and consequences of their actions, since the Hospital was counting on them to work in the wards. Ultimately, the students decided to boycott classes but fulfill their clinical obligations, a compromise that pleased both sides. Cook, for one, was inspired by the students' behavior. "Nursing school," she has realized over the years, "makes them come face to face with their mortality and the gut issues of life. They are a lot more mature than the average college student."

Compromises were not always reached. Revealingly, while physicians in and out of the Medical Center were imploring the School to concentrate more on the practical and less on the theoretical, students were demanding that it do the opposite. In 1967, in a letter distributed on street corners and posted on bulletin boards around the Medical Center, the class of 1969 proclaimed:

We entered the institution with the understanding that our principle affiliation existed with a university community. This is a fallacy. We are crippled by the residual of what was once a hospital school of nursing. While our education should have entertained an academic orientation, we find ourselves victimized by traditional clinical and classroom dogma. Failing to expose the student body to the totality of the educational experience, the knowledge and ideologies of multiple disciplines and various modes of self-actualization, our curriculum and environment deprive us of meaningful channels of expression other than those of medical foci.

To illustrate our need for a university-patterned program of study, the senior class offered the Department of Nursing a symbol of our dilemma, a sign to be placed upon the residence hall and to read — Columbia University Department of Nursing.

The administration rejected our gift. Dissatisfied with the credibility of its rationale for declination, the senior class concluded that the nuclear issues of our syndrome had to be heard. Our pleas for too long have fallen upon deaf ears; intervention at this point is critical.

Complaints from students about the School's antiquated ways were not new. Lois Mueller Rimmer '60 "seriously thought about scratching the whole thing and going back to college and majoring in history. There was very much of the 'old school' mentality. You had a real probationary period and you had to wear the dark uniform and black stockings and shoes. It was very regimented."

Bettie Jackson also recalls a curriculum that was too clinically oriented. "Once we got going full tilt," says the former student government president, "we worked in the Hospital twenty-eight hours a week. After the second semester, many students did a course titled 'Continuity of Care,' which we called 'Evenings and Nights,' because we actually ran the Hospital from midnight to eight in the morning, six shifts straight. Each of us was in charge of twenty-four patients. Then, each morning, we had class from nine to twelve. We would fall asleep listening to lectures on topics like biorhythms, of all things. It didn't make any sense." Clinical supervision, she claimed, was nil. "You had to call the supervisor every time you gave Demerol, but other than that, you were totally on your own."

Keville Frederickson '64, a transfer student from a midwestern nursing program, had a similar experience. "We never did nights at the University of Illinois," she says. "The reason we were on a clinical unit was to learn, and we had very specific objectives. Here I made the mistake to say, 'What are the objectives today?' They just looked at me. I never saw an instructor in the clinical setting at night. The whole mentality was learning by doing. I was shocked with the amount of clinical time, and with how devalued the intellectual part of nursing was, with the exception of Dorothy Reilly and a few other teachers."

These three discontents did not protest the School's academic shortcomings, however. "Students were more compliant in those days," notes Jackson, who joined the faculty soon after graduation. "I was thrilled to be at Columbia; it was a privilege. I wasn't in a position to question things."

But as youths around the nation started to question their elders, so did students at the School of Nursing. More and more of its enrollees were like Palmer Blakely '73 and Alexandra O'Shea '73, two of several Columbia nursing students profiled in a 1972 *New York Times* article. In her prenursing days, Blakely had campaigned for presidential candidate Eugene McCarthy, lobbied for local political reform, and marched in antiwar protests in Chicago and Washington. "You'll find as high a percentage of political activists here as in any law school," she was quoted as saying. Before coming to Columbia, O'Shea had dropped out of college to teach on an Indian reservation, but found that unsatisfying as well. "I didn't feel I was

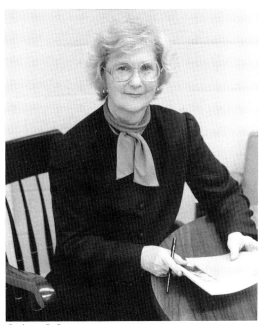

JoAnn S. Jamann

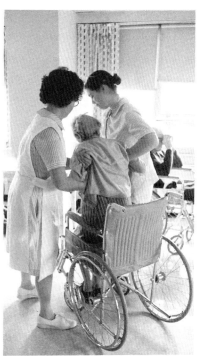

Above: *Nursing at Isabella Geriatric Center, clinical affiliate, 1981*

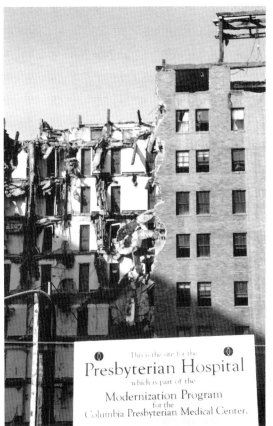

Left: *The last days of Maxwell Hall, 1984*

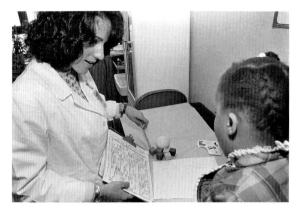

Left: *Graduate student Lisa Iannacci '77 assessing a preschooler at P.S. 223 in Jamaica, Queens, 1988*

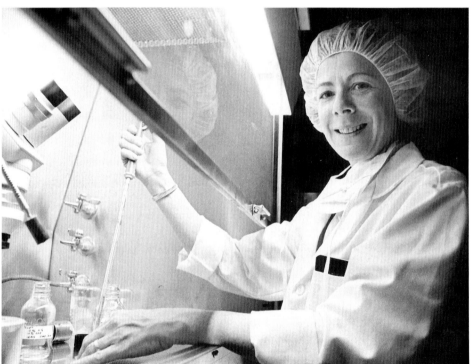

Above: *Faculty member Rae Janet Jacobs-Cohen, nurse and neurobiologist*

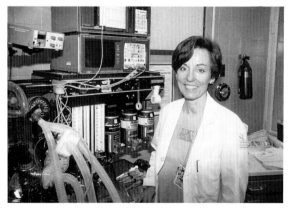

Left: *Assistant Dean for Student Affairs Theresa Doddato, nurse anesthetist, at Roosevelt Hospital, her faculty practice site, 1989*

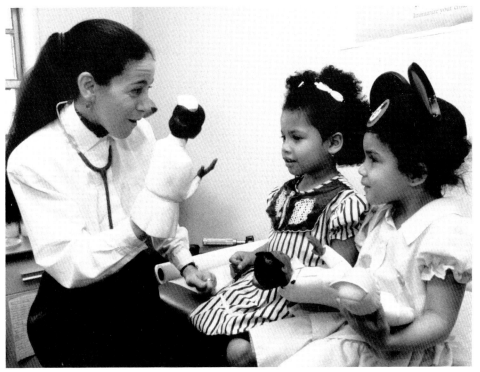

Above: *Judy Honig, pediatric nurse practitioner, at her faculty practice, a school-based clinic in the Bronx, 1990*

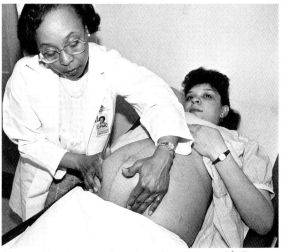

Above: *Faculty member Betty Carrington, Ph.D., nurse midwife, conducting research into manual methods of estimating fetal size and weight, 1987*

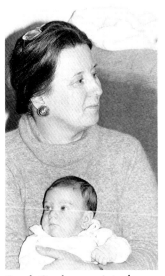

Sarah Cook, associate dean for academic and clinical affairs, 1988

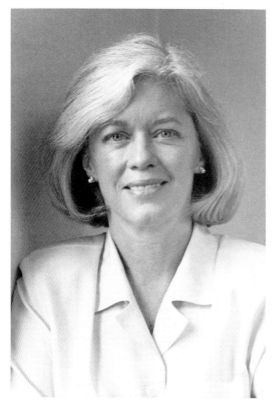

Dean Mary O. Mundinger

Below: *Dean Mundinger with 1990 commencement speaker, New York City Mayor David N. Dinkins, his daughter, Donna Dinkins-Hoggard '90, and granddaughter*

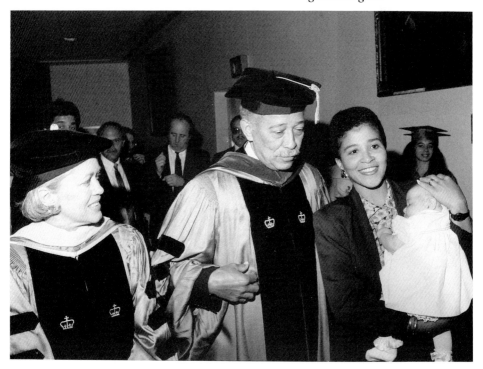

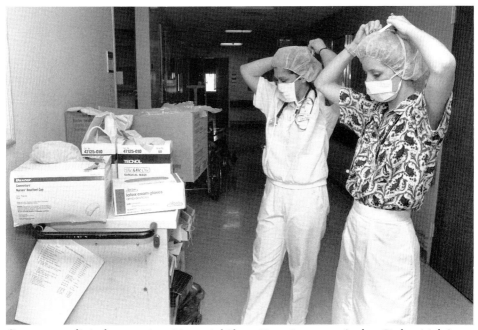

One-to-one clinical precepting: Memorial Sloan-Kettering nurse Andrea Dolan (right) with student Victoria Josof '91, 1990

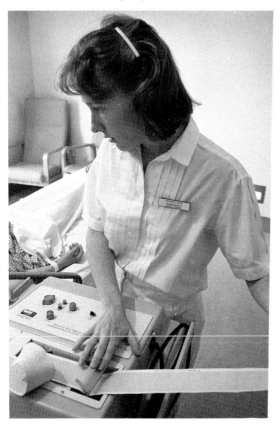

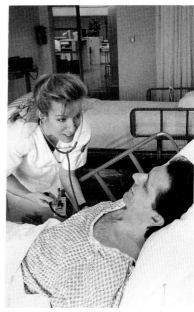

Above: *Susan Miller '89, 1989*

Left: *Kathleen McCooe '89, 1989*

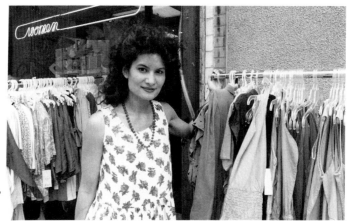

Bonnie Yim '91, former dress designer

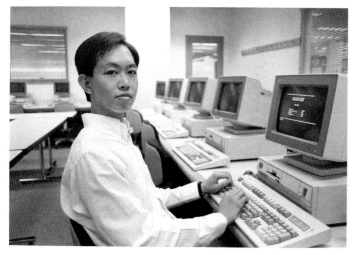

Eric Chong '90, computer science major

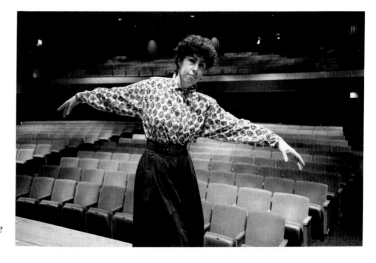

Leslie Kotin '91 ex-dancer and movement science major

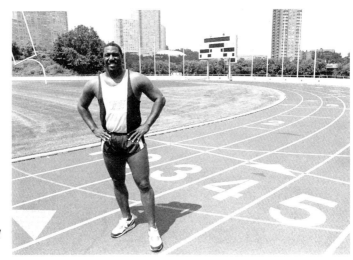

*Kevin Pugh '91,
former college
football star and
salesman*

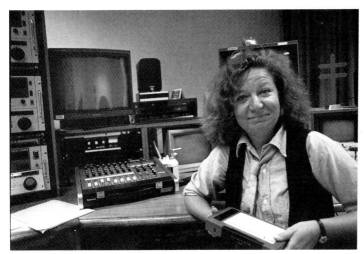

*Connie Milner '90,
former New York
area Emmy Awards
administrator*

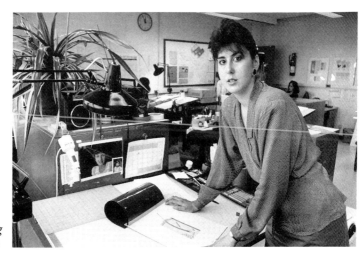

*Lee Stelter '91,
former advertising
account executive*

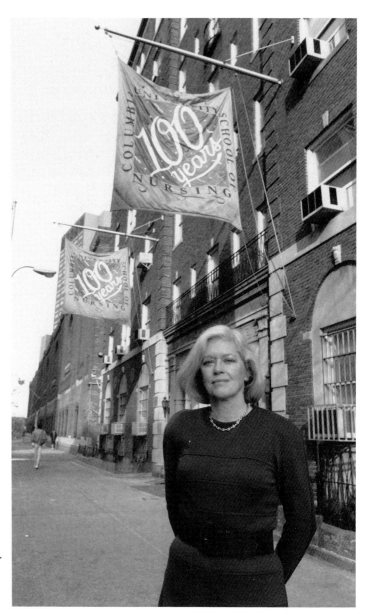

Mary Mundinger in front of the School's current residence, 1992

accomplishing anything," she remarked. "I decided there was a cultural conflict [in teaching Indians], and I have very strong feelings about the destruction of culture. I got mad at the government and decided that there were two things I could do: become President of the United States or work with people on a one-to-one basis."

The Blakelys and O'Sheas were quick to voice their complaints, particularly when their lofty ideals of nursing ran head on into the gritty realities of hospital practice. They found many people to blame, from chauvinistic physicians to "unnatural" nurses. The "ideal versus the real," as the general debate was labeled, became the topic of two student-faculty forums during the 1969-70 academic year and numerous *Alumnae Magazine* articles. Student leader Patricia Schadt '71 wrote,

> Students are expected to be always pleasant, efficient, and under control of the situation at all times. The student is taught to perform according to the expectations of the instructor. If a student cannot measure up to such standards she quickly wins disapproval from her [clinical] instructor, and her clinical grade suffers for it.
>
> This type of role-teaching struck the student forum participant as unnatural to one's own personality. She believes that trying to conform to such a stereotype stifles the individuality of the person. Unless a nurse can react humanly in situations, being able to cry with a patient if the need arises, or get justifiably angry with a patient, nursing care will become superficial and hypocritical...
>
> [Faculty] are afraid to let their feelings show with students, trying to maintain a superior, professional attitude at the expense of their individuality...
>
> To repress the communication of such needs to others and assume the air of perfect physiological well-being creates only frustration and loneliness for both faculty and students.

Irked by Schadt's comments, alumna Louise Schlicting '44, responded:

> As a student at Columbia-Presbyterian, and as a diploma school faculty member, I have known many teachers to "relate meaningfully" with students and yet maintain the "ideal nurse image." I have also known some who lost it trying to curry favor by communication of their own human needs. I feel grateful that our school still presents this image of being "pleasant, efficient and under control of the situation at all times." This does not preclude expressing empathy with the patient and most good experienced faculty members express it with their students too.
>
> Part of the value of being a Columbia-Presbyterian graduate is that many doctors and employers have learned over the years to expect us to maintain "superior professional attitudes" and at the same time to express our own warm, understanding personalities. Believe me, both can be done.

And Ardyce Hoover Peck '51 retorted, "To say we should cry with the patient is ridiculous ... I have been proud that I have been able to smile throughout whatever the situation has been." She recommended that students listen to their instructors and afterward, "Discard what you don't believe."

Some members of the faculty, on the other hand, found merit in the students' protestations. Frederickson, then an instructor in nursing, wrote, "The student nurse watches hospital staff breaking nurse care principles, cutting corners and placing patient needs at the end of the priority list. When these things occur, the student is unable to find or identify with a realistic hospital nurse as a role model. Therefore she may incorporate the 'ideal' of the instructor though this is not seen in actuality. Thus the dichotomy is formed between the staff and instructor, or ideal and the real. Also emphasizing this problem is the instructor, who sends double messages by teaching the optimal nursing care yet silently observing the execution of poor nursing."

And a sympathetic Mary Crawford offered,

> We have spent too much time teaching students an ideal kind of care and have failed to teach them how to attain this ideal. Our students must learn in their basic program the theory and principles of bringing about change. We must stop thinking that we must have an ideal situation in which to teach nursing. Every one of our students is going to be faced with less than an ideal situation. Are we going to teach her how to study the strengths of the head nurse, to build on those strengths in her efforts to improve patient care so that the head nurse will begin to recognize and utilize some of her strengths? Or are we going to turn her into an unhappy, destructive critic, roaming the country looking for the ideal her teachers kept talking about and never finding it?

But they were already too late, according to Schadt, who said:

> A random sampling of the senior class ... revealed that the majority of those interviewed do not intend to work as a nurse on a hospital staff for their careers. If anything, the picture they have formed of hospital nursing as students has disillusioned many about the role of the nurse as a hospital health team member. They point out that while their educational program encourages creative thinking and independence, the reality of working in the hospital does not lend itself to such ideals. The hospital nurse is seen working below her potential and being unable to initiate care on her own ...
>
> The disadvantages of hospital staff nursing, its meniality, its authoritarian hierarchy, and the internecine hostility among the various health professionals exist as formidable barriers against the young and educated idealistic nurse.

Administrative positions offered the best opportunity to foster change, the students believed, but they wanted to work with patients—"where the action is." As the sixties progressed, fewer and fewer of the School's new graduates stayed on at the Medical Center to start their careers. "Many graduates went elsewhere to look for work, to look for nirvana," says Sarah Cook.

Columbia nursing students weren't alone in their frustration, reported Robert Elliot, M.D., associate dean at P&S. While attending the 1968 American Nurses' Association convention, he noticed a great deal of dissatisfaction among current baccalaureate students and recent graduates. "The nursing educators just can't seem to believe that they are not teaching their young ladies how to nurse," he reported.

Veteran nurses like Joanne Yodice Heide '65 were not so alarmed. "I wonder if they [the students] realize that new graduates have always been anxious about confronting this ultimate test," she wrote some years later.

Cook does not question Elliot's assessment, but believes there was another dynamic at play. "Students and new graduates were shocked about real practice because they were not astute in the politics of health care—and neither were we in the faculty," she says. "We felt that if we presented data, the facts, that the physician and hospital administrators would listen. That was the dumbest and most naive conclusion that we ever came to."

Thus the School routinely produced graduates like Faith Harley Howarth '61, well-prepared clinicians but ill-prepared "politicians." "Female-dominated professions," she said in 1981, "even after many years of proving their worth…can't prove they are critical occupations in the way that would earn or mandate society's respect, recognition and reward. I didn't know all this in 1961…Innocence with a white cap. [I was] educated to think and analyze, plan and provide high quality, professional nursing care. Symbolically, I was clutching a white candle, in search of the suffering of the world who were patiently, yet eagerly awaiting me and my services in dark corners. In search of a niche into which all my knowledge would fit, be used, appreciated and valued, I went forth." The niche was not there. Like many other graduates of her time, she had to carve one of her own.

Further controversies pitted students against their elders, or at least progressives against traditionalists. One by one, the symbols and traditions of the Columbia nurse vanished. To the new generation, they were emblematic of the longstanding oppression of nurses and women. The uniform, for example, was replaced by a simpler, short-sleeved, wash-and-wear version, partly because facilities for cleaning, pressing, and starching the uniforms were inadequate and partly because the design was old-fashioned and cumbersome. The updated design was in turn replaced by a simple striped blouse. The famous stripes disappeared altogether in the early eighties.

The cap vanished, too. Student Brita Carhart '74 objected to the cap because it "seems to widen the gap between health workers: setting nurses on an elitist pedestal (second only to doctors) ... Psychiatric nurses wear no caps and I've yet to hear an uproar questioning their pride in nursing. Nurses in a variety of settings wear street clothes and are still identifiable ... Perhaps the cap is also just another (weakening) means of romanticizing nursing as it existed in the 19th century."

Bettie Jackson, a doctoral candidate in 1974, the height of the cap controversy, agreed. "Traditions that serve a purpose ... are obviously worthwhile," she wrote in the *Alumnae Magazine*. "The nurse's cap is not such a tradition. While it is true that a cap serves to identify a nurse, it also identifies a dental hygienist. And men in nursing don't wear caps. So the profession no longer truly has a distinguishing feature in the cap ... They are cumbersome when working with bulky patient care equipment and they are symbolic of the staid and old fashion ... It's about time we stopped hiding behind traditional garb and *distinguished our profession by our practice* ... Our practice, our modern competencies, based on sound scientific rationales, identify us."

Sylvia Carlson '47, a nurse at Long Island Jewish–Hillside Medical Center, noted that her employer let nurses choose whether or not they would wear a cap and that 99 percent did not. "In no way has it affected patient care or made our nursing staff 'less dignified,'" she said.

Many alumnae, however, particularly older ones, were deeply troubled (forgetting that Anna Maxwell never wore her cap and somehow prospered). Edna Nelson '55 wrote that she "took pride in the old-fashioned ... uniform ... It sort of reminded me of the many nurses before me who had followed certain of the old traditions, but because of the magnitude of the University, our sights and goals were always of the most high and most progressive. Progress is marvelous but some of the older traditions should not always be discarded."

Phyllis Loomis '46 replied that the idea of a capless nurse made her bristle: "I agree nurses should not require a cap to uphold their qualifications, but I do feel it is the crowning touch to a well-chosen profession."

"I love my 'P.H.' cap and all it has meant to me through the years," Helen L. De Witt '32 commented. "It reminds me with a warm glow of Helen Young and the 'Anna Maxwell' we never knew but always revered ... and some of the most wonderful people in the whole world. Tell the young lady

[Jackson] to wait until she is out in the world a few years longer, and she'll treasure her 'P.H.' cap." (De Witt wasn't far off the mark. Jackson recently commented, "There was something about the uniforms the graduate nurses and faculty wore that carried a certain aura of confidence and power that I regret nursing seems to have thrown out. There is an old-fashioned piece of me, which must come from my Columbia days, that feels there are certain ways that a professional nurse dresses and bears herself. It should instill in the patient a certain sense of confidence and trust.")

And Ruth Simpson '09 added, "I am one of those old fogies who think a nurse without a cap would be like a soldier without one—an incomplete uniform... The 'capping ceremony' is an event in one's nursing career and its abolishment would detract from pride in the profession."

Helen Pettit believes the uniform, if not the cap, will come back, "because it served a great purpose to the patient and the family and the visitors, distinguishing them from all the other hospital personnel."

Perhaps the wisest comment on the whole topic was delivered three decades earlier, at the 1942 commencement, by the Reverend Donald B. Aldrich of New York's Church of Ascension: "The only reason I can imagine for wearing [the cap] is that it does do one thing—it makes you remember that you have a head. And how in the days before you, you will have to use it."

Another uniform imbroglio arose in 1977 over a rule requiring the uniform to be worn at commencement. Unable to convince the student graduation committee to overturn the rule, thirty-six seniors (about a quarter of the class) and twelve instructors signed a petition stating, in part, "We feel and agree that the traditional white uniform is not always identified with professional nursing," which was sent to P&S Dean Donald F. Tapley, M.D. Tapley replied that majority opinion ought to rule.

The time-honored Dedication Ceremony was the next tradition to wither. The ceremony was started in the days of the Presbyterian Hospital School of Nursing to acknowledge the students' successful passage through the probationary period. It was a proud moment, when students shed the dull-gray beginner's uniform for the prestigious blue-and-white stripes. But by 1975 there was little enthusiasm or money for such a ceremony, usually an elaborate dinner with a speaker, music, and flowers. "Who in this day and age is enthused about traditions and ceremonies?" asked one junior. "I'm not dedicating myself to a profession. All I care about is what's happening between me and the patients." "Dedication? The whole ceremony is meaningless," added another. "I've decided that I want to be a nurse. I don't need to walk across a stage and light a candle to show that I am dedicated." (Ironically, the rituals originated with the students, albeit of an earlier generation. It was first called the Capping Ceremony, because successful probies were awarded the Presbyterian cap. Later, when the probationary interval was eliminated, the full uniform, save the white stockings, was given to beginning students. The ceremony was then renamed, with dedication to nursing as the theme.)

The ceremony meant something to Mary Mueller '75, however. "It's just not possible to simply enter through one door marked 'nursing' and exit with a B.A. through another," she contended. "Constant personal re-evaluations are part of nursing education. By the time the student reaches the midpoint of the second semester, the frustrations of nursing school are met head-on. It seems to me rather than barreling through angry, annoyed, disappointed, it is essential that there be a formalized something that says: 'Stop. Look where you've been ... where you're going ... what you want now ... what it means in terms of your personal goals.'" Mueller scrambled to arrange a ceremony for the juniors, but only 48 of 125 showed up. As in the past, each nurse was called up to the front to light a candle and sign a pledge book, but this one featured a new updated pledge written by 1969 graduates Joan Hagan and Parker Weisheit. The pledge read:

> We dedicate our professional lives to nursing care of quality. To achieve this ideal we must know ourselves, and know that we are an influential force in our relationships with patients and society. For ourselves we seek sensitivity, perception, judgment, creativity, honor, enlightenment, scholarship and, as in any relationship, the fulfillment of our own needs. This is our directive: a concern and a willingness to act not only for the individual but also for the community of peoples. Every person deserves to be respected as an individual, and as a member of a culture, to be provided with available health services, not only to live, but also to die, with dignity, and we will attempt to assure these rights. Ours is to make the ideal of quality in our care of people a reality.

Quite a contrast to the Nightingale Pledge, in which the nurse swore before God to "pass my life in purity ... [and] to abstain from whatever is deleterious and mischievous."

Student George Morton '76 also addressed the students' Holy Grail of "ideal" care in his address at the Dedication Ceremony: "We are here to dedicate ourselves to a profession, nursing — a profession whose values and ideals have taken on personal meaning for us. Columbia has generated another feeling — a feeling for which we were not prepared:

frustration." They were frustrated with the artificial clinical experiences, with lectures that did not meet their needs, and with exams that did not reflect the knowledge they had learned. "And, finally," he added, "we feel frustrated when we wonder whether the regimen we are going through will prepare us to be the kind of nurses we want to become."

"Does this mean the School and students have lost the sense of charm and tradition that you and I knew?" queried Susan M. Rockwell '64, editor of the *Alumnae Magazine,* in reaction to the ceremony.

"Yes, it probably does mean the school and students have lost the sense of charm that ... you knew," answered Louise Dodd '76. But it does not mean that we are not dedicated to the profession of nursing.

> We are no longer a lonely outpost perched on a hill, we are part of the hurting, teeming community. We can no longer venture very far into new surroundings without feelings of visual or verbal abuse. Maxwell Hall is a security risk—any stranger entering the front door is automatically suspect until properly identified.
> I find little charm in the $6,000-plus fees I pay each year to be a student ... I regard myself as a Columbia University student, not a Columbia University-Presbyterian Hospital student. The scope of education has broadened and subsequently many of the homey, charming aspects of a small school have fallen by the way ... I am committed to nursing ... But I don't wear it on my sleeve.

It could be argued that Dodd and her peers were *more* dedicated than their predecessors, at least in the sense that they were more likely to make a career of nursing and not retire because of marriage or parenthood. As Ruth Runge Marsh '53 noted, "After talking with many, many inactive nurses, I have concluded that their dedication to *family* comes before dedication to *nursing*." The last Dedication Ceremony was held in the late-seventies.

Never before had such a generation gap divided nursing. The children of the sixties and seventies, for example, were no longer willing to pay heed to the unstated rules of etiquette that governed nurse-physician relations, to stand when a doctor entered the room or let him enter the elevator first. These were symbols of nurses' oppression, they would say, symbols that belonged in the hospital's incinerator with the rest of the medical waste.

Earlier generations of nurses, in contrast, ignored the symbolism and focused on the practicalities. Former Director of Nursing at Presbyterian Margaret Eliot, for instance, lectured students to put up with the physician's ignoble behavior in order to get him out of their hair. "Look, he's only going to cause you trouble," she reportedly reasoned. "Don't let him get into your sterile dishes because he'll put the lid down and you'll have it all to boil over again. Don't let him go through the charts—hand him the charts and let him go."

Helen Pettit thought these nurse-physician interactions were "fun," an entertaining part of hospital nursing. She recalls how J. Bentley Squier, M.D., the famous urologist, would conduct rounds in tails on Sunday mornings and stop by the nursing stations to check supplies for dirt and dust. "What we went through to get everything fine on the surface — because there was no earthly way to clean everything," she says. "He was a bright man and had to know this was going on, and he must have laughed his head off. Why he or we kept it up I'll never know. Everybody got along fine and you didn't pay a lot of attention to the formalities except with certain powers that be."

To the new generation of students, however, the finely choreographed dance of etiquette between physicians and nurses was not an entertainment. It was a demeaning cultural artifice, a symbol of nurses' and women's oppression.

"Who created these students?" alumni must have wondered. "What happened to the traditional Columbia-Presbyterian nurse, who was forthright but discreet, defiant but ultimately deferential?" Society, of course, was to blame or to credit. But so was the School of Nursing. While the School remained a fairly conservative place, it apparently made no attempt to censor the progressive nursing outlook. On numerous occasions, prominent alumnae, faculty members, and guest speakers urged students to break traditions, vigorously and vocally.

In her welcoming address to the class of 1969, Virginia Henderson, the distinguished professor of nursing from Yale, remarked,

> Since nursing is necessarily affected by the era and the surrounding culture, nurses cannot ... escape the obligation of trying to change it ... This means we must be, to some extent, philosophers — people who "search into the reason and nature of things, who study society as a whole." ... We must also be statesmen or philosophers who act on their convictions.
>
> All the burning social questions that are discussed in the news media and in conversation ... affect nursing: How to stop war, how to control crime, how to provide equal opportunities regardless of sex, race, creed or color; how to protect the young and old, and how to heal the breach between youth and age ... Our potential influence as citizens is incalculable because of our numbers, our experience, our level of intelligence and training.

Six years later, commencement speaker Shirley Smoyak, Ph.D., professor of nursing at Rutgers, remarked, "How will you keep your balance — if tradition is no longer operative as in the past? The answer is very simple and direct — you set a new tradition for nursing, one based on practitioners who are sophisticated, have high self-esteem and are articulate, knowledgeable, energetic and self-directed, and who work with others in a colleagueship manner. Now that shouldn't be too difficult. From what I've heard, you have been functioning in that way already." She added that new graduates have the power to ask unsettling questions. "These are allowed of novices since they can't be expected to know ... The new nurse — in a new tradition — is a systems analyst. Change cannot be recommended in a haphazard manner. Nurses will have to be politically astute. Think of political expertise, as well as nursing expertise, when you are planning your continuing education."

The following year, Beth Berman '69 told the seniors, "You have become adults in a country that spends billions of dollars and thousands of lives in war abroad, yet cuts back jobs and closes medical facilities when financial crises arise at home." But, she noted, this is an era of "possibilities." The system could be changed, and it was within their power to act or not act.

The students listened and learned. "In a nutshell, we are given an education that should make it difficult to accept the status quo," student Louise Dodd noted. "We are change agents."

But by and large, the faculty and the administration did not get the message, possibly because *they* were the status quo. Tradition had served them well, so why change? Part of the problem was that many had known no other type of nursing. More than half of the eighty-four member 1967-68 faculty (full and part time), including the top five leaders, were Presbyterian or Columbia nursing graduates, and another ten had some sort of Columbia degree.

"As a faculty member, I was distressed because the students were fighting our battles, which we should have fought long ago," says Dorothy Reilly, Ed.D., probably the School's most progressive educator in the 1960s. "They wanted to know why more nurses were not on the Faculty of Medicine — the policy-making group — and who was speaking for us. They challenged the dean, asking what position she took. As a result of the student protests, there was a change and a lot of faculty came forward. It was something nobody had ever experienced before. In nursing, you sort of stayed in your little bailiwick and did your own thing." But the students of this era wouldn't have that. During the Columbia protests, Reilly notes, "many of the faculty were unsure where they should be or shouldn't be. The students cared less whether you were with them or against them, but they sure were upset if you didn't have a position."

Elsewhere, schools of nursing were advancing more rapidly, supporting more research, hiring more doctorally prepared faculty, opening more graduate programs. "There were creative people on the faculty," asserts Reilly, "but we were bound down by some of the clingers-on. "We were coming out from under momma — the maternalistic model."

Sarah Cook concurs: "When I first started teaching here, it would drive me crazy when I would bring up an idea in a meeting and I would get beaten down. People tried to conduct research because that was the thing academic nurses were supposed to do. But you completed your other responsibilities first, namely teach your class and supervise clinical experiences."

Individual faculty members, particularly "outsiders" like Constance Baker Ort, assistant professor nursing, started to worry. In a 1974 issue of the *Alumni Magazine,* she warned that "the very survival of nursing is dependent on our ability to systematically structure and verify the theoretical core of nursing knowledge, yet scholarship in nursing is very unpopular." Nursing, she added, needed to foster an atmosphere receptive to nursing science, synthesize the teacher-scholar and practitioner-scholar roles, and teach students to embrace scholarly work. But it would be many years before these goals were institutionalized at Columbia.

One of the most noteworthy changes at the School of Nursing during the 1960s was the enrollment of minorities. In years past, there were no Lester Maddoxes standing in the doorway denying entry to people of color, but neither were there policies or programs or scholarships that encouraged them to enroll. Consequently, the School's "color barrier" was not broken until the early 1960s, when the nation started to stir out of its long complacency toward racial inequality.

"It was the nature of the profession," believes Sarah Cook, "particularly the top levels of baccalaureate nursing education. For most of the School's history, there were innumerable people willing to come here, and they tended to be white and Anglo-Saxon. Others weren't excluded; they just didn't apply. Nor was there much effort to recruit other types of students."

"Among practically all groups of white nurses, whether involved in hospital work, private practice, educational institutions, public health associations, or professional organizations, located in the North or South, the predominant image of the black nurse was that of a moral and social inferior," writes Darlene Clark Hine in *Black Women in White*. Whether this attitude prevailed at the School of Nursing is hard to tell. However, Presbyterian Hospital, an institution originally intended for people of all colors, was not always as fair-minded as it professed to be. "When I was at Presbyterian," remembers Elizabeth Colmers Standen '40, "I had a black friend, a doctor at Vanderbilt Clinic, who couldn't get his pregnant wife a private room. I went out of my mind. Here was this beautiful plaque in front of the Hospital, which read 'Without Regard to Race, Creed, or Color,' and it didn't admit blacks in the private pavilion, there were no black attending physicians, no black nurses, and no black nursing students. It was the times, I guess. Nobody thought about it. But I believed every word the plaque said. What they taught us in School was antidiscrimination. Helen Young instilled in us the ethical, warm, loving part of nursing."

But on at least one occasion Young was a party to discrimination. When Margaret Lawrence, one of the first black women to enroll at P&S, applied for an internship at Babies Hospital in 1940, she was turned down by Rustin McIntosh, M.D., chief of pediatrics. According to Lawrence, "He said he was pleased that I had applied ... that I was well qualified and they had hoped to accept me for internship. But since there were no quarters for women interns at the doctors' residences, women interns had to stay at the [graduate] nurses' residence ... and the superintendent of nursing [Young] had said that they could not possibly accept Negroes in the nurses' residence."

Presbyterian Hospital was no further along the road to racial equality in the mid-sixties. In 1965 nurse Darline Bacon, who is black, was hired sight unseen, but when she appeared at the personnel office, she was told that the position had already been filled. It had not. Bacon persisted, landing a job at Babies Hospital, where the atmosphere was not much warmer. "I was the only black professional," she remembers. "There were no black doctors. The first day I was there a doctor slapped my hand. He didn't want me to touch his patients."

The first mention of race in the School's papers and publications had appeared in 1948, when the superintendent of Dixie Hospital in Hampton, Va., wrote a letter to the dean of P&S to ask if the Medical Center would participate in a fundraising campaign for black nursing students. "The admission policies of the University apply to [the School of Nursing], and as you know they are very liberal," Conrad responded on the dean's behalf. "The scholarship resources are open to all students in nursing, as those in other divisions of the University. We do not, there-fore, have any need for special funds as you suggest. It would not be practical for Columbia University to take part in a fund-raising cam-paign for one group of students in a special field."

Conrad apparently was not bothered that the School had never had a black student or faculty member (nor had most other schools of nurs-ing). And, by leaving the recruitment process be, she did nothing to improve the chances that the School would soon have any minorities. As before, the School's best recruiters were the all-white, upper-middle-class alumnae, who had minimal contact with young blacks or Hispanics.

Finally, in 1962, a black student, Imodale Kelfa-Caulker '65 from Ghana, found her way into the School of Nursing. Two years later, stu-dents and faculty, awakened by the civil rights movement, met to discuss racial issues in the country and at the School. Committees were formed to recruit minority students by working with guidance counselors and Future Nurses' Clubs in high schools and by writing magazine articles. While laudable, their efforts largely failed.

When, in 1966, Alvin W. Poussaint, M.D., of the Medical Committee for Human Rights, heard of the School's record in minority enrollment, he wrote to Elizabeth Gill, the School's leader for most of the decade: "I was shocked to read in the *New York Times* recently that you have *no* Negro nursing students enrolled. This is unbelievable in this day and age. Something is obviously wrong with your student recruitment program that reflects either conscious or unconscious racial bias."

Gill protested (perhaps a bit too much): "You will find we have admitted and graduated two Negro students before there was open concern in this matter. Two will be admitted this month* ... Additionally, we have employed several Negro faculty members. Many factors mitigate against Negro students seeking admission to collegiate nursing programs. Nurs-ing does not have the status or potential for financial gain that many col-lege bound students seek." Suggestions as to where one could locate well-qualified minority applicants were welcomed, she added.

In subsequent years, more minorities enrolled, but the School's makeup did not come close to reflecting that of society at large. Displeased with the School's progress, the Black Caucus of Columbia-Presbyterian Medical Center, an organization composed of employees, students, and house staff, wrote in 1970 to Mary Crawford, then the School's director, "We ... are appalled and deeply concerned over the lack of Black students in

* One of those students was Faye Wattleton, now president of the Planned Parenthood Federation of America.

the School of Nursing. In view of the fact that so many Blacks comprise the staff of the Medical Center and environs, not to mention the number of Black teaching patients, we feel that there should be a greater Black representation. We would appreciate knowing if any steps are being taken to alleviate this problem and would appreciate hearing from you." Because the letter lacked a personal signature (it had an address), P&S administrator Robert Elliot advised Crawford not to respond, and she did not.

By and large, the few black students who did enroll got a warm reception from their peers. Olga Brown-Vanderpool '70, the only black in her class, was elected class president. Patients, too, generally reacted well. On the wards, Brown-Vanderpool reports, the color of her uniform blinded patients to the color of her skin. "The uniform was very outstanding, so you got respect from the nurses and the aides and the patients," she says. "Even the students from other hospitals respected you for being a Columbia nursing student."

Over the years she has wondered why not one instructor stepped forth to become her mentor. "It seems to me that, coming close to graduation, some of the staff could have asked me, 'What do you want to do? Do you want to go on to graduate school? This is where we see you having an aptitude.' I do that routinely with nursing students, regardless of their color," says Brown-Vanderpool, now director of visiting nursing for the city of Stamford, Conn.

The faculty were embroiled in several purported bias incidents, exposing the administration's insensitivity to minority needs and concerns. After investigating the incidents, P&S Associate Dean George Lythcott, M.D., wrote to Dean Paul Marks, M.D.,

> I, frankly, don't know what we can do about the iceberg that underlies the attached tip … The Nursing School, it would seem, does not have a rational system for arriving at what ultimately become very important policy decisions (to the student), or at least a rationale that they can defend to objective observers … [T]he Nursing School administration is probably absolutely correct in the final decisions arrived at, but they are made to look bad when a confrontation occurs … I must add that a complete lack of sensitivity exists in some quarters of the Nursing School administration about the Black/White issue which I feel underlies their unwillingness to address the issue of a rational system; a type of indifference of apathy which I, of course, find incomprehensible in 1971.

The School's treatment of minority faculty members was also incomprehensible, according to Darline Bacon, who was hired to teach public health in 1967. By accident, she discovered that her salary was far lower than that of a less-experienced, less-credentialed white colleague. She immediately confronted Gill. "Her response was not that I didn't deserve a raise," Bacon recalls, "it was: 'How did you find that out? We don't discuss salaries here.'" Gill stalled, but Bacon (a veteran civil rights campaigner) persevered, winning a substantial, though still not equitable, raise. Throughout her stay, Bacon established cordial and sometimes close relationships with her colleagues, but most considered her oversensitive to racial issues. "My issue was that *they* were *insensitive*," she says, adding that the students were much more accepting. "They were the joy of my life."

On the surface, it looked as though the School of Nursing had started to confront its discrimination demons. In the autumn of 1970, Bacon, who had been on sabbatical the previous academic year, was appointed to the newly formed post of Recruiter of Minority Group Students. Bacon's task was to recruit minorities, find money for financial aid, and offer guidance and academic support. "It sounded to me as though they wanted to give the impression of recruiting without real commitment to bringing in students who had the academic ability but not the money," she claims. Bacon took the position anyway, but her fears were eventually realized. "I was told that if we found qualified students, we would find a way to get them in. That wasn't the case. It was farcical." She resigned before the year was out. "Not one student was admitted as a result of my recruitment. Not one."

Minority enrollment increased slightly with the beginning of the four-year curriculum in 1973 yet remained low until the 1980s.

Another "minority" group arrived on campus during this era. In 1970, Ramon Lavandero '72 and John Mladinich '72 became the first men to enroll at the School of Nursing in its seventy-eight-year history. (One man applied in 1968 but was turned down or decided not to attend.) As with blacks, men were neither discouraged nor encouraged to apply — and few did, to Columbia or any other nursing program. Men accounted for only 1 percent of the nation's active nurses in 1960. But slowly, men started to migrate to the profession, recognizing (thanks in part to the women's movement) the absurdity of occupational genderization.

Both Lavandero and Mladinich received a warm welcome from their classmates. "We welcome the boys and hope there will be more coming in the future," one female student remarked. In turn, one of the men said, "They sort of 'sister' us and make us feel a part of the group."

Lavandero was less pleased with the administration's laissez-faire response to men in nursing. He found it "inconceivable" that the University could integrate men into a historically female-dominated School "without further ado." "I sought the experiences I wished and, with more or less effort, obtained most of them. I encountered no concerted effort to constrain me," he conceded in the *Alumnae Magazine*. "Yet, no concerted effort was made to facilitate me ... The denial of having men in the nursing program had to be confronted. The faculty was at a loss. Sadly, those instructors directly involved were provided minimal or no guidance in dealing with their very real feelings about men in nursing which surfaced. Needless to say, the students involved received even less support." He predicted larger problems if the issue was not fully addressed. However, since few men enrolled in the ensuing years, the School safely ignored them.

But the leave-it-alone approach made life unpleasant at times for the men. "There were faculty who had great difficulty dealing with men in their classes," said Jerold Cohen '74. Men, he theorized, posed a threat of some sort. "Nursing had been the instructors' one and only choice of profession, unlike most of the male students. We didn't grow up wanting to be nurses ... They couldn't accept that." In the clinical setting, he added, the men were sometimes used for their brawn rather than their brains.

David Ekstrom '75, one of four men in his class, was also stereotyped. "A lot of time I felt I was being asked to represent the man's view," he said. "Being placed in that position was a pain in the neck." But, he contends, the faculty showed no animosity and gave him much support and encouragement. Actually, he believes he was treated better than his female classmates. His one distasteful encounter in the clinical setting was "a private duty nurse who told me outright: 'Get out of here; there's no reason you should be here.' She was horrendous."

Ken Zwolski '78 enjoyed "being somewhat of a pioneer." Like most other male students, he was embarking upon a second career and was older than the typical undergraduate. He was supported by his wife (a nurse) as well as his friends, who "thought it was a really hip thing to do. Maybe it had to do with my choice of friends to begin with." After graduation, Zwolski found that sexual bias could work in his favor. "The first time I'm on a floor," he said in 1983, when he was a faculty member, "a doctor will often come up and start consulting with me. They just start talking about a case, so I start talking back. It gives me a good opportunity to show that nurses know a lot, too."

When Craig La Russo '83 chose nursing as a career, his family was sharply divided. His father thought he was settling for second best; however, his brother, a medical student, was very supportive.

Richard Gallagher '86, a successful freelance medical writer in his mid-fifties when he enrolled, elicited all sorts of reactions. "My sister and brother were astonished that I would do such a thing. My brother is business-oriented and couldn't quite understand. My sister brought up the usual questions of homosexuality and questioned why I was throwing away a perfectly good freelance career." Those responses did not deter Gallagher, who relished the thought of playing against type. Whenever he was asked, "Why nursing?" he would reply, "I want to marry a rich doctor." Because of his graying hair and wrinkled face, he is not sure if the reactions he evoked were due to his age or his gender. "Other students would wonder whether to call me Mr. Gallagher or Richard. I've never figured out how the faculty took to me. I was older than most of them."

One alumnus reported he was repeatedly asked by patients, with a note of surprise, "Oh, you're a nurse? Will you go on to become a doctor?" In time he devised a stock answer, meant to startle them further: "Yes, I intend to get a Ph.D. in nursing."

While all this was occurring, the School moved as best it could to strengthen the curriculum. In the early 1960s the separate introductory courses in science and nursing were combined, culminating decades of efforts to integrate scientific theory into the curriculum. The teaching of basic science was further strengthened in mid-sixties, when the Public Health Service awarded the School a grant to determine which material in the biological and physical sciences should be incorporated in the introductory nursing course. In another PHS-funded study, researchers articulated a role for the clinical nurse specialist in neurology. Other investigators focused on obstetrics and pediatrics material in the undergraduate curriculum, which led to new courses in maternal-child health.

To improve the teaching of acute care nursing, two new courses were added to the third year of the curriculum, "Special Aspects of Surgical Nursing" and "Patient Care During the Twenty-Four Hours." Long-term illness was also given special emphasis in the senior year. Led by Elizabeth Gill, the faculty placed more stress on holistic care. "We began to think more about the whole patient," she said in 1986. "We made time to stop and talk with them, to get their views and find out what was troubling them. While I was a student and a head nurse, we were never encouraged to do that. Now students are encouraged at every turn."

Recognizing the broadening scope of the professional nurse, Gill's teaching staff expanded "Leadership in Nursing" to cover the role of the nurse practitioner. In a related move, the Alpha Zeta Chapter of nursing's National Honor Society, Sigma Theta Tau, was established at the School in mid-1960s with fifty-seven faculty, student, and alumnae members.

Beginning with the 1965-66 academic year, the graduate program was enriched with the addition of a second clinical speciality, psychiatric-community mental health nursing, a response to the post war development of new (mainly pharmacological) treatment modalities for mental illness. The program was directed by Anne Earle, Ed.D., assistant professor of nursing. Over two academic years and one summer (set aside for work experience), students studied such subjects as advanced psychiatric theory, psychiatric nursing concepts, educational processes in society, principles and techniques of research, epidemiology, biostatistics, and administration. Several courses were offered at the School of Social Work, the Graduate School of Arts and Sciences, Teachers College, the School of Public Health, and the New York State Psychiatric Institute. Eventually, clinical sites included the Psychiatric Institute, Harlem Hospital, the 159th Street Block Community Council, Reality House (a drug treatment center), the Visiting Nurse Service, the Grosvenor House (for senior citizens), and the Polo Grounds Housing project. The program was broadened in 1976 with the addition of a pediatric focus.

The undergraduate program won high praise in the late-sixties from the New York Board of Nurse Examiners, which was particularly pleased with the School's close relationship with Presbyterian Hospital. With so many dual appointments, the board wrote, "the faculty is constantly aware of (and may control) developments and changes in the practice of nursing." Further plaudits were given to the psychosocial seminars. "Perhaps one of the most valuable personal development experiences students now have is the series of small group psycho-social seminars which help them to determine their professional role. These seminars undoubtedly promote personal security for the student in her chosen field."

The School of Nursing was noted (less positively) for another reason: it was the longest upper-division collegiate program in the country — a decided recruitment minus. Most students who wanted to earn their baccalaureate in nursing from Columbia had to spend up to five years in college (two years in liberal arts at another institution, plus another three at the School of Nursing), which was costly in both time and money. A Columbia nursing degree, long one of the great bargains in academe, was by the 1960s a substantial financial investment. "It seems to me that you are pricing yourself right out of a future supply of students," complained one parent in response to yet another tuition hike and a first-ever annual fee for room and board. "To increase educational costs while realizing that the earnings of the nurses have not kept pace with those of other professions is quite a paradox," she continued. From her admittedly lay perspective, she (rightly) observed that "the number of hours of work they put in—days, evenings, nights—appear to be considerably beyond mere *training* requirements." Columbia's program was not the most expensive, but it was the lengthiest, a discouragement to students who had to finance their educations and thus wanted to get to work as soon as possible. Gill apologized to parents and alumnae for the high fees, acknowledging the "inconvenience and even downright hardship" they caused. However, she added, the fees did not begin to cover the actual cost of nursing education, which, because of the need for close clinical supervision, was almost four times the cost of other types of undergraduate programs.

The only solution was to shorten the curriculum. Starting in 1966, the regular program (for those with two years of college) was reduced by a full academic year to two academic years plus two summers; the short course for college graduates was reduced by one summer to two academic years plus one summer. Tuition was raised yet again, bringing the total yearly cost of a Columbia nursing education to $4,750. The program was abridged largely by slashing the well-padded clinical schedule (although evening and night duty was still required). Academically it was the same, if a little more concentrated. In the first year, the curriculum covered anatomy and physiology, epidemiology, pathophysiology, essentials of nursing care, general medical-surgical nursing, psychosocial aspects of patient care, philosophy and history of nursing, dynamics of teaching and learning, psychosocial developments in health and disease, nursing in the acute phase of illness, nursing in long-term illness, family behavior in crisis, and maternal-child nursing. The second year covered psychology, public health, community health, leadership in nursing, and independent study.

Also in 1966 the School announced that it would soon admit graduate nurses who wished to improve their academic credentials by earning a baccalaureate in nursing. Applicants with only forty-six liberal arts credits (fourteen fewer than normal) would be accepted, if they completed the remaining credits concurrently with their nursing studies. As many as twenty-four credits would be awarded to candidates who passed clinical competency tests. The response was phenomenal. Over 600 registered nurses made inquiries; however, only one had enough credits to enroll. Guidance and counseling was provided to over one hundred promising candidates over the next year.

The shortening of the program in the mid-sixties not only saved students time and money, it also moved the School closer to another goal: the establishment of a four-year, combined liberal arts–nursing curriculum, operated in conjunction with Columbia's School of General Studies and the University's affiliate, Barnard College. For the first time, in 1973, students enrolled as freshman as candidates for the baccalaureate in nursing (the general scheme in collegiate nursing schools).

There were several reasons for the reorganization. As Crawford told the alumni, nurses must receive a "quality liberal arts education" in order to prepare them to meet "modern nursing's constant demand to adjust to advances in medicine, psychology, and sociology." By bringing students under the Columbia umbrella for their entire undergraduate term, the School could ensure the quality of that education. Of equal importance, the extended curriculum gave students more time to grow accustomed to the role of the nurse and, simultaneously, to view other intellectual horizons. The existing two-year schedule was so packed with nursing material that students commonly wondered if there was life beyond 168th Street. Another impetus for the change was that the School was attracting fewer and fewer junior transfer students. The enrollment of newly minted high school graduates, it was hoped, would reverse this trend. (Transfer students and those with previous degrees were still accepted, but the School intended to phase out the two-year program.)

Under the new plan, which was designed with the assistance of Margaret Tyson of Teachers College and coordinated by Associate Professor of Nursing Constance Cleary, the freshman and sophomore years were mainly, but not exclusively, devoted to the study of liberal arts at either Barnard or the School of General Studies and included required courses in biology, chemistry, psychology, sociology, and English. Concurrently, students were introduced to nursing theory and practice, beginning with a course in community health, which emphasized health promotion and the acquisition of manual and observational skills. Fifteen different community agencies were used for clinical assignments. Nursing content in the sophomore year shifted to family health, with an accent on illness prevention. Several different maternity services were used for hands-on experience.

In the program's second half, the emphasis switched from liberal arts to nursing and from wellness to illness. Juniors delved into the care, cure, and rehabilitation of patients in a variety of settings, honing their problem-solving and clinical skills. Finally, as seniors, they addressed the synthesis and professionalization of practice, with an opportunity to concentrate in primary care, acute care, or health maintenance in either long-term or geriatric care. Seniors also learned the fine points of team leadership and collaboration with other health professionals.

"I would like to see the baccalaureate student learning the role of the patient care coordinator ... " said Mary Crawford.

> Nurses will have to carry a much greater share of the load in health teaching, in screening for illness, in coordinating the multitude of different health workers who will be involved in giving acute care, and in providing restorative or rehabilitative care to those with chronic illness...
>
> Many institutions are experimenting with the nurse clinician, a nurse with a master's preparation in a particular clinical area of nursing. Hospitals are experimenting with the use of the baccalaureate graduate in the patient care coordinator role. This is the head nurse minus the management activities but also with a new philosophy. She is responsible for giving care to a specific group of patients in a particular setting, 24 hours a day, 7 days a week ... She is responsible for assessing patient needs and deciding who can best care for each patient. In some cases, she gives direct care herself. In other cases, she assigns that care to a technical nurse, a practical nurse, or an auxiliary worker...
>
> We can no longer employ baccalaureate degree graduates, diploma graduates, associate degree graduates, and practical nurses to do the same job.

The program was supported administratively, financially, intellectually, and clinically by P&S affiliates St. Luke's Hospital and Roosevelt Hospital, which were closing their respective and respected diploma programs but wished to continue some connection to nursing education. (Harlem Hospital, which was seeking to upgrade its diploma program, also was considered as a participant, but political and philosophical differences could not be resolved.) Additional financial support belatedly arrived in 1974 in the form of a Public Health Service curriculum development grant of almost a million dollars. The grant was used to define new roles in nursing; devise new educational technologies (e.g., computer-assisted learning) and novel methods of independent, self-paced learning; and to promote shared learning experiences with other students in the health sciences.

The four-year plan got off to a modest start in the 1973-74 academic year with a freshman class of thirty-four. Most were housed in St. Luke's Eli White Residence Hall. By and large, students were pleased, citing in particular the variety of experiences and the opportunity to share in typical college life. Enrollment gradually climbed, and in 1975-76, an unexpectedly large percentage of those who were sent acceptance letters took the School up on its offer. "We have considerably oversubscribed, hoping that someone will marry, another will move away, someone will fall off a horse, or whatever," joked Elin Ozdemir, director of admissions.

The atmosphere was less joyous in years to come. Hopes for enrollments as large as one hundred per class never materialized. There simply was not enough interest at the secondary school level. Recruiters received little assistance from guidance counselors, who generally were not favorably disposed toward nursing. "We find in general there remains the image of a nurse as a subservient member of the health care team," explained Ozdemir. "They are inclined to counsel the able student toward pre-med ... [showing] little understanding of the vigorous academic studies and employment of skill required to earn the Bachelor of Science in Nursing." Recruitment suffered for other reasons: fear of the big city and the exorbitant cost of a Columbia education — it was safer and cheaper to study elsewhere for two years and then transfer into the nursing program. "Families were not yet ready to pay that much tuition for somebody who wanted to be a nurse," says Helen Pettit. Moreover, prospective enrollees probably heard through the grapevine that nursing students were seen as outsiders on the main campus. (Nursing students didn't live in Columbia housing and, because of tight schedules, they often had to attend their liberal arts classes in uniform, which didn't go over well with their nonconformist nonnursing classmates.) Ultimately, Columbia's experiment failed, ending in 1980. Crawford and her advisors had misread the educational marketplace (see Chapter 20).

As the School's leaders during this critical transitional period, Elizabeth S. Gill '37 (1961-68) and Mary I. Crawford (1968-76) must shoulder substantial responsibility for the School's limited progress. Gill, by nature and by training, was not one to deviate from the norm. She was literally a product of the old school. Gill was born in 1903 in Belmont, Mass., and largely raised in New York City. She attended Elmira College in upstate New York, graduating in 1927 with a degree in social science. "I do not recall that she was outstandingly brilliant, but her values were always in the right spot," reminisced one of her college professors, Georgia Harkness, in 1968. "It was during a decade when we heard so much about 'flaming youth,' with the rejection of much of what was traditional in moral standards. It was a day not unlike our own. Elizabeth in a quiet way helped to keep the college on an even keel." Her mother passed away during this time, but Gill reportedly handled the loss well.

She remained in Elmira after graduation, securing a post as secretary of the Girls Reserve of the YWCA. Louise C. Woermbke, a member of the Reserve, recalled, "We girls looked to Elizabeth Gill as the epitome of all that we wanted to be one day." Gill's heart, however, was in nursing. Despite family objections, she mustered the courage to enroll at Presbyterian in 1934. After earning her diploma, Gill remained at the Hospital as a staff nurse and quickly ascended to night supervisor in ophthalmology and head nurse in medicine. She joined the School's faculty in 1941.

To scores of students, she was the consummate teacher. "I think some of the skills she learned with the YWCA served her in good stead," says Helen Pettit. A member of one of several classes to select Gill as their faculty advisor, Mary Relief Rumely Munn '44, remembered, "One of the first days someone asked a question. Her reply was: 'I don't know, but I'll look it up and tell you tomorrow,' instead of stalling or pretending to know. That sold us all on Miss Gill." Her lectures were liberally sprinkled with fascinating historical tidbits and anecdotes, which made learning a pleasure instead of a chore. "I had high regard for Elizabeth," says Bettie Jackson, a student at the end of Gill's career. "It's hard to put my finger on why. She must have left a tremendous impression upon me as being strong and kind, a standard bearer, a matron."

With characteristic modesty, Gill once said, "[As a teacher,] I have received more than I have given."

Early on, Gill earned a reputation as an expert pharmacologist. Among her publications were the section on pharmacology in the 1951 version of the *Quick Reference Book for Nurses,* the *Laboratory Manual of Microbiology for Nurses,* which she coauthored with James T. Culbertson (1947), and *Pharmacology and Therapeutics* (1952), which she revised with Charles Solomon. The National League of Nursing Education Committee on Tests and Measurements called on her to help develop its exams in pharmacology.

In 1958 she earned a master's degree in nursing education from Teachers

College. Three years later, she was given the directorship of nursing education and nursing service at Columbia-Presbyterian Medical Center. Dual appointments had fallen out of favor at many teaching institutions, mainly to distance nursing schools from hospital interference and clinical obligations, but also because the job had become overwhelming. When the deans of the country's leading nursing programs were asked to recommend candidates to succeed Eleanor Lee, most warned that it would be extremely difficult to find anyone who could be proficient in both roles. But the Faculty of Medicine ignored their warnings. So did Gill, who eagerly accepted the challenge. As she explained years later, the dual role was a vantage point that allowed one to "see what students needed in both clinical experience and academic experience."

In some ways, Gill did manage to balance the demands of her two masters. For example, to ease Presbyterian's chronic nursing shortage, she instituted a plan to license students as practical nurses once they finished certain rotations so they could be hired by the Hospital on their days off. In other ways, she tilted in favor of the University. She brazenly ended weekend duty for students without consulting Presbyterian (as required by the agreement in effect between the University and the Hospital), knowing that it would sour her relationship with officials there. Moreover, Gill resisted a Presbyterian-supported proposal to lower the School's standards. The Hospital, fed up with the chronic nursing shortage and the School's diminishing clinical contributions, pushed for a multilevel nursing school within Columbia, offering the whole gamut of degrees, from the associate's to the master's. "The faculty fought it tooth and nail," recalls Dorothy Reilly. "We felt that as a university program we should be preparing nurses for their baccalaureate and master's. I remember the faculty saying, 'If any other school in the University offered that kind of program, okay, but they were only asking nursing to offer the associate's degree. Would they do that with the medical school if they needed more physicians?'"

Still desperate for nurses, the Hospital sought instead to start a school for licensed practical nurses and asked for the School's assistance. Again, the faculty balked, unable to comprehend why the Hospital would support a new program — and a retrogressive one at that — when the baccalaureate program was in financial trouble.

Troubled by the faculty's opposition, Augustus C. Long, president of Presbyterian's Board of Trustees, wrote to University President Grayson Kirk, "If we don't have the wholehearted support of our senior nurses then the program will fail. It seems to me that the time has come when we have a project that is supported by the University, the Hospital, the doctors and everyone but the two senior nurses, then we will have to insist on the cooperation of these nurses or find new ones."

Kirk responded: "I am assured by Dr. Merritt that Miss Gill and Miss Pettit will do everything possible to support and encourage this new program... [W]e must bear in mind that regardless of what the personal views are of our nursing professors, they are to some extent under obligation to support, at least publicly, the stated policy of their professional national and regional associations, both which have made public resolutions in favor of gradual elimination of L.P.N. training schools... Their loyalties to the Medical Center are firm and strong, and we should have no worry in that connection."

Recognizing the program's inevitability, Gill and Pettit reluctantly offered their support. Thus, Presbyterian persevered, opening its diploma program (named the Edna McConnell Clark School of Nursing after its major benefactor) in September 1968. But so did the University, thanks to Gill and her staff, fending off serious attempts to drag the School backward.

After the Clark skirmish, relations between the School of the Hospital were never quite the same. In the heat of battle, Presbyterian withdrew support for an ambitious expansion and renovation of Maxwell Hall, which was desperately needed to meet the needs of a growing student body and faculty. (In subsequent years, the two parties fought over the rights to various funds, including the School's endowment. Matters were largely settled in the early eighties. But the animosity remained.)

"We had to wean the Hospital from the idea that student nurses were there to run the Hospital but [rather] to get an education," said Gill, summing up those years. "That was not nursing and nurses here would not succumb to that. The doctors appreciated our ideas, but it was a little hard for some of them to take."

But to some, Gill was not nearly aggressive enough. It was not her temperament "to rock the boat," said one faculty member. "It was too bad because the school was ready [for a change]." According to Keville Frederickson, "Gill was upset about airing problems in public." For instance, she blanched when one of her senior faculty members wrote a controversial letter-to-the-editor on health care.

Gill's critics also point to her treatment of Dorothy Reilly, who brought a scholarly approach to nursing that was not appreciated, as some tell it, by Gill and other traditionalists at the Medical Center. "The sixties was a battle for professional recognition [at Columbia-Presbyterian],"

Reilly says. "We also were battling the fact that we were mostly women. The macho attitude there was extremely prevalent."

After a year's sabbatical in 1965-66, Reilly returned to Columbia and soon was awarded her doctorate in nursing education — the first for a faculty member at the School of Nursing. It was an occasion to be celebrated; instead, she was shown the door. Reilly left, she says, because "I was told there was nothing more for me there after I got my doctorate." Sarah Cook suspects that the physicians "leaned on" Gill to dismiss Reilly and that Gill acquiesced. "Gill saw herself as director of nursing and head of the school at the behest of the physicians."

In subsequent years, under Mary Crawford, other teachers were internally exiled for the crime of pursuing an advanced degree, according to Frederickson, who earned her doctorate in 1974. One by one they left the School to find a more academically minded home. "I think that's where Columbia got into difficulty," she believes.

Gill retired in 1968, around the time of the Reilly and diploma program controversies, settling in Chatham, Mass., where she shared a home with Florence Vanderbilt, longtime director of residence at Maxwell Hall. In 1982 she received the Distinguished Alumnae Award of the Alumni Association. She currently resides in Rosemont, Pa.

Gill was succeeded by Mary Crawford, Ed.D., the first nonalumna since Anna Maxwell to lead the School of Nursing. More than a few instructors were pleased the Faculty of Medicine had finally turned to an outsider, a counterweight to the School's heavy inbreeding, a pioneer who might challenge nursing's traditionally subordinate relationship to medicine at the Medical Center. That Crawford was also the first director to hold a doctorate only added to her promise.

Crawford was born in 1921 in Lakewood, Ohio. The child of a physician–hospital administrator, she enrolled at the University of Michigan intent on a career in physical education. "I soon realized I didn't like it," she recalled. "While attending school, I worked as a nursing aide in a Cleveland hospital and found the work most gratifying. I decided to become a nurse to help the war effort." After graduation, she entered the Frances Payne Bolton School of Nursing at Western Reserve University, finishing in 1945. For five years, she worked as a head nurse and instructor in Western Reserve's teaching hospitals. She then returned to school, earning a master's from Teachers College in 1952 and a certificate in nurse-midwifery from the Maternity Center Association in 1953. Crawford briefly taught at Yale, but it was her work with Teachers College and MCA that established her reputation. With the college she participated in a pioneering demonstration project that prompted Johns Hopkins to establish the first hospital-based nurse-midwifery program. And under the aegis of MCA, she helped design Columbia's graduate program in maternity nursing, the first of its kind. In 1956 she joined the Columbia faculty (and the staff of Sloane Hospital). She was promoted to coordinator of maternal-child health in 1961.

Three years later Crawford resigned to pursue a doctorate in nursing research at Teachers College. Two papers resulted from her dissertation, including, "Physiological and Behavioral Cues to Disturbances in Childbirth," published in the *Bulletin of the American College of Nurse Midwifery*. Toward the end of her studies, she was given a joint appointment with Teachers College and the School of Nursing to explore the relationship between the preparation of teachers and practitioners in nurse-midwifery and to strengthen collaboration between the two institutions in graduate education. Her crowning year was 1968, when she was awarded her doctorate and the dual directorship of nursing at Columbia and Presbyterian. Her appointment elicited congratulations as well as hints of sympathy. People were thinking, she said, "You're in for a terrific beating. I wonder if you really know what you're getting into."

As the Medical Center's chief nurse, she wanted to cultivate more graduate programs for the clinical specialist, improve nurse-physician cooperation, and, most of all, eliminate disparities between the "ideal" and the "real." "Those of us working along the lines of ideal care," she wrote, "have really not settled down and faced the problems of how to develop our concepts in the real situation. We cannot continue to deny reality, but must face the reality of the day by day hospital nursing service problems and study the forces and factors that either facilitate or impede comprehensive nursing care services."

If anyone was equipped to forge a new educational paradigm for nursing it was Mary Crawford, hailed as a pioneer and visionary in nurse-midwifery education and practice. She seemed to have no qualms about challenging physician dominance of health care, at least as it pertained to obstetrics. Moved by the physician shortage and the nation's unacceptably high infant mortality rate, she concluded in a 1968 study, "The obstetrician cannot be tied up providing care which can be done by a less skilled person. This person may be less skilled in the treatment of complications but highly skilled in the promotion of positive health, in the application of preventive measures, in the early detection of disease ... The [nurse-midwife] is the sentinel of the mother, sorting out the high risk maternity cases for special care by the doctor. She conducts the normal delivery and summons help in the event of an emergency."

Crawford appeared to be the embodiment of the academic nurse—a teacher, clinician, researcher, administrator, speaker, writer, consultant. She was active in the American College of Nurse-Midwifery (which she served as president), the New York State Nurses' Association, the Council of Deans of Nursing, the National League for Nursing, and the American Nurses' Association. "Everybody touted Mary Crawford as this savior on a white steed," remembers Bettie Jackson. "Here was this doctorally prepared nurse. She was not a Columbia graduate. She was viewed as a breath of fresh air. And she was given a big fancy office in Atchley Pavilion [where Presbyterian housed its top administrators and private physician practices]. So we began to sense there were changes in the role of nursing's leader in the organization."

And Crawford spoke the right words. "Above all," she told the Presbyterian managers, "we need nurses who can provide leadership," who are flexible and adaptable, who understand different cultures, who can motivate and teach patients, who possess sharp assessment skills. "Most of all these nurses must be able to ensure that the patient does not get divided into a multitude of pieces by all these different people giving care."

"At the doctoral level," she wrote to P&S Dean Paul Marks early in her term, "the School of Nursing has the potential for preparing nurses with a strong background in the sciences and in research, capable of finding the means for extending the impact and the effectiveness of the contribution of nurses to health care. At the master's level the School of Nursing has the potential for preparing the nurse clinician in all clinical areas...These nurses will carry consultative responsibility in the whole broad spectrum of health care."

And Crawford recognized the growing tensions between the generations of nurses. "Nurses who have become somewhat set in their ways feel threatened by the vocal young generation because they have neither learned to be very vocal themselves or have become skilled in the art of persuasion," she said. "They depend on rigid rules for their security and use these rules as their defense mechanism against the logical arguments of the younger generation. Our younger nurses want to give patient care today but they want to give ideal care to one or two patients. They have not faced up to how to provide the best care for all."

The highlight of Crawford's administration was a novel series of multidisciplinary seminars in psychosocial aspects of patient care. The idea originated in the early seventies with Bernard D. Schoenberg, M.D., associate dean for allied health affairs at P&S, who envisioned a Medical Center–wide school of allied health, uniting all of Columbia's health sciences programs. If nurses, physicians, dentists, and physical and occupational therapists are to work side by side as graduates, he reasoned, they ought to study side by side as students, sharing such courses as anatomy and physiology and human development. Moreover, he thought all students needed more assistance with adapting to the stresses of clinical care and more insight into the psychological and sociological aspects of the healing arts. In nursing, clinical experiences focused primarily on pathology and treatment, often skirting important secondary issues. For example, in the obstetrics rotation, there was relatively little discussion of student attitudes toward sex or student reactions to such emotionally wrenching issues as birth and death and incurably ill babies—all of which would affect their performance as practitioners. Following Schoenberg's lead, P&S won a large grant for a number of experimental educational projects, including seminars involving faculty and students from the various disciplines (medical students never participated, however, because of reported scheduling constraints). "It was a glorious Camelot of an experiment in comprehensive collaborative education, an attempt to integrate didactic and affective learning," says Sarah Cook. Though the seminars did not survive the decade, the content was eventually folded into the rest of the nursing curriculum.

Aside from the psychosocial seminars, under Crawford there were no revolutionary changes, no new educational paradigms. Despite her scholarly credentials and her best intentions, the curriculum retained its heavy clinical focus, research continued to be a secondary pursuit, no new graduate programs materialized, and the faculty remained too insular and under-credentialed. (In 1976, Crawford's final year, 15 percent of the staff, full and part time, was prepared only at the baccalaureate level—a substantial drop from the 25 percent proportion she had inherited, but not up to University standards.) The School still had little, if any, representation on important University governing bodies. (As of 1973, there were no nursing representatives on the fourteen-member executive council of the Faculty of Medicine, only three nurses on its 116-member faculty council, and no nurses in the University Senate.) And the School failed to win its independence. Legally, it was still considered the Department of Nursing under the Faculty of Medicine, and the associate dean (nursing) reported to the dean of P&S, who had the last word on nursing's curriculum and finances. When the Health Sciences campus underwent an administrative reorganization in 1973, she lobbied for a change in this chain of command. "Nursing faculty around the country have been convinced that the program offered at Columbia was no more than a glorified diploma program in nursing, an apprenticeship program that does not meet the standards of academia," she told P&S authorities. And to University President William McGill, she said, this "will seriously jeopardize our chances of recruiting qualified faculty and would probably result in the loss of accreditation." She preferred a chain of command in which the School's leader reported directly to the newly created post of vice president for Health Sciences. But the Faculty of Medicine prevailed, appeasing Crawford by granting the Department of Nursing permission only to *identify* itself publicly as the School of Nursing.

To be fair, Crawford faced enormous fiscal and administrative constraints. The School was dealt a series of crushing economic blows in the early seventies, including a mandate from the Joint Board of Trustees to put the School in the black within two years; the complete curtailment of financial support from the Hospital (which had lost third-party reimbursement for nursing education); a University-wide budget cut of 10 percent and freeze on faculty salaries; the withdrawal of New York State Department of Mental Hygiene funds supporting four faculty members; and the failure of the federal government to provide adequate support for nursing education. (Consequently, the School closed Maxwell Hall's cafeteria, infirmary, and—luxury of luxuries—maid service for students.)

"The majority of the time of the Associate Dean for Nursing over the past four years has been spent in coping with the problems of administering a School of Nursing 'in limbo' and in preparing proposals over and over again for solving the administrative and financial problems of the School of Nursing with no final decisions forthcoming," wrote Crawford in 1974. "This severely limits the amount of time available for guidance of faculty and students."

In Crawford's defense, a former high-ranking faculty member argues, "Crawford's dual position was impossible because of the attitudes of P.H. and P&S [administrators]. God couldn't have succeeded."

Crawford's instructors were similarly overwhelmed. Members of the understaffed faculty spent an average of thirty hours per week in direct student contact and untold hours preparing for classes, grading papers, and participating in School committees and professional activities. With such a crowded schedule, who had time or energy for research?

"I would like to be sure that we are not losing our potential leaders due to our own rigidity, thus losing creative people." Crawford told the Presbyterian Board of Managers. But at the School, that is exactly what was happening—partly because of Crawford's own inflexibility. Like others of her generation, she did not know how to react to the increasingly restive and socially aware faculty and student body. When some of them adopted a relatively radical stance in reaction to the Kent State killings (which sparked one of the student walkouts), "Miss Crawford was so upset," says Keville Frederickson. "Her social issues were between 165th and 168th Streets." So, it seemed, was her vision of nursing. "There was a whole group of faculty who loved Columbia and would have stayed had there been a change in administrative philosophy," adds Frederickson.

But Crawford remained at the School until 1976, when a Medical Center task force recommended a split in the governance of education and service. By then work had taken on a new meaning for Crawford; it had become a self-prescribed therapy for the cancer ravaging her body. "She was struggling very hard," recalls Helen Pettit, "which she felt was keeping her alive. She was very bitter when she was asked [by the University] to step aside." Crawford retained her clinical post at Presbyterian, retitled vice president for nursing. She died at the Hospital in 1979 and was succeeded by Martha Haber '49.

What does one make of the School's record in the 1960s and early 1970s? Was it dated and in decline? Or still vibrant and in touch with the times? One indication was enrollment, which remained fairly stable through the seventies, even while more and more professions—with far better salaries and working conditions and opportunities for advancement—opened to women. But, ominously, the quality of applicants began to erode. (Filling the classes with capable young women was not yet a problem. But it would be a crushing one soon.)

Another measure was the value of the Columbia nurse in the open marketplace. "People wanted to hire our graduates," contends Dorothy Reilly. "I have to say we turned out excellently prepared nurses. And I don't mean only clinically."

"How come the School turned out so many of us who went on to prominent positions?" asks Keville Frederickson, a product of this era. "There had to be something in that."

Bettie Jackson agrees: "Columbia produced incredible practitioners with a commitment and a fervor that is still alive today." She is still in awe of the responsibility placed upon students back then, and of the way they responded. "When the blackout happened in sixty-five, there was never a question about what we would do as nursing students. We went to the Hospital and went to work. Nobody needed to organize us, to tell us what to do…The reason that I'm still a nurse, that I have very strong feelings about the mission of nursing, has to come from the School of Nursing."

A third measure, and one that cannot be easily dismissed, comes from a 1974 National Science Foundation survey of deans of nursing, which rated Columbia among the top four professional nursing schools in the country.

Either the School was doing something right or it was coasting along on the strengths of a considerable but crumbling foundation. Its performance over the next decade would tell.

20

Once Grand and Glorious

Many of my classmates have had second thoughts about
becoming nurses...Disillusionment may spread and
reach a peak—both nursing and the School of Nursing
have not proved as expected.

Maureen Casey '83 (1980)

HISTORICALLY, ONE CAN JUDGE the status of the School of Nursing by the
nature of its lodgings. A century ago the first pupils and instructors were
relegated—like unwanted guests—to Presbyterian Hospital's attic. Soon
they were welcomed into the therapeutic family (as minor dependents) and
awarded rooms of their own, in graceful Florence Nightingale Hall.
Nursing's ascent continued through the 1920s, earning it a prominent place
in the nation's first medical center. Maxwell Hall, nursing's new residence
in Washington Heights, was grand and glorious, perched on a grassy bluff
high above the Hudson River. Under Columbia's banner, the School evolved
further still, and the Hall was enlarged and refurbished.

Slowly over the years, the luster faded, as neither the University, which
occupied the Hall, nor the Hospital, which owned it, could agree about the
building's fate. Blueprints for renewal in the 1960s turned to dust. Maintenance suffered as the Hospital washed its hands of its wayward child but
not of its valuable real estate. Indeed, the Hall was eventually demolished
to make way for a mammoth new tertiary-care facility, and the School was
hurried off to an incompletely renovated, old apartment house recently
purchased by Columbia. The choice of quarters was dictated by the chronic
and critical shortage of space at the Medical Center. Still, the symbolism
of the move could not have been clearer: The School had outgrown its hospital origins but still did not warrant a home in academe.

Maxwell Hall's demise coincided with the administrations of Helen Pettit and JoAnn Jamann. Pettit, like her predecessors, attempted to update the School, adding here and there bits and pieces of the professional model. Jamann, the School's eighth leader, brought a more scholarly approach and an outsider's perspective. However, neither of these deans quite found the right blend of practice, research, and education. Despite their best efforts, the walls came tumbling down.

Helen F. Pettit was born in Brooklyn in 1914. As a young child, she wanted to be a nurse, and nothing else. "When family and friends were sick, I liked to take care of them," she recalls, matter-of-factly. But the future was not so straightforward. After high school, she was sent to Florida to study at St. Petersburg Junior College, which her family owned and operated. Within a year, her studies, as well as the college, fell victim to the Great Depression. Family obligations brought her back to Brooklyn, but only temporarily. After a year or so, she was encouraged by her loved ones to study nursing and was asked only to stay close by. Presbyterian Hospital fit the bill, and she enrolled in the Class of 1936.

Pettit started her career, like so many other alumni, at the Medical Center, beginning as a staff nurse at Sloane Hospital. Within four months, she was a head nurse, spending, to her great satisfaction, roughly half her time teaching. With some reluctance, she earned a baccalaureate in education at Teachers College (1940), which led to a faculty appointment at the School of Nursing. Pettit taught in all levels of the program, quickly establishing a reputation as a "great teacher" and a "hard taskmaster." As colleague Constance Cleary recalled, "She was always fair but firm."

In ten years, Pettit rose to the rank of assistant professor, contributed to two faculty publishing projects (*Essentials of Nursing* and *The Quick Reference Book for Nurses,* the second and third editions of which she edited), earned a master's in education from New York University (1952), and conducted a semester-long study of public health teaching in nursing schools around the country. In the early fifties, she was the obvious successor to Eleanor Lee, director of education, who was elevated to the School's top post. It was a timely promotion, allowing Pettit to oversee the School's groundbreaking experiments in graduate maternity nursing education and psychosocial seminars, as well as a study of mental health nursing education. Concurrently, she served as assistant director of the nursing service at Presbyterian. In 1958 she was appointed full professor.

Outside of the Medical Center, Pettit was active in numerous professional organizations, serving as chairwoman of the education division of the Southern New York League for Nursing, field accreditation visitor for the National League for Nursing, member of the board of directors of the American Hospital Association and Stony Wold Sanatorium, and president of the New York State Board of Nurse Examiners. She also worked with the American Heart Association, the Visiting Nurse Service of New York, the Foundation of Thanatology, and the New York State Nurses' Association.

To Pettit and her contemporaries, proper decorum had as much to do with good nursing as proper skills and techniques. "Grooming was important [to her]—all students were required to appear fully dressed in their uniforms, highly starched, winter and summer, didn't matter if it was 105 degrees outside, no knee socks below the second floor," said colleague Constance Cleary. When students asked for permission to have men in their rooms in Maxwell Hall, claiming the same right to privacy they would have at home, Pettit responded: "But at home you have a living room and a place to entertain. In your room, all you have is one chair and one bed." In general, noted the editors of the *Alumni Magazine*, she was constantly "dreaming dreams but always there, generous with her time, offering encouragement and opportunities for advancement."

Nevertheless, a portion of the faculty grew concerned when she was appointed acting associate dean—a virtual stepping stone to the School's leadership, since the University had never mounted a serious outside search for a nursing director and was not inclined to stage one now. Pettit was available and, better yet, old-guard Presbyterian: predictable and trustworthy. Nine instructors petitioned the University to broaden its search for a new leader, "preferring one who is *educationally* and *experientially* prepared to assist us in realizing the School of Nursing's potential for excellence." For symbolic and practical reasons, they wanted a leader with impeccable academic credentials, doctorally prepared and research-minded. Pettit, whose highest degree was a master's and who had minimal research experience, did not measure up in their eyes. She got the appointment anyway.

Pettit's primary goal and major accomplishment as associate dean for nursing was to expand the graduate program, which at the start of her tenure included only two tracks, maternity nursing and psychiatric-community health nursing. Over the next five years, her faculty initiated programs for pediatric, adult, geriatric, and perinatal nurse practitioners as well as for nurse anesthetists (with Roosevelt Hospital). In keeping with tradition, the programs were clinically focused — a wise choice in a market bereft of graduate programs accentuating patient care. Two additional graduate tracks, acute care of the adult and the child, were plotted during these years. And under Pettit, faculty member Lucie Kelly, Ph.D., started the School's first dual master's degree program with the School of Public Health, which prepares nurses to be expert clinicians and administrators or planners.

Despite the rising cost of tuition, graduate enrollments remained fairly stable in the late seventies. Master's recipient Marcia Harriman *'81* was not alone in saying, "The best testimony I can give to Columbia is that I paid for this education myself, and I got my money's worth."

Plainly, a different message was being disseminated by baccalaureate recipients, helping to depress undergraduate enrollments to unsustainable levels. High school seniors had decided that a Columbia nursing degree was not worth the investment. They were not alone. People throughout the University began circulating complaints about the quality of nursing education at Columbia (Teachers College included). Some wondered if the baccalaureate program was necessary. Others, seeing no coherent plan for advanced training, speculated that the University was squandering its limited resources on duplicative graduate programs. Many questioned why the School was so isolated from its educational and clinical affiliates, especially Presbyterian. "When I came back to Presbyterian Hospital in 1979," commented Martha Haber, vice president for nursing, "I was concerned that the staff did not see themselves as part of the educational process." To those who still saw the School as a proving ground for Presbyterian's nursing service — and there were many — the School's apparent separatism was tantamount to treason.

The chorus of complaints eventually reached the ears of Paul A. Marks, M.D., vice president for Health Sciences, who in 1978 convened a special committee to weigh nursing's future at Columbia. Curiously, Pettit was asked to head the investigation. She had been a part of nursing's inner circle for as long as anybody could remember, hardly an impartial observer. To be sure, the School's predicament was decades in the making, but Pettit was two years into her own administration and had had ample opportunity to chart a new path for nursing. Apparently, Marks was content with the status quo and had formed the committee only to mollify critics. With Pettit in charge, the committee might stir change but certainly not revolution.

Predictably, the committee's 1979 report essentially endorsed the existing step-by-step approach to academic nursing. "It is logical," wrote committee members Pettit, Constance Cleary, and Anne Earle, "that private universities with nursing schools in tertiary care settings that provide the opportunity for interdisciplinary learning, joint appointments (between practice and education, as well as between disciplines), and a research environment, concentrate on graduate education and research."

Echoing an earlier recommendation of the nursing faculty, the committee suggested that the School should terminate the four-year undergraduate curriculum in favor of the old two-year format and gradually phase out baccalaureate study altogether. Pettit mourned the end of the four-year curriculum, which occurred in 1980, believing it could have worked had the University given it more time and resources. "You don't establish traditions on two campuses overnight," she now says, referring to Columbia and its clinical affiliates, St. Luke's and Roosevelt hospitals, major partners in the program. Because of underfunding, the affiliates "didn't have the people who were qualified to help the students," she adds. "A lot of people thought that did not matter, but we discovered we just couldn't turn people loose in clinical settings and not have the underpinnings."

But the program was undermined by larger forces. Columbia, one of the more expensive nursing schools, costing $7,570 per year, simply couldn't compete in a state glutted with baccalaureate programs. The School had a far easier time competing in the growing market for advanced degrees, where its strong patient-care focus and trove of academic resources were unmatched. Furthermore, the federal government was more inclined to support graduate nursing education (convinced that baccalaureate nurses were sufficiently abundant). At the tuition-driven School of Nursing, where two-thirds of the student body relied on financial aid, the availability of government largess meant all the difference in the world.

Thus, the committee envisioned a School dedicated primarily to advanced study, offering, in addition to its traditional degrees for clinical specialists and nurse practitioners, a new specialty master's for registered nurses with baccalaureates in nursing or other disciplines; a new nurse generalist master's degree for college graduates with no nursing experience; and joint-degree programs with other disciplines. Doctoral study was also advised, though not immediately.

Moreover, the committee recommended that the School recruit more research-minded faculty and make scholarly inquiry a priority of all instructors and students, offer more continuing education programs for working nurses (particularly those at the University's clinical affiliates), create more cooperative educational ventures with its clinical affiliates and other schools in the health sciences, and encourage more faculty participation in practice issues and the formulation of health care policy. "Fully utilizing the resources of the Health Sciences Campus and the University as a whole, the School of Nursing can become a noted Center for Advanced Practice, a model of interdisciplinary practice and research," the committee concluded. "With the added dimensions of public health, administration, and education ... Columbia University is in the enviable position of having an unlimited potential for continued development of excellence in nursing."

The call for a more scholarly School of Nursing sounded impressive but rang hollow. It was a wish list for some future administration, not a workable blueprint for the present. The creation of a truly academic program would have required a substantial reallocation of University resources, which was not about to happen, and new sources of income (e.g., research grants, faculty practice earnings), which the report had not addressed.

Thus, the recommendations stirred no one, except for current freshman and sophomores. Despite promises that their studies would not be affected, they felt they had been abandoned, that their degrees would be tarnished. "If they cut your program, it sounds like there's something wrong with your school," reasoned sophomore Clare Ipolito '82. "If we had known beforehand, we would have gone to another school." Freshman Maureen Casey '83, treasurer of the student government, bemoaned the loss of a clinical experience in family health. "A program without a sophomore year is not the program I chose when deciding which college to attend," she wrote to Pettit. "The sophomore year is part of what made Columbia's nursing program so attractive and outstanding to me. No other program I investigated offered its students so early an opportunity to experience their chosen profession. The importance of the early clinical must not be overlooked, and none should know this better than the faculty itself."

Pettit, sympathetic but unswayed, replied, "As much unhappiness and disbelief as there is, we don't think [the shortened curriculum will be] poor." P&S Dean Donald Tapley added, "It's a calculated move toward improving the school. Lower degrees are out, higher degrees are in." He also noted that the new curriculum would attract a more committed student body: "One of the problems [with students] coming out of high school is that this is a career choice many kids are not really prepared to make."

A little more than a year after the report was released, Helen Pettit retired, justifiably content that she had made a substantial contribution to the School of Nursing, the focus of her entire adult life. (Today, from her secluded lakefront home in Sherman, Conn., she remains active in School and alumni affairs.) The task of implementing her recommendations went to JoAnn S. Jamann, Ed.D., an outsider and an academician.

The 1980s began with great promise. For the first time, it seemed that the University was serious about welcoming the School of Nursing into the academic community. Jamann was designated a full dean, giving her parity with principals of other Columbia programs. The School itself was given greater autonomy, which Health Sciences administrators finally had recognized was essential to nursing's rehabilitation. "The impression among several consultants ... was that the Nursing School was within the Medical School, and consequently, did not have full responsibility for academic programs nor a budget that was identifiably separate from that of the School of Medicine," explained Thomas Q. Morris, M.D., a P&S administrator and member of the search committee that selected Jamann. "That relationship, therefore, was considered to be a major deterrent not only to recruitment of a nationally recognized leader in nursing, but also to academic development and growth within the Nursing School itself."

"The reputation of the School was that it was dominated by medicine," confirms Jamann, "and there was no way that nursing was going to be autonomous, as it should be, working with medicine rather than under medicine." In fact, the School's profile in the academic nursing community was so low as to be nonexistent. "It wasn't really well known outside of the New York area," she recalls. "The nursing school that was identified with Columbia was Teachers College."

Like several other nursing leaders, Jamann thought twice about accepting the University's invitation to become dean and professor of nursing at Columbia. But the opportunity to work in an environment with so much potential for nursing, and to return to the Northeast, was irresistible.

JoAnn Jamann, who was born in DuBois, Pa., in 1932, first studied and practiced nursing at Robert Packer Hospital in Allentown, Pa. Not quite content with staff nursing, she enrolled at the University of Pennsylvania School of Nursing, earning a baccalaureate in 1962 and a master's in 1965. In academia, she found her niche. She remained at the university for another eleven years as a member of the faculty, the last four as coordinator of the graduate division. Her most noteworthy achievement was to open a doctoral program in nursing science, a novelty in its day. Jamann earned her own doctorate, in higher education administration, from Lehigh University in 1974. She soon moved on to Rush-Presbyterian-St. Luke's Medical Center in Chicago, where she started another doctoral program and served as associate dean and assistant vice president.

Jamann, a nationally recognized authority in gerontology nursing education and doctoral nursing education, seemed an ideal choice to be the School's first dean. She was clearly of nursing's modern era: a doctorally prepared nurse, a seasoned administrator, comfortable in her role as a colleague of physicians and scientists in an academic medical center. A minor point perhaps, but she was also the School's first married leader. Nursing, to her, was a professional career, not a substitute for marriage or a route to marriage, and not a religious calling. In the public's mind, repressed Nurse Ratcheds and oversexed Hot Lips Houlihans and devout Florence Nightingales were still commonplace, a perception that no doubt spilled over into the academic community. Jamann played against type.

"Her experience will be invaluable as she leads the School of Nursing to pre-eminence in service, research and training," proclaimed Columbia President Michael Sovern. Despite everyone's best intentions, preeminence would not be the denouement of Jamann's term.

"It was a hopeful time," she recalls. "The faculty wanted to change. The [University] administration wanted to change. Columbia had the resources, the desires, to be a clinically oriented leader in nursing. But it wasn't very long after I arrived that they started this business about building the new hospital and where they were going to place it. Maxwell Hall became a horrendous complication to deal with. Energies were consumed by a non-academic, nonprofessional problem."

Jamann had the misfortune to arrive at a time of great flux throughout the Medical Center and the University. "During my tenure," she reports, "we had four different vice presidents of the Health Sciences, three different financial officers, three different configurations of the provost's office, and two different leaders at Presbyterian Hospital. It was not that people weren't willing to listen and be supportive—they had to learn their own jobs and the politics, and before they could learn it they would be gone. There was never a solid year in which you had the same top-level administrative team working together."

One of those administrative reconfigurations brought in Paul Goldberger, M.D., as university provost and vice president for health sciences. A basic scientist from the National Institutes of Health, Goldberger doubted nursing's potential for academic rigor, the School's leaders were convinced. He soon relinquished his Health Sciences post, but he continued to thwart nursing's advance from the Morningside campus, the nurses report. (Had this new administrative structure, which brought nursing back under medicine, existed when Jamann was offered the job, she would have declined it.)

Jamann quickly discovered that Goldberger's views were not the only antiquated things at Columbia-Presbyterian. Within the School, Jamann found an administrative model that was "ten years behind the times," a crippling shortage of computers for management and teaching, and a skills laboratory with medicine cabinets and other items dating to the 1920s. Moreover, much of Presbyterian Hospital, the School's primary clinical site, was obsolete. It was a world-class hospital trapped in a half-century-old design. "The Medical Center itself had not moved as rapidly as other service centers," Jamann believes.

Jamann also had to contend with a mercurial and labyrinthine accounting system, made all the more complicated by the University's decision to separate nursing's budget from medicine's. She welcomed financial autonomy, though not until the current record-breaking decline in enrollments (and revenues) started to ease. (From 1977 to 1985, undergraduate enrollments fell by 57 percent, from 413 to 176. Graduate enrollments dropped less precipitously, but more and more of those enrollees were studying part-time and paying partial tuition; at one point, half of the specialty majors were economically unsustainable.) Near the end of her term, Jamann was further constrained by a University-wide budget crisis, which froze salaries and hiring and dampened faculty morale.

Nevertheless, Jamann was confident that the School's fortunes would soon reverse. The decline in enrollments, she reasoned, was largely a result of one-time or reversible events: the closure of the four-year curriculum and an untimely drop in nursing applications nationwide (a natural fluctuation of interest in nursing). That the University did not share her optimism rankles her still. "The long-range planning, if they had looked at it, showed that enrollment would go down for a few years and then it would come back," she says.

Revealingly, Jamann failed where she had succeeded so well in the past, in doctoral education. She reportedly hindered her own efforts by not following procedures to the letter, yet it probably did not matter. "The proposal was essentially approved by the Medical Center, but it sat at the [University] provost's office," she says. "Goldberger was the single most important factor in stopping the doctoral program." The University—or at least influential parts of it—still could not envision clinical nurses as academicians. (In truth, the faculty had not distinguished themselves as researchers and had not published many papers. But other nurses had, and there was no reason, given the right environment, that Columbia nurses could not do the same.)

An atmosphere less conducive to progress was difficult to imagine. Nonetheless, Jamann's tenure was notable for several accomplishments. One of the first was to reorganize and decentralize overall operations. "By the sixties, nursing as a whole had started to move toward the professional model," she says. "I tried to increase the management skills of the faculty and to get them involved in making decisions about appointments and performance evaluations, which were all centralized." Decentralization had many benefits, not the least of which was to ease the administrative burden of senior faculty, who should have been spending their non-teaching time in scholarly activities or mentoring less-experienced colleagues.

Scholarship received another boost when Jamann appointed a director of nursing research, Bettie Jackson '67, and raised funds for clinical research from the Rudin family of New York. Jamann also hired more doctorally prepared faculty. The School had its share of highly credentialed instructors in the past, but they tended to be younger and less inexperienced, and rarely were they given the time or resources to launch a research career. "They cut their teeth here and left," says longtime faculty member Sarah Cook. "The School, consciously or unconsciously, had a revolving door hiring policy."

To ingrain the idea that research was part and parcel of nursing, undergraduates were given an earlier introduction to research theory. On the graduate level, Jamann's faculty instituted the School's first core curriculum, with shared courses in nursing theory and research, uniting strong but unintegrated specialty programs. Exemplary student research projects were highlighted in a new interdisciplinary research day, shared with students in occupational and physical therapy.

The academic atmosphere was further enriched with the creation of the Columbia University Nursing Consortium, an attempt "to mirror the kind of relationship that the school of medicine had with its clinical affiliates," wrote Jamann. The idea was to cultivate a community of nurses at the School's varied educational and clinical affiliates — the School of Public Health, Teachers College, Presbyterian Hospital, the Psychiatric Institute, Morristown Memorial Hospital, Overlook Hospital, St. Luke's-Roosevelt Hospital Center, Harlem Hospital Center, Mary Imogene Bassett Hospital, the Visiting Nurse Service of New York, and the Isabella Geriatric Center — lowering barriers that separated educators and practitioners and researchers. Accordingly, the School arranged dozens of joint appointments, giving clinicians formal educational responsibilities and teachers formal clinical responsibilities—a modernized version of the old diploma school model. The consortium was also intended to strengthen nursing's voice in the making of health care policy. Regrettably, few consortium members actively participated.

Recruitment was the focus of another multi-institutional arrangement.

To entice more young people into nursing, the School initiated a dual-degree program with eleven liberal arts institutions, among them Fordham, Middlebury, Providence College, and Marymount Manhattan. In five years —three years at a participating college and two at Columbia—students could obtain baccalaureates in the liberal arts and in nursing. For those desiring a full liberal arts education and a career in nursing, the arrangement saved both time and money.

Unfortunately, no recruiting gambit could counter the dismal public image of nursing. In the Reagan era, nursing, with its low salaries and even lower prestige, became a pariah profession. Bright young people, by and large, entered law or business or banking, esteemed fields that promised instant, tangible rewards. Nursing schools like Columbia, with high tuition and low financial aid, could promise only a mountain of debt, demanding work, and a modest economic return.

The School's saving grace was that it could still promise a personally rewarding and socially useful career. Intriguingly, as Reaganism took root, a small cohort of professionals, young and old, migrated to nursing, dissatisfied with what yuppiedom had to offer. Minorities, too, enrolled in record numbers. Although these newcomers to nursing were not enough to revive the School, they were an encouraging harbinger of things to come.

Jamann astutely adopted several measures to encourage nontraditional students. The key was curriculum flexibility; with such a diverse student body, no single approach could satisfy all. For those who needed to return to the work force as soon as possible, the School offered a year-round curriculum that enabled students to earn the baccalaureate in just sixteen months. For undergraduates who needed income during their studies, the School offered a new "learn-earn" option called SNAP (Student Nurse Assistant Program), based at St. Luke's-Roosevelt Hospital Center, in which students worked part-time during the summer and attended weekly nursing seminars.

Flexibility was even more critical for master's candidates, more and more of whom were part-time students and full-time nurses. To accommodate this group, courses were offered twice yearly and consolidated, where possible, into a consecutive two or three days. Another learn-earn option, called PREP (Practice, Research, Education Program), made it easier for full-time employees of Presbyterian or St. Luke's-Roosevelt to earn master's degrees in acute care or medical-surgical nursing. Within PREP, students could satisfy most of the clinical requirements (one-quarter of the total credits) in their practice setting, learning under the guidance of a experienced preceptor. PREP shortened the usual long haul of part-time study and, equally important, allowed participants to apply new knowledge directly to practice and to incorporate clinical research into their everyday routine —the basics of the professional model. The cost of PREP was borne by the employers, who earned a more capable, more satisfied employee from their investment.

The availability of these options, as well as two new clinical specialties, kept graduate enrollments relatively stable. Following Helen Pettit's lead, in 1981 Jamann started a new major in acute care of the adult or child, a response to the increasing acuity of the average inpatient's condition and the increasing complexity of nursing care. A second major, oncology nursing, was introduced in 1984 with Memorial Sloan-Kettering Cancer Center. In this program, one of the first of its kind, nurses learn all aspects of cancer care, ranging from screening to prevention, acute care, rehabilitation, and chronic care.

Finally, to publicize the varied efforts of the students, faculty, alumni, and clinical affiliates, Jamann started a journal, *SNC* (an acronym for the "School of Nursing at Columbia"). (Later, under Mary Mundinger, the journal was redesigned and renamed *The Academic Nurse,* reflecting the School's increased professional emphasis.)

Throughout her administration, Jamann was plagued with the extracurricular complication of Maxwell Hall. While she felt obliged to fight for the School's longtime home, she concluded early on that the battle was hopeless—Presbyterian Hospital owned the land, and that was that. Furthermore, to fight for the Hall, the logical (though not the only) site for a proposed tertiary-care facility, was to oppose Presbyterian's modernization and, by extension, the School's. Much of the Hospital was outdated (designed for 1920s health care), disjointed, and costly to operate. Presbyterian planners believed that nothing short of a $500 million renewal was needed to guarantee its preeminence in health care.

Nonetheless, the destruction of the Hall was painful to witness. For weeks on end, workers clawed at the graceful residence, tossing chunks of history to the ground below. At one point, the half-gutted building took on the look of an old newsreel from Hiroshima. Old nursing hands were warned not to look, as if fallout from the rubble would scar their rich memories of life and work on the bluff overlooking the Hudson. "I was very upset to see Maxwell Hall go down," said Laurie Verdisco '58, associate clinical professor of nursing. "It was my home for three years as a student. I guess I'm not convinced wholeheartedly that it had to go."

Professor Ann Earle added, "I feel a loss of tradition, even though I'm not an alumna. And we lost a good view. Just having a log in the fireplace at Christmas was a good tradition. The formality of Maxwell Hall is gone. There's also been a loss of privacy, which may only be temporary as we move into more of the [new] building. I'm not certain we got an even trade-in."

Others saw in the Hall's ruin a metaphor of the School's overall plight. "Maxwell Hall is a symbol of nursing here, of Anna Maxwell's fight to preserve a spot for nursing, to make it a critical part of the health care system," exclaimed Charmaine Fitzig, Dr.PH., associate clinical professor of nursing. "We, as nurses, are rarely recognized for our contribution to the Medical Center and health care. It's like the Barney Clark operation [the first implantation of a total artificial heart]. Nursing did 90 percent of the care for the gentleman. But who wrote up the studies and got the attention of the press? How can anyone not consider nursing an integral part of health care? That's sad. I hope we maintain some of the old, in terms of Maxwell's struggle for status, which we're struggling for now." On the other hand, Fitzig welcomed the stimulus for change. "It's a passage from one stage to another," she added.

Helen Pettit, whose entire adult life was centered at Maxwell Hall, was surprisingly unfazed. "The building had deteriorated badly," she explains. "There was no health service, no food service, a mixed student group. People who were upset when it was torn down were not there to see how bad it was." However, she does understand their reactions, noting that "the School filled an emotional void for a great many students."

Geri Wood, associate in nursing, added, "For people who've been here a long time, Maxwell Hall did have a lot of tradition steeped in its walls. As a newcomer, I found it oppressive. It was dark, dingy, and dirty. The new offices are cleaner and brighter and give us a sense of cohesiveness. It facilitates communication within divisions of the School. We may have less space, but it has a lot of potential."

Equally disturbing was the School's hasty and uncoordinated removal, which disrupted operations and upset students and faculty. For a time, the recruitment office was the Hall's lone tenant. "People had to crawl through windows to get in and out sometimes," remembers Jamann. "It was awful." And little was done to oversee the retrieval of archival materials and memorabilia. People grabbed what they could. With demolition underway, alumni who lived nearby sneaked in to gather a few leftover items. One can only guess what went down with the Hall, or what disappeared into the homes and offices of Medical Center employees.

A further aggravation was that the School's new home was not quite ready for occupation. When students and staff were moved into the "Georgian

Apartments," a seven-story building located at 617 West 168th Street just across from Presbyterian's main entrance, they were greeted by peeling paint, leaky plumbing, weary elevators, and ever-present repairmen. At least the building, erected in 1914, had potential. In time, it could be a comfortable home, though never as elegant as Maxwell Hall.

Elegance was in short supply in the Medical Center neighborhood. By the seventies, urban blight had crept up from Harlem to Washington Heights, undermining this once-stable working-class enclave. Concerns about safety gave applicants yet another reason to study elsewhere. The area's ambience was further threatened in the mid-eighties when the city opened a shelter for the homeless in the mammoth National Guard Armory next door to the Georgian. Each day in peak winter months, as many as 800 men, including many with psychiatric and substance abuse problems, were housed on 168th Street. Like many others, the School questioned the wisdom of congregating so many homeless in one site, but it quietly accepted their right to shelter and, in neighborly fashion, participated in health care programs for the men.

Jamann does not blame anybody in particular for the problems surrounding Maxwell Hall. "There were so many problems at the Medical Center that they—the administrators—didn't really see the magnitude of the effect it would have on the School of Nursing," she says.

Not long after the move, five years into her term, Jamann resigned. Frustration or demoralization had nothing to do with it, she insists, with little apparent bitterness. "Deans ought to be people in mid-career," she explains. "They should do it for maybe five, ten years and then move into senior professorships." Jamann is currently working as a consultant and a volunteer visiting nurse for homebound elderly in rural South Carolina.

Although JoAnn Jamann did more to move nursing toward academe than her recent predecessors, she bequeathed to her successor, Mary Mundinger, a school in deep trouble. Would-be nurses were reluctant to pay the price of a Columbia nursing degree. Experienced academicians were unwilling to join a faculty where scholarship was secondary to teaching, in a Medical Center that showed little apparent respect for nursing, in a decaying neighborhood and an expensive city.

Once again, people throughout the Health Sciences campus were grumbling about the quality of the faculty (which had only two tenured members: JoAnn Jamann and Lucie Kelly), about the clinical abilities of recent graduates, about an unfocused curriculum, about the inefficiencies and high costs of clinical supervision, and about the School's isolation from the general health care community. In 1986 Provost Goldberger ordered yet another review of nursing. But this one was different. Nurses were a minority on this multidisciplinary committee, which seemed destined to proffer one of two equally repugnant recommendations: turn back the clock or turn off the lights.

21

The Academic Nurse

> Unless there is a major change in the curriculum such
> that there is a complete integration of students into the
> Hospital's activities, the School is dead in the water.
>
> *Member, Task Force to Review the*
> *Columbia University School of Nursing (1987)*

> Unless the School develops a tenured faculty of research
> scholars it is not viable.
>
> *Mary Mundinger, Dean*
> *School of Nursing (1987)*

ECONOMICALLY ANEMIC AND PHILOSOPHICALLY ADRIFT, the School of Nursing at mid-decade faced the chilling prospect of extinction. In recent years, Cornell, Duke, and Boston universities had closed their prestigious nursing programs, so it was not unthinkable that Columbia would do the same. University budget-cutters were poised to cull the weakest of the academic herd (as the esteemed but insolvent School of Library Service, slated to close in 1992, soon would discover). All they needed was a gloomy report from Goldberger's task force on nursing.

What the University got was a gloomy assessment of *academic* nursing. Forget all this business about scholarship, the task force said, and concentrate on the training of nurses. More specifically, it advocated an end to the baccalaureate program, mainly to bring nursing in line with the University's overall philosophy that the master's should be the first professional degree. And it stated that the School should distinguish itself, as it had in the past, by "focusing on education and care," not on research or doctoral-level study. "A leadership position for the School of Nursing," wrote task force leader Kathleen Mullinix, vice provost for the University, "would involve the development of new models of teaching such that students would receive the majority of their training at the bedside and at other 'care-delivery' sites of hospitals (primarily Presbyterian) and would emerge from our program as competent deliverers of care." Without such a focus, one member commented, the School would be "dead in the water."

Although the task force indicated that research and doctoral study might be appropriate in the future, it seriously questioned whether the body of nursing knowledge was "substantive and unique" and thus worthy of advanced study. (The task force did not explain how nursing could establish its own body of knowledge without such study.) It also argued that nurses, like physicians, could always pursue doctorates in other disciplines. Finally, it doubted that current student nurses had the mettle to become "first-rate academics," that the School could recruit appropriate faculty, or that nurse researchers could successfully compete for limited research funds.

The recommendations were not supported unanimously. Four members of the eleven-member task force—a social worker, a Health Sciences administrator, and two nurses (faculty members Sarah Cook and Eura Lennon)—refused to sign the majority report. The School, they argued in a report of their own, was antiquated and inadequate *because* of its orthodox, care-focused curriculum. What the majority viewed as a life preserver, the minority viewed as an anchor chained to the past. The only thing that would be preserved in the majority's scheme would be nursing's second-class status at the Medical Center. In the dissenting report, written by Cook, the minority countered, "It is not appropriate for a University based School of Nursing to exist solely for provision of staff for its major clinical affiliate"—which seemed to be the intent of the majority proposal.

Provost Goldberger, to no one's surprise, sided with the majority and pressed Acting Dean Mundinger to accept its recommendations. She did —to a point. Fully aware that to reject them out of hand was to give the provost an excuse to shut down the School, she agreed to the general intent of the recommendations (i.e., to phase out undergraduate study and delay scholarly goals until resources were available) but not the specifics. With support from the highest authorities at P&S and the University (other than Goldberger), Mundinger and her colleagues started to devise and implement a far more progressive vision of nursing education, which came to be known as the Columbia Model, a unique weave of partnerships between education and service. They were intent on reestablishing the School's reputation for clinical excellence and on nurturing a scholarly atmosphere by adopting the three-point professional model: practice, research, and education. "The faculty has essentially been one dimensional—that is, teachers," she explained at the time. "Though they committed themselves 100 percent to the welfare and education of students, they didn't establish a research base. Secondly, most had given up their practice positions to teach full time, so they lost touch with practice. That's critical, especially now, because practice is changing so rapidly. Soon after leaving clinical practice, one is teaching nursing from a perspective that is no longer valid ... Nobody else [at the Medical Center] is unidimensional. Everybody else is engaged in research or practice as well as teaching. We can't survive if we aren't similarly productive."

While the model did not blatantly violate the task force guidelines, it effectively rendered them moot. Before long, Goldberger was gone and the School was convincing naysayers that scholarship and nursing education were not mutually exclusive. Within a year or so, enrollments were up (countering a national trend) and operating deficits were erased. Undergraduate study was retained, but mainly as a stepping stone to graduate study. And the beginnings of a scholarly faculty were assembled. In 1988 Mary Mundinger's appointment was made permanent—an obvious vote of confidence in her vision of academic nursing from University authorities, if not her faculty. Mundinger's changes were so sweeping, so radical in comparison to traditional Columbia nursing dogma, that most of the instructors were forced to or decided to leave. Short-term stability, one alumna notes, had to be sacrificed in the name of long-term stability. Not surprisingly, many alumni were startled by the events.

At the heart of the Columbia Model is the country's first universal faculty practice plan in nursing, which requires instructors to engage in research or "scholarly" practice, depending on their academic credentials. Those with doctorates, called "research scholars," are required to conduct research in nursing or a related field, and they are given the time and resources to do so. "That's the only way to be current," believes Richard Garfield, Ph.D., assistant professor of nursing and public health and director of research. "It means that faculty will be teaching a little less, but they will give a lot more when they teach."

Thus far, the School's research scholars have studied care of the frail elderly, case management of diabetics, various aspects of AIDS, suicide prevention for adolescents, family stress and dysfunction in times of crisis, neural crest cell development, and patterns of ethical practice in nursing, among other topics. Demonstrating the School's ability to become a significant participant in Columbia's academic community, Mundinger and Garfield were awarded a million-dollar grant from the Kellogg Foundation to craft a model approach for academic medical centers—starting with Columbia-Presbyterian—to the care of poor, medically underserved, inner-city communities. The investigators' final report will address emerging health care issues, such as the need for increased home care, continuity of care, and access to care; suggest a research agenda to provide data for new primary care initiatives; delineate the resources and linkages required to deliver quality care in large urban communities; and recommend changes in the training of health professionals. The grant also set the tone for the Mundinger administration, signalling that it would adopt a more eclectic approach to nursing. Larger issues of health policy would not be ignored.

Complementing the research scholars are "clinical scholars," nondoctorally prepared faculty who participate in an outside clinical practice that is salaried, secondary to their teaching responsibilities (consuming up to two days per week), and, most important, scholarly. Moonlighting as a staff nurse, for example, is not acceptable. The position must offer opportunities to develop or test nursing theory or practice. Thus far, faculty members have practiced in women's shelters, geriatric day care centers, pediatrics clinics, student health services, public schools, operating rooms, labor and delivery areas, anesthesia services, emergency departments, and critical care units, to name a few. They have been involved in virtually every facet of health care — primary care, consulting, staff development, orientation, quality assurance, patient teaching and counseling, accreditation site visits, ethics rounds, nursing unit design, and search committees for heads of medical departments.

"It's natural for nurses to be practicing," says Assistant Dean for Student Affairs Theresa Doddato, whose faculty practice is based at Roosevelt Hospital, where she is educational director of nurse anesthesia services. "After all, the focus of the profession is patient care. Like artists and performers, who must constantly practice in order to keep proficient, we must do the same thing if we are to maintain and promote excellence in the practice aspect of our profession."

Faculty practice has already proved successful, according to Cheryl Holly, Ed.D., former associate dean for student affairs, who has studied the practices of fifteen instructors. In the journal *Nursing Connections,* she reports that such practices are broadening faculty perspectives, enhancing classroom and clinical instruction, boosting faculty self-esteem, improving patient care, and widening the School's influence. Moreover, income from the various practices and research projects is lessening the School's precarious reliance on tuition income and extending resources for faculty salaries.

Clinical scholars report that they are "now sharing anecdotes from their practices with the students, rather than using examples that were a few years old," writes Holly. "Many faculty had students with them in their practice sites. The majority of faculty indicated that they spent a considerable amount of time in curriculum revision based on a better understanding of contemporary practice." One instructor commented, "I find it difficult to teach something I've not personally done or observed. I have much more credibility because I practice. Clinical credibility is necessary if we purport to be master clinicians."

Not surprisingly, some instructors have experienced difficulty cultivating both halves of the teacher-practitioner role. "Many felt pressured by their own need to do excellent work in both the practice site and the school, and were, therefore, putting in more than the negotiated amount of time," Holly writes. This has impinged upon time for supervising and counseling students, communicating with peers, and participating in various academic activities. A few instructors have complained of having to serve "two masters" and of continual exhaustion. The problem, Holly suspects, is that some faculty have not merged their dual roles into an "integrated whole," a result of "inconsistent, unclear, or widely differing expectations between the work sites and individual faculty." Role integration is likely to improve with time, especially as faculty become wiser negotiators of practice responsibilities. Nonetheless, Holly has found general satisfaction with this added academic dimension. "Faculty indicated that they enjoyed the flexibility and autonomy associated with their practice, and that they would not accept a job without a practice component," she concludes.

Hand-in-hand with faculty practice has come another innovation — clinical precepting—which has transformed the way undergraduates are introduced to bedside care. The faculty concluded that traditional clinical supervision, in which a group of six to ten students is guided by a lone instructor, does not give novices enough individual attention and hands-on experience to prepare them for the acutely ill patients and complicated technologies that now predominate. Merely one generation ago, fifty nurses were needed to deliver round-the-clock care for one hundred patients; today, ninety-one nurses are needed. "[Traditional supervision] didn't work very well," says Mundinger. "Students didn't get socialized into real practice. That's where nursing culture shock came from. When the students graduated and went into practice, they hit this invisible wall of the real responsibility of patient care—and many quit nursing because of it." Furthermore, the old system was costly, requiring tremendous amounts of faculty time.

Fortunately, the faculty discovered the germ of a solution in the existing system. To extend their reach, instructors had been eliciting the assistance of staff nurses who showed an aptitude for teaching and a desire for an expanded role. This impromptu collaboration seemed to improve teaching as well as patient care and staff morale. "We decided it would make more sense to formalize this arrangement," says Sarah Cook. Today, for the first time in any school of nursing, every first-semester student is assigned to a clinical preceptor for the initial patient care experience. Faculty remain on-site, offering instruction as needed, conducting weekly student seminars, and serving as liaisons among students, preceptors, and administrators.

A basic tenet of clinical precepting, Cheryl Holly writes, is that "the senior practitioner in the field—the staff nurse—is best able to instruct the student in the complexities and fast pace of nursing practice while contributing to the socialization of these new nurses to the work environment." The arrangement could be described as an academically focused "cognitive apprenticeship," in contrast to the task-focused "craft apprenticeship" characteristic of traditional nursing education.

"We guarantee that beginning students have basic skills before they come to the unit so they can make some sort of contribution," explains Cook. Students return to the same unit for their final clinical experience, at which point they are highly skilled and productive. The hospital also profits by socializing the students to its particular institution, gaining a leg up on other potential employers—no small benefit when it costs thousands of dollars to recruit and orient each new nurse.

A further benefit is that precepting is less disruptive to nursing units. "The managers feel they aren't being 'invaded,'" notes Elizabeth Rolston, university affiliation coordinator at Lenox Hill Hospital, one of the first sites to participate in clinical precepting. "It's just one student working with one preceptor." Consequently, clinical affiliates have been able to open up new clinical areas to student nurses. "This is the first time students have been placed in our open-heart, intensive care, and cardiac care units," says Rolston.

Participating institutions include the Presbyterian Hospital and its urban community hospital, the Allen Pavilion; St. Luke's-Roosevelt Hospital Center; Lenox Hill Hospital; Memorial Sloan-Kettering Cancer Center; Mt. Sinai Medical Center; and Lawrence Hospital (Bronxville, N.Y.). Overall, the School uses more than hundred clinical sites throughout the metropolitan area to prepare undergraduate and graduate students.

For their contribution, preceptors are entitled to an adjunct faculty appointment with Columbia, access to certain continuing education programs and university resources, an expanded clinical role, and the opportunity to serve as a role model—all incentives to keep good nurses in nursing and at the bedside. Most preceptors are pleased with the arrangement. "I like the program because I like to teach," says Lenox Hill preceptor Philip Jacobs. "I like to think that I'm helping them get a good start in their careers, because if they have a good knowledge base coming in and learn how to organize, their first exposure to the work environment after graduation won't be as traumatic... They won't go into practice with as many false hopes and won't end up disillusioned."

Preliminary analyses confirm the faculty's expectations of clinical precepting. "Both first- and second-level students enjoyed the independence of the precepted experience, feeling involved with the unit, seeing good nurses in action, and being able to interact with those nurses," reports Anne Peirce, Ph.D., assistant dean for undergraduate studies and assistant professor of nursing, in "Precepted Students' View of Their Clinical Experience," a survey study of twenty-two undergraduates published in the *Journal of Nursing Education*. Beginning students felt that precepting offered a well-rounded, hands-on introduction to bedside care, while advanced students felt it offered realistic practice opportunities. Precepted students have commented: "I have learned the difference between short-cuts and compromise"; "This experience has taught me the importance of organizing and prioritizing"; "Now I know how nursing is really practiced and what will be expected of me when I graduate"; and "Now I am anxious to begin work and be part of a team and develop greater autonomy."

Interestingly, students seem to develop a different relationship with staff preceptors than with faculty instructors, a relationship more concerned with professional competence than with personal style. "Preceptors are chosen for their clinical expertise and that is how the students appeared to judge them," Peirce writes. "Instructors on the other hand were judged not only on clinical expertise but on a variety of other personality characteristics. The instructors' direct link to the educational system may be part of the reason why this difference exists, so too may be the maternalistic manner in which many nursing schools operate."

Perhaps Peirce's most compelling finding is that clinical precepting "may hasten the professional growth of students." Traditionally supervised students in their last clinical course reportedly progress through three stages of professional development. In the first two, they gain self-confidence, but only in the third do they articulate a clinical focus, achieve independence from their instructor, and feel like real nurses. "In the present study," writes Peirce, "only the first-level students exhibited attributes of the [early developmental stages.] The second-level students reported functioning on a par with staff nurses, being comfortable in their clinical setting, and exhibited no dependence upon the preceptor staff." Thus, it does appear that one-to-one supervision lessens the "reality shock" of new nurses.

One key to successful clinical precepting is finding and developing the right preceptor. Would-be preceptors are identified by the nursing education departments of participating hospitals. The nurses must be highly skilled and meet the minimal requirements for an associate faculty appointment (a baccalaureate in nursing, two years' experience, current licensure); certification in a specialty area is desired. According to Priscilla Loanzon, Ed.D., assistant professor of nursing, who has studied preceptor development and certification, most nurses who meet these criteria are confident of their clinical expertise, but not their teaching expertise. Thus, all preceptor candidates attend a special orientation workshop covering the School's history, philosophy, theoretical framework, and curriculum as well as clinical teaching strategies, selection and evaluation of student assignments, and feedback techniques.

Another component of the Columbia Model is accelerated study leading to the master's degree. Two distinct tracks are offered, one for students with a baccalaureate in another field and one for registered nurses who have yet to earn a nursing baccalaureate. The former track, named the Entry-Into-Practice Program for Non-nurses, is designed for the increasing numbers of disenchanted workers from all sorts of professions who are coming to the School in search of a more rewarding career. They are an unusually accomplished and motivated lot, intent on establishing an advanced practice as clinical specialists or nurse practitioners or administrators or educators. At the same time, they generally cannot afford to spend too much time out of the work force; many have families and mortgages and other obligations. The School's solution is an accelerated program in which students earn both the baccalaureate and a specialty master's in three to three-and-a-half years. What distinguishes Columbia's accelerated program from others is a midpoint break for full-time practice. "The graduate faculty felt very strongly that students should have a period of time when they work as registered nurses," says Sarah Cook. "So Dr. Mundinger came up with a program that in sixteen months prepares students for entry into practice." Then, as registered nurses, they begin full-time work and part-time graduate study. Finally, in the third stage, the emphasis reverses to full-time study and part-time work.

One of the program's main attractions is that students are treated as master's-degree candidates at the onset; graduate-level theory is presented in the first semester, and all clinical experiences are geared toward their desired area of specialization. (They still are awarded baccalaureates, which are required to sit for state registration examinations and licensing.)

In a related program, promising students are given an opportunity to trade future service for current tuition support. On one side is the would-be student, hard-pressed to pay for another degree (federal financial aid is not available for second baccalaureates); on the other, the hospital, endlessly seeking high-quality nurses and spending a fortune in the process. "So we evolved a plan in which the hospital pays for the entry-into-practice [baccalaureate] component of the student's education," Cook relates. "In return, the student guarantees that, as a graduate registered nurse, he or she will work for that institution for an equal amount of time." The arrangement articulates perfectly with the accelerated curriculum, which requires the student to work after the baccalaureate phase. "We also guarantee that the student has most of his or her clinical experiences at the sponsoring hospital, which professionally socializes the student to that institution," she adds. (The student is sent to the School's other clinical affiliates for experiences that the participating hospital cannot provide.) Everyone benefits: the School gets a student and a tuition payment it might have lost; the student an opportunity to study for an advanced degree at the "cost" of having to work at a prestigious health care institution for about a year and a half; and the institution a high-quality Columbia nurse, already socialized to its ways, at a lower-than-normal cost. Presbyterian Hospital and Memorial Sloan-Kettering Cancer Center are currently participating.

Although Presbyterian remains a valued clinical affiliate, relations between the School and the Hospital still are strained, largely because of differences in practice philosophy. While the School's thrust has switched to advanced nurse practice, the Hospital's has not, according to Mundinger. She suspects that Presbyterian soon will adopt a progressive approach in order to keep up with the changing health care scene, and she looks forward to more clinical partnerships with this "natural" affiliate.

Left untouched by the curriculum renewal is the philosophically compatible accelerated master's program (AMP) for registered nurses. In AMP, which slightly predates the Columbia Model, registered nurses without a nursing degree follow a streamlined path to the master's, in some instances in as little as two-and-a-half years, even while working part time. Credit is awarded individually for previous nursing and educational experience. The idea is to offer highly qualified and motivated nurses more reasonable opportunities for clinical advancement, which theoretically should keep them satisfied and in the profession.

Although Columbia undergraduates in nursing have always been bright and capable, today's student nurses are different. They're older and wiser, seasoned professionals with clearly articulated goals. Among the recent enrollees are a computer scientist, a football player and salesman, a physician and mother of three from the Dominican Republic, a dress designer, an administrator of the New York area Emmy Awards, a television health and science reporter, an advertising account executive, an Off-Broadway actress, a financial consultant, a taxi driver, a specialist in movement science, a Peace Corps health educator, and an architect.

Connie Milner '90, the Emmy Awards administrator, was a typically untypical student nurse. Milner gravitated to nursing only recently, transformed by the experience of caring for her mother, who was stricken with Alzheimer's disease. "For a year and a half," she recounts, "I tried to keep her out of a nursing home. I nursed her, I learned how to give injections, how to change the bed while she was still in it, how to wash her, how to safeguard the house. I quit my weekend job to stay with her from Friday night through Monday morning. The strange thing was, by Monday I felt so good; there was something to this. I actually improved the quality of one person's life in my own small way. In the eight years I worked at the Emmy Awards, with the glamour and the gowns ... , I never felt that way for one minute." Milner's mother died, but in the process a nurse was born.

Faced with such accomplished and diverse people, the faculty have been forced to rethink its ways and means. "With junior transfer students, either purposefully or unconsciously, you tend to set up a program that smacks of maternalism," says Cook. "It's a combination of having to deal with late adolescence and attitudes from the old apprenticeship programs that still remain. But now, we are dealing with different students — adult learners — who don't take nicely to being treated like children ... They are mature, focused, motivated adults who know what they want and where they are going."

The School has also come to be filled with "nontraditional" students — men and minorities — who accounted for one-third and one-quarter, respectively, of new enrollees in 1990. According to Cheryl Holly, "Nursing, like teaching, has always been a route for upward mobility for the lower classes. First it was the Irish and the Italians. Now, that's changing to blacks and Hispanics." The precipitous rise in minority enrollments is also a result of increasing support from private foundations and other forms of financial aid. It is harder to explain the growing number of men, but apparently the age-old stigma of male nurses is dissipating, at least among caring, educated, and mature men.

Immigrants are also adding to the School's cultural mix, lured to the United States by its rich educational and employment opportunities in nursing. In recent years, a number of Filipinos, Russians, Botswanians, and Dominicans have enrolled, many of whom have studied or practiced nursing or medicine in their native lands.

To support these varied students, the School has created an Office of Multicultural Affairs, which is directed by Pat Shonubi, assistant professor of clinical nursing, an experienced nurse and minority counselor. Shonubi's office delivers a variety of support services, ranging from open-agenda group meetings to seminars on study skills, time management, and writing.

According to Sarah Cook, minorities (and many adult learners) also must be taught to "work the system" better. They commonly do not know how to get the most out of a large, complicated organization, such as the School of Nursing, which is part of a major university and a massive medical center with countless affiliations. Cook explains, "It's the same phenomenon we see in the neighborhood of Columbia-Presbyterian. The health services may be there, but the people often don't know how to gain access to them. It's not that they aren't capable, they just don't know how the system works ... It's very difficult to make the adjustment from a successful work-life to nursing school ... even if you have a master's degree in philosophy or science."

Faculty, too, must make adjustments, she adds. "In recent years, we've been examining what people have to do or know to become a nurse and what kind of students we have here ... One thing we've looked at is the use of facilitative teaching rather than punitive teaching. In other words, the teacher has a responsibility to find a way to let students learn; it's not only the students' responsibility to change their style of learning. Several faculty members have felt this way for a long time, but it's been difficult to articulate and approach."

Dean Mundinger has been only partly successful so far in improving the faculty mix. Interestingly, not one faculty member is a baccalaureate graduate of the School of Nursing, quite a contrast to the times not long ago when virtually every instructor was an alumna. As for minority faculty, "I wish we had more," she says, "but they are a scarce commodity. They are highly recruited and can choose wherever they want to go. A nurse with a doctoral degree can teach in a nursing school or in public health, medicine, sociology." And a nurse with an advanced clinical degree can find higher salaries in nursing service, Cook adds. "It's not a matter of discrimination or bias, but simply market conditions."

In the meantime, says Mundinger, the School is doing its best "to make sure that this is an enriching place for minority faculty, and that all faculty have an attractive role." The School is also preparing the next generation of minority teachers by bringing more minorities into the profession. "Within six years from the time they walk in here as beginning students, they could be clinical faculty members," she explains. "That's a short lag time compared to most other professions."

If the faculty is not culturally diverse, it does not lack experience in working with diverse cultures, a benefit of the School's location in the middle of the ethnic mosaic that is Washington Heights and New York City. "Our faculty are all in practice," remarks Mundinger. "They're not in some ivy-covered office building thinking about what book they'd like to read next and how they would incorporate it in a lecture. They're out there taking care of different types of people. Their anecdotes in class have to do with a wide variety of cultural interactions."

In 1986 Mary Mundinger said, "We need to be very careful that those who come here with a career goal of high-level nursing education get what they pay for — something different from a non-university-based program. We must make use of our access to the School of Public Health, the College of Physicians & Surgeons, the library, the research opportunities — the things that make it worth the premium they pay to come here." Judging by the steady rise in the quantity and quality of applicants willing to pay Columbia's pricey tuition (more than $14,000 a year), Mundinger has succeeded. Flush with new enrollees and diversified sources of income, the School is financially stable, actually better off than most other components of the University. In recent years, the endowment has more than doubled, to $11 million, and financial aid to students has quadrupled. Adding style to the School's substance, Mundinger has essentially completed the Georgian's renovation, decorating several rooms with treasured Maxwell Hall memorabilia.

Today, nurses can study to become clinical specialists in six areas (critical care, nurse anesthesia, nurse midwifery, oncology, neonatal/perinatal care, or psychiatric/mental health nursing) or primary care practitioners in five areas (adult, family, geriatric, neonatal, or pediatric nursing). The core curriculum features courses in nursing theory, advanced role development, health policy and management, curriculum development and teaching, advanced physiology, pathophysiology, family theory and therapy, and theories of psychosocial development, and research.

In addition, nurses can choose to study for dual master's degrees with the School of Public Health or, in a new program, with the School of Business. The latter program, in two-and-a-half years, prepares nurses to become advanced clinical practitioners and executive nurse managers in a variety of health care settings.

Any moment now, the School will win final approval for a clinically focused doctoral program in nursing science. Not surprisingly, the current proposal, crafted by Cheryl Holly and Anne Peirce, has aroused opposition from some scientists at the University who still argue that nursing does not constitute a defined body of knowledge. Nonetheless, barring any last-minute complications, the first doctoral candidates might enroll as early as the fall of 1992, which would be a fitting start to the School's one-hundredth academic year. "We've spent a lot of time educating people about what we are and what we do, and that's starting to pay off," says Sarah Cook.

Certain to add to the School's national reputation are four new or proposed endowed chairs. The first, the Chair for Health Policy, is the only one of its kind in a school of nursing. According to the dean, the chair is not necessarily for someone involved in legislative affairs. "We think of health policy in a much broader context. The person who takes this chair will engage in research that influences how public resources are allocated, with a specific focus on explicating the value of nursing." For example, the researcher might examine the cost effectiveness of case management for elderly people who live at home. "The new chair adds to the School's emphasis on health policy and brings us one step closer to activities of the School of Public Health and the College of Physicians & Surgeons. It will make us more of a major player in health policy issues at the Medical Center and beyond."

Another innovation is the coming Chair in Pharmaceutical Nursing Therapy. "Nurses in thirty-eight states now have prescription privileges," the dean reports. "This chair is devoted to developing nursing's use of this new authority in practice, research, and education."

The School is currently working to endow the Anna C. Maxwell Chair, which will honor the accomplishments of the School's founder and highlight the School's traditional clinical focus. The fourth chair (as yet unnamed) is a gift of the Columbia University – Presbyterian Hospital Alumni Association. Funds for this chair come from the capital growth and interest on donations from generations of alumni. "It is truly the legacy of 100 graduating classes," notes Alumni Association President Keville Frederickson.

Although no single individual is responsible for the School's renewal, Dean Mary O'Neil Mundinger deserves a large share of the credit. Mundinger, who was born in Fredonia, N.Y., in 1937 (fittingly, the year the School joined the University), holds a baccalaureate in nursing from the University of Michigan (1959), a master's in administration of community nursing services from Teachers College (1974), and a doctorate in public health from Columbia's School of Public Health (1981). Her career began with a Head Start program in Oxford, Ohio, where she was health director, followed by a stint as a public health nurse in Ithaca, N.Y. Switching gears, she became director of nursing education at United Hospital in Port Chester, N.Y. and a faculty member at the Lienhard School of Nursing at Pace University in Pleasantville, N.Y.

Mundinger joined the School of Nursing in 1982 as director of graduate studies. From this post, she oversaw the creation of programs in family, acute care, and community nursing and laid the foundations for two more, in geriatric and oncology nursing. During the 1984-85 academic year, as a Robert Wood Johnson Health Policy Fellow, she served as a staff member for Senator Edward Kennedy's Senate Committee on Labor and Human Services. She returned to Columbia in late 1985 as assistant dean at P&S, continuing her policy work. The following year, she was appointed full professor and acting dean at the School of Nursing, then full dean in 1988.

An expert on home care and care of the frail elderly, Mundinger is the author of *Autonomy in Nursing* (1980) and *Home Care Controversy: Too Little, Too Costly, Too Late* (1983), both of which garnered book-of-the-year honors from the *American Journal of Nursing*. She has also served as associate editor of *Nursing Outlook* and editorial reviewer for Aspen publications. Mundinger, who is married and the mother of four grown children, is a Fellow of the American Academy of Nurses and the National Academy of Practice and a member of policy committees of the Institute of Medicine and the National Academy of Sciences.

From her prematurely silver-white hair to her forthright manner to her original vision of nursing, Mundinger is a modern-day incarnation of the School's founder. Like Anna Maxwell, she has confronted a conservative, self-protective health care establishment, forcing it to reassess nursing's potential. Like Maxwell, she has proved that there are alternatives to existing practices, that nurses need not be second to anyone, as practitioners or as scholars. Exactly one hundred years ago, Maxwell dreamed of bringing nursing "to the level of a profession"; today, Mundinger is realizing that dream.

Nevertheless, Mundinger is far from content. Hidden in the rosy enrollment picture is a disturbing trend: Not enough of the School's students, now numbering about 450, are new to nursing. Word of new opportunities in the field is spreading to non-nurses, though slowly. Thus, the student body largely consists of nurses who, in Mundinger's words, have returned "to school because they have found the practice site so hostile, so difficult, and so unappealing." Clearly, if the profession is to attract and retain nurses it must make the predominant clinical setting (still the hospital) more amenable to nurses. Salaries have risen substantially in recent years, yet they are only one issue. "We also have to change the structure and rewards of work, the image of nursing, and the professional reputation of nursing in order to make it attractive," says Mundinger. "Most forward-thinking directors of nursing service in hospitals are looking for ways to structure patient assignments to give nurses more accountability, more autonomy, and more follow-through, so that they actually have responsibility for an identifiable group of patients over a period of time, as a physician does." However, she adds, directors of nursing cannot do this alone. Hospital administrators must cooperate by reorganizing the practice setting so that nurses "can do the highest-level work for which they are prepared. Instead, employers are cutting out the infrastructure below nursing; aides, dietitians, central supply workers, even pharmacists are disappearing. Nurses are expected to work harder, and an increasing amount of that work is unsatisfying, below their abilities."

Furthermore, says Mundinger, physicians must learn to treat nurses as colleagues, not subservient caregivers. "That doesn't happen after you get an M.D. after your name. It happens while you're getting socialized into the profession. Let medical and nursing students work together in the same classrooms and clinical sites, so when they first enter practice, the collegial connection is already established. It can be an attractive, satisfying connection for both physicians and nurses. Physicians will feel better about sharing care responsibilities with nurses." To this end, Mundinger has strengthened ties to the College of Physicians & Surgeons and other educational components of the Medical Center. Encouragingly, P&S is in the midst of its own curriculum revolution, one that will emphasize team teaching and collaborative practice between medicine and nursing.

With the Columbia Model of Nursing Education, Mundinger and her faculty believe they have satisfied the University's demands for academic rigor *and* clinical excellence. "Such innovation does not threaten the traditional concept of nursing, but rather restructures practice and educational settings to maintain quality health care," notes Cheryl Holly. "Nurses educated and practicing within the framework of the Columbia Model are not only expert caregivers but administrators, teachers, problem solvers, and diplomats as well. Viewed from this perspective, the Columbia Model has the unlimited potential to change the face of nursing practice."

And much more, says Joseph A. Califano, Jr., secretary of the Department of Health, Education and Welfare under President Jimmy Carter. In a stirring address at the School's Centennial Convocation on September, 11, 1991 (proclaimed Columbia University School of Nursing Day by New York City Mayor David N. Dinkins), Califano celebrated the Columbia Model "as the premier example of what a school of nursing should be." Graduates of such a school, he said, are ideally situated to partake in what he called "America's Health Care Revolution." If Califano had his way, he would overthrow a system that spends almost $2 billion a day on health care ("more than enough") yet continues to ration care by "our wallets." Of all the people who have a role to play in this revolution, he said,

> few of us have a greater responsibility than the American nurse...It's time to give nurses more to do, to face the reality that the physician monopoly over the practice of medicine, once a professional imperative to protect patients from quacks and charlatans, is now rooted as much in economic self-interest as in consumer protection. Failure to relax that monopoly denies the American people many benefits of modern technology. For such technology ... opens to trained nurses the ability to perform many procedures once reserved for physicians, just as competently and less expensively...
>
> If we are going to attract the best and brightest to nursing, we must offer them the opportunity to use their talent and training to its full capacity. That means opening the door of modern diagnosis and treatment to qualified nurses... [which will free physicians] to stay abreast of rapid changes in technology and pharmaceuticals and to concentrate on the more complex features of medical practice...

No one who is overweight, who smokes, who doesn't exercise, who shows signs of inordinate stress, should be able to see any nurse without being informed of the risks, and getting some good advice — and where appropriate, a referral for special help ... Nurses — wherever they are, in doctor's offices, hospitals, patients' homes, schools, corporate offices, rural clinics — have an extraordinary opportunity to counsel patients...

This is no time for nurses to sit in the back of the medical bus ... As we approach the twenty-first century, the cost of decades of indulgence in health care has caught up with us. We can no longer afford to buy our way out of our difficulties. We must work our way out and think our way out. That's why we need nurses to be American health care revolutionaries.

Only time will tell if the Columbia Model and Columbia nurses are helping to foment this revolution. Hardly a month goes by without a visit from a nursing educator from places near and far — from Manhattan to Michigan, from Armenia to Australia, from Spain to Sweden, from Asia to Iceland — seeking new perspectives on academic nursing. No one else has adopted the model wholesale — what is right for Columbia is not necessarily right for everyone — but portions of it are surfacing here and there. And dozens of nurses prepared under the Columbia Model are advancing through the health care system — practicing, teaching, researching, publishing, consulting.

There are those, of course, who see no need for a revolution in health care or for a new model of nursing education. Faculty members have departed, alumni have complained, educators have disapproved, physicians have protested, and administrators have criticized — all perhaps fearing that the School has abandoned its clinical focus, its supposed reason for being. "The reason students come to Columbia ... will be the same in the future as it was in the past — premier clinical training," counters Mundinger. "Students here get high-level supervision and tremendously broad opportunities to learn about clinical care. It's not better at any other place I know of. We're not going to lose that in developing research."

If anything will be lost, the faculty seem to be saying, it will be the notion that nursing is for women only, for second-rate thinkers, or for subservient caregivers. For one hundred years, through the hands and hearts and minds of 8,300 graduates (82 percent of whom are still alive), the Columbia University School of Nursing has been refuting those ill-informed notions. Long ago Anna Maxwell told an audience of new graduate nurses, "The field is wide; you must set no limits to your usefulness." Today, the field is even wider. "The opportunities in nursing have never been better," says Mary Mundinger, "particularly with the move toward community-based care and away from expensive high-tech care. Never has a career in nursing been so inviting. Nurses are in short supply. Nursing leadership is critically needed. We have an opportunity to highlight our contributions in ways we've never had before. It's a promising time for nursing."

Bibliography

BOOKS

Austin AL: *The Woolsey Sisters of New York: A Family's Involvement in the Civil War and a New Profession, 1860-1900.* Philadelphia, American Philosophical Society, 1971.

Ashley JA: *Hospitals, Paternalism, and the Role of the Nurse.* New York, Teachers College Press, 1976.

Clappison JB: *The Training Camp for Nurses at Vassar College.* Lake Mills, Iowa, Graphic Publishing Co., 1964.

Davis F (Ed): *The Nursing Profession: Five Sociological Essays.* New York, John Wiley & Sons, 1966.

Delavan DB: *Early Days of the Presbyterian Hospital in the City of New York.* New York, published privately, 1926.

Dock LL: *History of American Red Cross Nursing.* New York, Macmillan, 1922.

Flanagan L: *One Strong Voice: The Story of the American Nurses Association.* Kansis City, American Nurses Association, 1976.

Goldmark JC: *Nursing and Nursing Education in the United States and Canada.* New York, Macmillan, 1923.

Hine DC: *Black Women in White: Racial Conflict and Cooperation in the Nursing Profession, 1890-1950.* Bloomington, Ind., Indiana University Press, 1989.

Jamieson EM, Sewall MF, and Suhrie EB: *Trends in Nursing History: Their Social, International, and Ethical Relationships.* Philadelphia, W.B. Saunders Co., 1966.

Kaufman M (Ed.): *Dictionary of American Nursing Biography.* New York, Greenwood Press, 1988.

Kelly LY: *The Nursing Experience: Trends, Challenges, and Transitions.* New York, Macmillan, 1987.

Lagemann EC: *Nursing History: New Perspectives, New Possibilities.* New York, Teachers College Press, 1983.

Lamb AR: *The Presbyterian Hospital and the Columbia-Presbyterian Medical Center 1868-1943: A History of a Great Medical Adventure.* New York, Columbia University Press, 1955.

Lee E: *History of the School of Nursing of the Presbyterian Hospital, New York, 1892-1942*. New York, G.P. Putnam's Sons, 1942.

Lee E: *Neighbors 1892-1967: A History of The Department of Nursing, Faculty of Medicine, Columbia University 1937-1967 and its Predecessor The School of Nursing of the Presbyterian Hospital New York 1892-1937*. New York, Columbia University-Presbyterian Hospital School of Nursing Alumnae Association, Inc., 1967.

Lightfoot SL: *Balm in Gilead*. Reading, Mass., Addison-Wesley Publishing Co., 1988.

Maxwell AC and Pope AE: *Practical Nursing: A Text-Book for Nurses*, (Third Edition). New York, G.P. Putnam's Sons, 1914.

Melosh B: *The Physician's Hand: Work Culture and Conflict in American Nursing*. Philadelphia: Temple University Press, 1982.

Melosh B: "Apprenticeship Culture and Nurses' Resistance to Professionalization." In *Alternate Conceptions of Work and Society*. Proceedings of the 1988 Deans' Summer Seminar of the American Association of Colleges of Nursing.

Parsons SE: *History of the Massachussetts General Hospital Training School for Nurses*. Boston, Whitcomb & Barrows, 1922.

Peto M: *Women Were Not Expected*. West Englewood, N.J., published privately, 1947.

Rappleye WC: *The Faculty of Medicine 1910-1958*. New York, Columbia University, 1958.

Reverby S: *Ordered to Care*. Cambridge, Cambridge University Press, 1987.

Riddle MM: *Boston City Training School for Nurses: Historial Sketch*. Boston, published privately, 1928.

Robinson V: *White Caps: The Story of Nursing*. Philadelphia, Lippincott, 1946.

Rosenberg CE: *The Care of Strangers: The Rise of America's Hospital System*. New York, Basic Books, 1987.

Rothman, SM: *Woman's Proper Place: A History of Changing Ideas and Practices, 1870 to the Present*. New York, Basic Books, 1978.

Zinn H: *A People's History of the United States*. New York, Harper Colophon Books, 1980.

JOURNALS & MAGAZINES
(chronological order)

Thompson WG: "The Overtrained Nurse." *New York Medical Journal*, April 28, 1906, pp. 845-849.

Cameron ME: (Review of) *Practical Nursing: A Text-Book for Nurses, and a Hand-Book for all who Care for the Sick*, by Anna Caroline Maxwell and Amy E. Pope. *American Journal of Nursing* 1908:88-90.

Bewley MA: "Visiting Nursing as a Part of the Training School Curriculum." *American Journal of Nursing* 1908:890-895.

Hegan ET: "The Russian Revolution from a Hospital Window." *Harpers Monthly* Vol. 135 (1917), No. 808, pp. 555-568.

Maxwell AC: "The Private Nurse and Twenty-Four Hour Hospital Duty." *American Journal of Nursing* 1917:191-194.

Maxwell AC: "Struggles of the Pioneers." *American Journal of Nursing* 1921:321-329.

"Anna Caroline Maxwell, R.N., M.A." *American Journal of Nursing* 1921:692-697.

"Tributes to Miss Maxwel." (Editorial) *American Journal of Nursing* 1921:683.

"A Brilliant Event." (Editorial) *American Journal of Nursing* 1922:407-409.

"Anna Caroline Maxwell, R.N., M.A., 1851-1929." *American Journal of Nursing* 1924:187-194.

Lee E: "The Block System of Instruction." *American Journal of Nursing* 1931:935-939.

Lee E: "A Year's Survey of Ward Teaching." *American Journal of Nursing* 1932:445-451.

"You Bet They're Legionnaires." *American Legion Monthly* April 1934.

"History and Manual of the Army Nurse Corps." *Army Medical Bulletin* Number 41; Special Issue: October 1, 1937.

Jones TM: "Modern Florence Nightingales from Columbia's Newest School." *Columbia Alumni News* April 26, 1940, pp. 5, 12.

Conrad ME and Reddig RF: "Nursing and Health in the Family: A School of Nursing Reports." *American Journal of Nursing* 1940:1020-1021

Dwyer SM: "A Base Hospital in England." *American Journal of Nursing* 1941:877-884.

Peto M: "Tea in England." *American Journal of Nursing* 1943:653-4.

Kirk NT: "Girls in the Foxholes." *American Magazine* May, 1944.

Conrad ME: "Preparing the Nursing for Her Professional Responsibilities." *American Journal of Nursing* 1949:110-112.

"Nursing Care for Patients — Dilemma 1959." *New York Medicine* November 5, 1959; pp. 881-896.

"The Shortage of Bedside Nurses." *New York Medicine* April 5, 1960.

Cooper P: "Nurse, be the nurse your hospital trained you to be." *Bulletin of the American College of Surgeons* March-April, 1968, pp. 71-72.

"National Commission for the Study of Nursing and Nursing Education: Summary Report and Recommendations." *American Journal of Nursing* 1970:279-294.

Group TM and Roberts JI: "Exorcising the Ghosts of Crimea." *Nursing Outlook* 1974;22:368-372

Baer ED: "Nursing's Divided House — An Historical View." *Nursing Research* 1985;34:32-38

Cook SS and Finelli L: "Faculty Practice: A New Perspective on Academic Competence." *Journal of Professional Nursing* January-February 1988, pp. 23-29.

Brennan H and Dooley M: "Where Have All the Nurses Gone?" *Columbia* December 1988, pp. 14-19.

Holly CM: "Attacking the Nursing Shortage from Within: The Columbia Model." *Nursing Connections* Winter 1989, pp. 19-27.

Cannadine D: "The Administering Angel." *New Republic* August 13, 1990, pp. 38-41.

NEWSPAPERS
(chronological order)

"A Manufactured Sensation: The Charges Against the Presbyterian Hospital Are Not Supported." *World* November 5, 1891.

"The Charges Fall Through: Presbyterian Hospital Vindicated—The Wild Baublings of an 'Opium Fiend' Disproved." *Mail and Express* November 5, 1891.

"Fatal Jump From a Hospital Window." *World* February 10, 1897.

"New Nurses Home Will Cost $300,000." *New York Herald* February 12, 1901.

"Suit Over Nurses' Home." *New York Herald* March 3, 1901.

"Neighbors Oppose Building." *New York Tribune* April 12, 1901.

"Is A Nurses Home Offensive?" (Editorial). *World* May 18, 1901.

"Mrs. Vanderbilt in New Charity, Provides Nurses." *New York Evening Telegram* February 15, 1904.

"Peculiar Rules for the Nurses." *New York Herald* September 12, 1904.

"Hospital Will Move: Presbyterian Institution Buys New Site." *New York Herald Tribune* February 10, 1909.

"Presbyterians Buying More Land." *Evening Mail* February 13, 1909.

"Haig Cites Nurses for Bravery." *World* December 29, 1917.

"From the Presbyterian, N.Y." *Thermometer* (Vassar Training School), Vols. 1 and 2, January 1919.

"Great Medical Center is Ready to Function." *New York Times* March 11, 1928.

"Presbyterian Hospital is Now in New Building." *New York Herald Tribune* March 27, 1928.

"Anna C. Maxwell, Noted Nurse, Dies." *New York Times* January 3, 1929.

"Miss Maxwell." *New York Times* January 4, 1929.

Editorial, *New York Herald-Tribune* January 5, 1929.

"Training of Nurses: American and English Methods." (Letter to editor) *London Times* August 25, 1931.

"The Training of Nurses: English Methods." (Letter to editor) *London Times* August 28, 1931.

"She Remembers Best Christmas in France." *World Telegram* December 20, 1932.

"A School for the Nurse: The Medical College of Columbia Takes a New and Significant Step." *New York Times* November 24, 1935.

"Nursing Department is Set Up At Columbia; New Division Will Give Bacherlor's Degree." *New York Times* January 1, 1937.

"Columbia Gives Top Ranking to Nursing." *New York Evening Journal* January 4, 1937.

"Mrs. Chase is the Best Patient That Any Hospital Ever Had." *New York Sun* January 5, 1939.

"Defense and Nursing Education: National Preparedness Program Stresses Significance of State Nursing Education Convention." *New York Sun* October 15, 1940.

"Nurses Sail to Serve In Greece: Hospitals There are Reported Greatly Understaffed," *New York Sun* March 19, 1941.

"Sunken Steamship's 170 Americans May Be Prisoners on Nazi Raider." *New York Sun* May 19, 1941.

"Battle Creek Woman Answers Red Cross Call." *Battle Creek Enquirer and News* November 23, 1941.

"Nurse Education Held Inadequate." *New York Times* October 9, 1948.

"Student Nurses Preview Careers on Tour of Country Health Centers," *New York Times* March 16, 1950.

"Clock Turned Back in Honoring Nurse." *New York Times* March 15, 1951.

"Value of Hospital Nursing Schools." (Letter to the editor) *New York Times* October 5, 1966.

"Miss Helen Young, Nursing Official, Long Association with Old Greenwich, Succumbs in Harkness Pavilion at 92." *Village Gazette* (Old Greenwich, Conn.) December 1, 1966.

"Nurses Shortage May Double by '70." *New York Times* February 15, 1967.

"Colleges Favored by Nursing Group." *New York Times* May 13, 1967.

"Nursing Education: New Independent Commission Set Up to Make Comprehensive Study of Needs." *New York Times* May 15, 1967.

"Eleanor Lee, 71, Nursing Director." *New York Times* June 1, 1967.

"Miss Eleanor Lee." *Falmouth Enterprise* June 2, 1967.

"Program with Nursing School Approved by Barnard Faculty." *Columbia Daily Spectator* December 14, 1971.

"Nursing, Maligned and Pitied — and Yet It's a Growing Field." *New York Times*, 1972.

"Cuts in Funding to Force Nursing to End Programs." *Columbia Daily Spectator* February 5, 1973.

"Nursing Program Enrollment to Nearly Double Next Year." *Columbia Daily Spectator* March 27, 1974.

"Jane St. John, 92; Served as a Nurse in 2 World Wars." (Obituary) *New York Times* April 2, 1977.

"Nursing: Second Chance for Career in Mid-Life." *New York Times* April 2, 1977.

"Dr. Mary I. Crawford, Former Vice President of Nursing at Hospital." (Obituary) *New York Times* April 4, 1979.

"Nursing degree cut to 2-year program; students are surprised and dismayed." *Columbia Daily Spectator* November 30, 1979.

"New Dean Named: Columbia Meets Nursing Challenge." *Columbia University Record* November 4, 1988.

"Big gain in Nursing Students Lifts Hopes Amid a Shortage." *New York Times* December 28, 1990.

"The Feminist Disdain for Nursing" (Op-Ed page) *New York Times* February 23, 1991.

"Pioneering Nursing School to Celebrate Centennial." *Columbia University Record* September 6, 1991.

"Chronicle: Choir doesn't sing for its supper." *New York Times* September 11, 1991.

COLUMBIA-PRESBYTERIAN MEDICAL CENTER ARCHIVES

(Including Columbia University School of Nursing; Columbia University–Presbyterian Hospital School of Nursing Alumni Association; College of Physicians & Surgeons, Office of Central Files; Hammer Health Sciences Library, Special Collections; Presbyterian Hospital, Office of Public Interest.)

Miscellaneous Documents
(chronological order)

Excerpts from annual reports, New York Post-Graduate School of Nursing, 1887 and 1891.

"The Presbyterian Hospital in the City of New York, Training School for Nurses" (program announcement), 1892.

Application questionnaire, Presbyterian Hospital Training School for Nurses, 1892.

Presbyterian Hospital and Columbia-Presbyterian Medical Center Annual Reports, 1892-1991.

Student files, Presbyterian Hospital and Columbia University School of Nursing (microfiche), 1892-1991.

"Constitution and By-Laws of the Alumnae Association of the Presbyterian Hospital Training School for Nurses, New York," circa 1897.

Maxwell AM: "Report to Training School Committee of the Presbyterian Hospital," 10/31/98.

"American National Red Cross Relief Committee Reports, May 1898 - March 1899."

"Report of the Alumnae Association of the Presbyterian Hospital Training School for Nurses, 1899-1906."

"The Presbyterian Hospital in the City of New York, Rules for Nurses, 1903."

"Bulletins" and "Announcements" of Presbyterian Hospital and Columbia University School of Nursing, 1906-1991.

World War I Diary of Elspeth Gould, Class of 1909.

"Charter, Constitution, By-Laws and Rules and Regulations of The Presbyterian Hospital in the City of New York," 4/14.

"Concert for the Benefit of the Pension Fund of the Presbyterian Hospital Training School for Nurses" (program), 1/31/17.

"Visiting Nursing Service Four Months' Undergraduate Course, Beginning February 1, 1918."

"Teachers College Bulletin, Report of the Dean," 11/9/18.

"Outline of Plan for affiliation with the Presbyterian Hospital School of Nursing, Teachers College, Department of Nursing and Health," 4/19.

Tyler GB: "Sideshows of World War I, 1918: A New York Presbyterian Hospital Girl's Experience in France and Belgium with the Army Nurse Corps Base Hospital #116 and Mobile Unit #9, U.S.A." (unpublished manuscript, not dated).

Class of 1920 scrapbook.

Sample "Form for Obstetrical Affiliations," early 1920s.

Sample "Student Nurse Report," early 1920s.

Sample "Summary of Student Nurse Record, Academic Report, Department of Nursing and Health, Teachers College, Columbia University," early 1920s.

Sample "Field Report, Nursing Department of the Henry Street Settlement," early 1920s.

"Columbia University School of Nursing, Tentative Outline of Plan, 1921."

"Rules Controlling the Use of Privileges Granted the Students' Association of the Presbyterian Hospital School of Nursing," 1921.

"Propositions Regarding Pupil Self Government in Trainings School for Nursing," circa 1921.

"Student Handbook," Presbyterian Hospital-Columbia University School of Nursing, 1922-1971.

Organization Committee of the School of Nursing (minutes), 2/23/22, 3/22/22, 4/19/22

"Without Regard to Race, Creed or Color" (Presbyterian Hospital fundraising brochure), 1924.

Scrapbook, L'Ecole Florence Nightingale, Bordeaux, France, presented to Anna Maxwell (not dated).

Biography of Anna Maxwell (Presbyterian Hospital in the City of New York, Building Fund, press release), 1/13/25.

Maxwell AC: "Struggles of the Pioneers in Nursing" (transcript, radio addresses), 1/28/25, 2/11/25.

Joint Administrative Board, Columbia-Presbyterian Medical Center, Bulletins, 9/18/25, 9/30/25, 10/17/25, 1/22/26, 2/22/26, 4/14/26, 4/26/26, 5/4/26, 5/11/26, 6/2/26, 7/13/26, 7/20/26, 11/1/26, 1/22/27, 1/31/27, 4/8/27, 6/23/27, 6/30/27, 10/11/27, 11/2/27, 11/9/27, 12/8/27, 11/30/27, 1/31/28, 10/8/28.

"The Pupil Nurse in the Out-Patient Department: A Study of the Nurse and Nursing Services in the Out-Patient Department," National League of Nursing Education, 1925.

Maxwell AC: "Message to Class of 1927," Newport Hospital School for Nurses, 6/30/27.

"Report of Schools of Nursing." Albany, The New York State Education Department, The University of the State of New York, 1927.

"The Presbyterian Hospital in the City of New York School of Nursing Probationer's Outfit," 1928.

"Anna Maxwell" (recollections of Edwin B. McDaniel, M.D.), circa 1929.

"House Regulations for Anna C. Maxwell Hall," 9/1/29.

"Anna C. Maxwell, R.N., M.A." (biographical booklet), circa 1930.

Rappleye WC: "Memorandum on Nursing Education," 5/9/33.

School of Nursing Yearbooks (some titled, "Stripes" or "Starch and Stripes"), 1936-1991.

"Memorandum on the Proposed Department of Nursing of Columbia University," 5/26/36, 7/2/36.

"Department of Nursing, College of Physicians & Surgeons, Columbia University" (brochure), circa 1937.

"Columbia-Presbyterian Medical Center, Air Raid Procedure, General Memorandum #1," 12/20/41.

"Black Out and Air Raid Regulations — Maxwell Hall," 6/1/42.

"Incidents in the Life of Anna C. Maxwell" (slide show script for 50th Anniversary Pagent), 1942.

Scrapbook, Bryn Mawr College Summer School of Nursing, 1942.

"New Defense Regulations," 9/15/43.

"Report of the Bryn Mawr College Summer School of Nursing," 1943.

"Addresses at the Closing Ceremonies, Bryn Mawr College Summer School of Nursing: Margaret E. Conrad, Dean of the Summer School; Alta E. Dines, Chairman, Committee on Nursing, American Red Cross," 9/13/45.

"News Bulletin of the Ladies Auxiliary of the Presbyterian Hospital Units." 2/43, 9/43, 4/44, 12/44, 5/45.

"Memorandum on Graduate Education," 3/20/44.

Western Union Telegram from Surgeon General Thomas Parran to Margaret E. Conrad, 5/11/44.

"Background Material for U.S. Cadet Nurse Corps Speech," Division of Nurse Education, U.S. Public Health Service, Federal Security Agency, Washington, D.C., 5/13/44.

"Army Nurse Corps Fact Sheet," Office of the Surgeon General, Services of Supply, War Department, 1/15/45.

Valentine J: "Report of Survey of Presbyterian Hospital School of Nursing and of Programs for Affiliating Students in the Presbyterian Hospital, City of New York, May 29, 31 and June 4, 1945."

Nicoll C: "Final Report on the Red Cross Volunteer Nurses' Aides at Presbyterian Hospital From 1942 Through 1945," circa 1945.

Naffiziger HG: "The Nursing Problem" (questionnaire), University of California Hospital, San Francisco, 5/15/46.

Steinbeck J: "Vanderbilt Clinic" (booklet), Department of Public Interest, Presbyterian Hospital, 3/47.

"Report of Survey of the School of Nursing of the Columbia-Presbyterian Medical Center, New York, N.Y., November 24 & 25, 1947, and January 13 & 14, 1948."

"Report of the Committee to Study Nursing Problems," 5/19/48.

"Catalogue to Contents of Anna C. Maxwell's Cabinet," circa 1950.

"Nursing Survey," Public Interest Department, The Presbyterian Hospital, 10/1/51.

"Resolution of the Medical Board [of Presbyterian Hospital]," 6/20/50.

"Summary of the Minutes of the Meeting of the Board of Trustees of The Presbyterian Hospital in the City of New York," 6/26/50.

McIntosh R, Parke JS: "Nurses and Doctors Crossing the Street in Uniform" (Presbyterian Hospital administrative bulletin), 8/31/50.

Lamb AC: "Recollections of Anna Caroline Maxwell: The Sixtieth Anniversary of Her Founding of The School of Nursing of The Presbyterian Hospital" (booklet), circa 1952.

"Report of Visit to the Department of Nursing, Faculty of Medicine, Columbia University, Presbyterian Hospital School of Nursing, New York City," The University of the State of New York, State Education Department, Board of Examiners of Nurses, Albany, New York, 12/53.

"Record of Individual Nurse Member" (Eleanor Lee), National League for Nursing, 7/7/56.

"The Report of the President's Committee on The Educational Future of the University." Columbia University, New York, 1957.

Reilly DE: "Nursing Student Responses to the Clinical Field." Department of Nursing, Faculty of Medicine, Columbia University, 1958.

Curriculum vitae: Helen Pettit, 11/24/59.

"These Things Miss Young Told Us (Probationers)," circa 1960s.

"Report on Public Health Nursing Field Work in Basic Baccalaureate Programs," Columbia University in the City of New York, Department of Nursing of the Faculty of Medicine, 5/60.

"Department of Nursing, Faculty of Medicine, Columbia University, Executive Committee Minutes," 5/7/62, 11/8/62, 2/6/63, 3/6/63, 3/20/63, 3/27/63, 9/25/63, 1/5/65.

Reilly DE: "College Graduates Choose A Nursing Career." Department of Nursing, Faculty of Medicine, Columbia University, 1963.

Press release and recommendations, Surgeon General's Consultant Group on Nursing, U.S. Depatment of Health, Education, and Welfare, Public Health Service, 2/24/63.

"Report of Visit to the Department of Nursing, Faculty of Medicine, Columbia University, Baccalaureate Program in Nursing," The University of the State of New York, The State Education Department, Division of Professional Education, Albany, N.Y., 10/65.

"Lillian Wald of Henry Street" (booklet). New York, Committee for the Election of Lillian D. Wald to the Hall of Fame for Great Americans at New York University, 1965.

Curriculum vitae: Elizabeth S. Gill, 1/66.

"Helen Young 1874-1966, Tributes and Remembrances By Those Who Knew Her" (booklet). New York, Columbia University–Presbyterian Hospital School of Nursing Alumnae Association, circa 1967.

"Progress Fund Meeting, Department of Nursing, Faculty of Medicine, Columbia University" (minutes), 4/20/67.

Gill E: "Memorial Service — Miss Eleanor Lee," 6/2/67.

"Familiar Faces, Familiar Voices: 75th Anniversary" (slide show transcript), 1967.

"Proposed Clinical Investigation: 'The Effect of Supplementary Postnatal Kinesthetic Stimulation of the Maturational Level of the Female Newborn' — Anne M. Earle, Assitant Professor of Nursing," 8/10/67.

"Memorandum of Meeting Regarding the Establishment of a School for Practical Nursing at the Medical Center," 12/13/67.

"Memorandum of Interview with Mrs. Marcia Britten," 12/19/67.

"Role and Preparation of the Nurse-Midwife in the Maternity Care in the United States: An Exploratory Study," Department of Nursing Education, Teachers College, and Department of Nursing, Faculty of Medicine, Columbia University, 11/67.

Elliot RHE: "Memoranda of First, Second, and Third Days at A.N.A. Convention in Dallas Texas," 5/68.

"Comparison of Charges to Student Nurses at Various Universities," 10/2/68.

"In Search of An Education" (protest letter), Class of 1969, 5/5/69.

"Nurse-Midwifery Service in Presbyterian Hospital" (memorandum from Charles M. Steer, M.D., to Members of the Executive Committee of the Medical Board of the Presbyterian Hospital), 12/16/69.

File memoranda, H. Houston Merritt, M.D., 5/1/70, 5/4/70.

"Memorandum of Hearing held in Dean Merritt's Office on Wednesday, May 13, 1970 Regrading Grievances of a Black Graduate Student enrolled in the Nurse Midwifery Program."

"Proposed Clinical Investigation: Hospital Teaching of Patients with Heart Failure — Patricia K. Bucholz and Shirlee Ann Stokes," 10/1/70.

"School of Nursing — Five Year Plan," 1971.

"Revised Curriculum Proposal for Four Year Integrated Baccalaureate Program Offered by the School of Nursing of the Department of Nursing of the Faculty of Medicine, Columbia University," 1971.

Crawford MI: "School of Nursing - Columbia University" (status report), 6/10/71.

Crawford MI: "Speech Delivered to the Board of Trustees," 3/29/71.

"Meeting on December 7, 1972 to Review Plans for Recruitment, Admissions and Curriculum for the Four Year Nursing Program to Begin September, 1973."

Crawford MI: "School of Nursing Evaluation: A Report by the Associate Dean," 9/26/74.

Ozdemir EB: "Report to the Faculty Council, School of Nursing, Office of Admissions," 10/27/75.

Mahoney EA: "Report of Undergraduate Curriculum Committee," 11/24/75.

"Nursing at Columbia University" (recruitment brochure), circa 1974.

"Why Nursing?" (recruitment brochure), circa 1977.

"School of Nursing Admissions Report," 1978.

"Columbia University Master's Programs in Clinical Nursing Practice" (recruitment brochure), 9/78.

Pettit H: "Tribute to Mary I. Crawford" (memorial service, Presbyterian Hospital Chapel), 4/4/79.

"Projecting the Future of Nursing at Columbia University: Report of the Special Committee Appointed January 1979 by Dr. Paul A. Marks, Vice President for Health Sciences," 10/79.

Press release announcing appointment of JoAnn Jamann, Office of Public Information, Columbia University, 12/8/80.

"School of Nursing, Columbia University, 1981-82 Fact Sheet," 12/81.

"Alternate Report to the Provost Review Task Force: Columbia University School of Nursing," 6/87.

"Report to the Provost of the Task Force to Review the Columbia University School of Nursing," 10/9/87.

Mundinger MO: "The School of Nursing," 1987.

Mellett H: "Authority for Nursing Practice: Nurse Practitioners in New York State, An Historical Analysis" (doctoral dissertation, Division of Health Administration, School of Public Health, Columbia University), 1988.

"Columbia University–Presbyterian Hospital School of Nursing Alumni Associate, Inc., Directory, 1989." White Plains, N.Y., Bernard C. Harris Publishing Co., Inc., 1989.

"Faculty Scholars: Columbia University School of Nursing, 1988-89" (booklet), 1989

"Columbia University School of Nursing Officers of Instruction" (minutes), 11/26/90.

Califano, JA, Jr.: "America's Health Care Revolution: The Nurse as a Revolutionary" (School of Nursing Centennial Convocation address), 9/11/91.

"Office of the Mayor of the City of New York, Proclamation: Columbia University School of Nursing Day," 9/11/91.

Journals & Magazines

Quarterly Magazine (1906-1965) and *Alumnae/Alumni Magazine* (1965-1991), Columbia University–Presbyterian Hospital Alumni Association.

P.H., the Quarterly of the Student Association of the School of Nursing, of the Presbyterian Hospital, New York, Vol. 1, Nos. 1 & 2, 1923.

Student Prints (Presbyterian Hospital School of Nursing student publication), 4/38, 6/38.

Vital Signs (Columbia University, Department of Nursing, student publication), 9/7/51, 9/21/51, 10/5/51, 10/26/51, 11/9/51, 12/7/51, 1/19/52, 2/8/52, 9/26/52, 10/24/52, 12/15/52, 2/12/53, 3/31/53, 6/61.

Stethoscope, Presbyterian Hospital, 1946-1990.

SNC (1980-1986) and *The Academic Nurse* (1987-1991), the Journal of the Columbia University School of Nursing (and backup files).

Letters & Memoranda
(chronological order)

Abbreviations:

MEC	Margaret E. Conrad '20	HFP	Helen F. Pettit '36
MIC	Mary I. Crawford, Ed.D.	WCR	Willard C. Rappleye, M.D.
EL	Eleanor Lee '20	DS	Dean Sage
PAM	Paul A. Marks, M.D.	DFT	Donald F. Tapley, M.D.
ACM	Anna C. Maxwell	AKW	Anne K. Williams '15
HHM	H. Houston Merritt, M.D.	HY	Helen Young '12

ACM to Laura Hesselberg '98, 5/22/94, 6/23/97
ACM to Gertrude Smith '01, 12/28/97
Conyers Prichett '03 to ACM, 12/19/99
B.C. Powell to ACM, 7/10/99
Rev. W. E. Dozier to ACM, 7/5/99
Dorothy Taylor '22 to ACM, 6/10/19, 8/15/19
Mrs. William K. Vanderbilt to ACM, 9/3/20
Gladys Thivierge '20 to ACM, 1/10/21
Nurses of the L'Ecole Florence Nightingale to ACM, 10/21
Gladys Thivierge to HY, 6/14/23
Delphine Wilde '26 to HY, circa 1923
DS to William Darrach, 1/21/24
William Darrach to DS, 2/12/24
William Darrach to Nicholas Murray Butler, 2/12/24
Isabel M. S. Stewart to DS, 2/20/24
Jeanette Archer '26 to Big Sisters of P.H., 2/21/25
HY and ACM to DS, 6/4/25

ACM to Miss Scott, 9/24/25
Classes of 1926, 1927, 1928 to HY, 1926
ACM to DS, 2/25/26, 4/19/26, 4/10/27
Isabel M. Stewart to WCR, 5/27/32
WCR to Executive Committee of the University Council, 12/15/32
John F. Bush to HY, 11/16/34
WCR to EL, 12/27/34
DS to WCR, 8/1/35
DS to WCR, 1/21/37
G. Alivizatos to General Director, Near East Foundation, 4/28/37
Laird Archer to HY, 6/24/37
Paul C. Fahrney to DS, 10/20/37
AKW to HY, 11/10/38
AKW to Annie W. Goodrich, 11/10/38
Annie W. Goodrich to AKW, 12/4/38
MEC to WCR, 2/19/40
E.C. Miller to MEC, 3/4/40, 9/2/41, 9/8/41, 3/23/42, 5/13/42, 6/4/42
Angelique Contostavlou to Laird Archer, 4/24/40
AKW to HY, 6/23/40
AKW to HY, 7/1/40
Clarence O. Cheney, M.D, to HY, 9/24/40
AKW to HY, 9/24/40
HY to Clarence O. Cheney, M.D, 9/28/40
Clarence O. Cheney, M.D, to HY, 10/5/40
Margaret Eliot to Clarence O. Cheney, 10/7/40
Sheila Dwyer to HY, 11/40
AKW to HY, 1/14/41
HY to AKW, 1/20/41
Katherine Saliari '41 to E.C. Miller, 4/7/41, 6/30/41
MEC to WCR, 7/30/41
T. Stuart Hart to EL, 8/2/41
Eugenia K. Spalding to MEC, 5/8/42
AKW to HY, 6/19/42
MEC to WCR, 3/15/45
MEC to WCR, 8/28/45
MEC to WCR, 1946
MEC to WCR, 1/24/46
WCR to Charles P. Cooper, 1/31/46
Anne Richardson to Lucile Petry, 1/31/46
Charles P. Cooper to WCR, 2/4/46
MEC to WCR, 6/12/46.
MEC to Mrs. Henry C. Taylor, 4/26/48
MEC to W.C. Walton, 9/27/48.
Margaret Eliot to John S. Parke, 7/6/49
John S. Parke to MEC, 1/27/50
MEC to John S. Parke, 2/13/50
John S. Parke to MEC, 2/20/50
MEC to WCR, 5/20/50
MEC to John S. Parke, 5/20/50

Senior Administrative Group, Department of Nursing, to Executive Committee of the Board of Trustees of the Presbyterian Hospital, 6/12/50
MEC to Kate Davison, 6/13/50
Representatives of the Student Government of the School of Nursing to Charles P. Cooper, 6/19/50
Representatives of the Supervisors and Head Nurses to the Board of Trustees of the Presbyterian Hospital, 6/22/50
MEC to WCR, 8/1/50
Annie Goodrich to MEC, 8/25/50
EL to WCR, 12/18/52
WCR to EL, 12/19/52
EL to Patricia A. Nutter '53, 12/24/52
WCR to Adrian M. Massie, 6/15/53
WCR to Carl Munson, 7/2/53
EL to WCR, 3/1/57
EL to WCR, 3/19/56
WCR to Stanley Salmen, 3/14/58
EL to HHM, 11/11/58
HHM to EL, 11/18/58
Anne Sengbusch to HHM, 3/23/60
Rhoda Reddig to HHM, 3/26/60
Florence M. Gipe to HHM, 3/28/60
Elizabeth L. Kemble to HHM, 3/28/60
Mary S. Tschudin to HHM, 3/31/60
Faye Crabbe to HHM, 4/4/60
Helen L. Bunge to HHM, 4/11/60
Ruth Sleeper to HHM, 4/12/60
E. Jean M. Hill to HHM, 4/22/60
Jean E. Boyle HHM, 4/27/60
Emily C. Cardew to HHM, 5/6/60
Sophie A. Greenberg to Board of Trustees, Columbia University, 5/7/63
Stanley Salmen to HHM, 6/23/65
Vincent J. Tesoriero to HHM, 6/30/66
Eleanor C. Lambertsen to HHM, 8/15/66
Alvin F. Poussaint to ESG, 8/18/66
ESG to Alvin F. Poussaint, 9/13/66
Dorothy E. Reilly to Douglas S. Damrosch, 10/7/66
W.E.S. Griswold to ESG, 4/21/67
E.T. Cleary to A.J. Binkert, 7/18/67
E.T. Cleary to HHM, 7/28/67
Augustus C. Long to Grayson Kirk, 12/14/67
Grayson Kirk to Augustus C. Long, 12/21/67
Roanne Dahlen '61 to HHM, 1/4/67
George A. Perera to Roanne Dahlen, 1/5/67
Douglas S. Damrosch to HHM, 11/3/67
ESG to HHM, 11/8/67
ESG to HHM, 1/25/68
MIC to HHM, 1/7/69
HHM to MIC, 2/5/69

Charles M. Steer to MIC, 4/9/69
A.J. Binkert to MIC, 5/29/69
Joseph E. Snyder to B. Derby, 4/30/70
Black Medical Students to George I. Lythcott, 4/29/70
George Lythcott to HHM, 4/30/70
Black Medical and Nursing Students of the College of Physicians & Surgeons,
    Columbia University to HHM, 5/6/70
MIC to Donald Swartz, 5/7/70
B.R. Derby to MIC, 5/11/70
HHM to Ross T. Hamilton, 5/22/70
The Black Caucus of Columbia-Presbyterian Medical Center to MIC, 7/6/70
MIC to Frederick B. Putney, Ph.D., 10/19/70
MIC to PAM, 10/16/71
George I. Lythcott, M.D., to PAM, 10/27/71
MIC to PAM, 12/10/71
PAM to MIC, 1/15/72
MIC to PAM, 1/25/72
MIC to William J. McGill, 4/24/73
Martha Haber to William J. McGill, 5/22/73
HFP to PAM, 6/21/73
Margaret G. Tyson to PAM, 7/2/73
PAM to Margaret G. Tyson, 7/7/73
Margaret G. Tyson to PAM, 7/18/73
Charmaine Fitzig, Keville Frederickson, and Elizabeth Carter to PAM, 8/2/73
DFT to PAM, 1/22/77
PAM to MIC, 2/12/74
Members of the Faculty of the School of Nursing to DFT, 6/30/76
Students of Class of 1977 to DFT, 5/1/77
William J. McGill to PAM, 7/7/78
PAM to Committee on the Future of Nursing at Columbia University, 1/10/79
HFP to DFT, 4/27/79
PAM to HFP, 12/21/79
PAM to Committee on the Future of Nursing at Columbia University, 1/3/80
Thomas Q. Morris, M.D., to DFT, 1/31/80
Members of the Faculty of the School of Nursing to HFP, 5/6/80
Maureen Casey to HFP, 6/11/80
Kathleen P. Mullinix to Robert F. Goldberger, 10/9/87

School of Nursing Commencement Addresses
William H. Draper, M.D. (1894)
S. Weir Mitchell. M.D. (1905)
Henry Fairfield Osborn, Sc.D., LL.D., D.Sc., "Science and
    Sentiment," (1907)
W. Gilman Thompson, M.D., "The Educational Value of the Trained Nurse,"
    (1911)
C. Irving Fisher, M.D. (1913)
Theodore C. Janeway, M.D., "Ideals in Medical and Nursing Education,"
    (1914)
James R. Sheffield (1915)

Chauncey Brewster Tinker, Ph.D., Litt.D., "The Quality of Mercy," (1927)
John Miller Turpin Finney, M.D. (1928)
Mrs. August Belmont (1929)
Samuel S. Drury, D.D. (1930)
Harry Emerson Fosdick, D.D. (1932)
Nicholas Murray Butler (1933)
John W. Davis (1934)
Robert R. Wicks, D.D. (1935)
George E. Vincent, Ph.D., LL.D. (1936)
Lewis Perry, LL.D. (1937)
Arthur Lee Kinsolving, D.D. (1938)
Maitland Alexander, D.D. (1939)
James W. Wadsworth (1940)
Walter Lippmann (1941)
Donald Bradshaw Aldrich, D.D. (1942)
William Allan Neilson (1943)
Thomas I. Parkinson (1944)
Henry Sloan Coffin, D.D., L.L.D. (1945)
Annie W. Goodrich (1946)
Oliver C. Carmichael, Ph.D., LL.D. (1947)
Dwight D. Eisenhower (1948)
Bruce Barton (1948)
Millicent McIntosh, Ph.D., L.L.D. (1950)
Paul Austin Wolfe, D.D., S.T.D. (1951)
William E.S. Griswold (1952)
James A. Pike, J.S.D. (1953)
Aura Severinghaus, Ph.D. (1953)
Grayson Kirk (1954)
Oveta Culp Hobby (1955)
Wilder Penfield, M.D. (1956)
Harry J. Carman (1957)
Margaret Arnstein '38, M.P.H., Sc.D. (1958)
Ray E. Trussel, M.D., Ph.D. (1959)
Jacques Barzun (1960)
Aims C. McGuiness, M.D. (1960)
Dana W. Atchley, M.D. (1961)
Aura Edward Sevringhaus, M.D. (1962)
George A. Perera, M.D. (1963)
Yale Kneeland, Jr., M.D. (1964)
Willard C. Rappleye, M.D. (1965)
George H. Humphreys II, M.D. (1966)
Lucile Petry Leone, M.A., "Over the Horizons in Nursing," (1967)
Lawrence C. Kolb, M.D. (1968)
Francesca Castronovo (1973)
Nancy M. Sargis (1973)
Charmaine Fitzig, M.S., Dr.P.H. (1974)
Shirley Smoyak, Ph.D. (1974)
Marianne Marcus (1981)
David N. Dinkins (1990)

OTHER ARCHIVES

Nursing Archives, Mugar Library, Boston University, Boston, Mass.
Anna C. Maxwell's application to Boston City Hospital Training School for
   Nurses, 1878.
Schlessinger Library, Radcliffe College, Harvard University, Cambridge, Mass.
Eleanor Lee papers.

INTERVIEWS

Darline Bacon
Olga Brown-Vanderpool '70
Sarah Sheets Cook
Keville Frederickson '64
Bettie Springer Jackson '67
JoAnn S. Jamann
Lucie Young Kelly
Mary O. Mundinger
Helen Pettit '36
Dorothy Reilly '42
Alice Bliss Smith '19

Index

PHOTO CREDITS

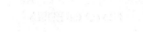